MALE INFERTILITY

Edited by **Anu Bashamboo**
and **Kenneth David McElreavey**

Male Infertility
Edited by Anu Bashamboo and Kenneth David McElreavey

Published by InTech

Janeza Trdine 9, 51000 Rijeka, Croatia

Publishing Process Manager Martina Blecic

Technical Editor Teodora Smiljanic

Cover Designer InTech Design Team

Additional hard copies can be obtained from orders@intechopen.com

Male Infertility, Edited by Anu Bashamboo and Kenneth David McElreavey
p. cm.
ISBN 978-953-51-0562-6

For EU product safety concerns:
IN TECH d.o.o., Prolaz Marije Krucifikse Kozulić 3, 51000 Rijeka, Croatia,
info@intechopen.com or visit our website at intechopen.com.

Meet the editors

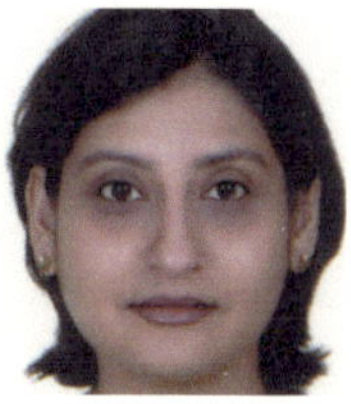

Dr. Anu Bashamboo is currently a staff scientist at the Institut Pasteur, Paris. She received her M.Sc. in Zoology (Genetics) from Aligarh Muslim University and her Ph.D. from the National Institute of Immunology, New Delhi, India. During her career she has authored and co-authored numerous articles and has served as an invited speaker in various international congresses and symposiums.

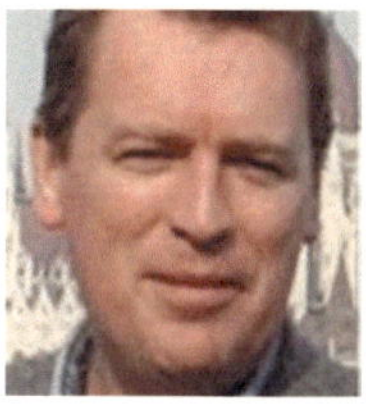

Dr. Kenneth David McElreavey received the B.Sc. in Microbiology (1985) and the Ph.D. in Hematology (1991) from The Queen's University of Belfast, U.K. Since 2008 he has been appointed as a Director of Human Developmental Genetics Unit at the Institut Pasteur, Paris. Other than actively participating in numerous international conferences and symposiums as an invited lecturer, Dr. McElreavey has also authored over 140 publications in international peer-reviewed journals.

Contents

Preface

In recent years there has been an increasing concern about possible decline in reproductive health with an estimate of one in seven couples worldwide having problems conceiving. Despite high and increasing rates of human infertility, our understanding of the genetic pathways and basic molecular mechanisms involved in gonadal development and function remains limited. A genetic contribution to spermatogenic failure is indicated by several families with multiple infertile or subfertile men. In some of these families an autosomal recessive mutation appears to be responsible whilst in others an autosomal dominant mutation with sex-limited expression is likely. In other families the genetic cause is known to involve either chromosomal anomalies or Y chromosome microdeletions. However, only a significant minority of the cases of male infertility and subfertility may be explained by the genetic causes. This raises the question of environmental contribution to male infertility and subfertility.

Prospective cross-sectional studies have indicated a general birth cohort decline in sperm quantity and quality as well as an increase in incidence of Testicular germ cell cancer during the last 50 years. These phenotypes, together with undescended testis and anomalies of the male external genitalia are termed "testicular dysgenesis syndrome" (TDS) and may have a common aetiology resulting from disruption of the gonadal environment during fœtal life. The rapid, often synchronous, rise in the incidence of TDS suggests an environmental aetiology possibly in genetically susceptible individuals. Emerging data suggest that exposure of a developing male foetus to a number of environmental factors, including but not limited to endocrine disruptors, can negatively regulate testicular development and function. Several studies show that this detrimental effect of environmental toxins on male germ cells may be epigenetic resulting in aberrant DNA methylation of key genes. Several reports suggest that the epigenetic landscape may be altered in some men with reduced sperm counts but relationship between these changes and infertility remains unclear.

The increase in incidence of male infertility is associated with an increase in demand for infertility treatments. These include intracytoplasmic sperm injection (ICSI) and in vitro fertilization (IVF). In some European countries, such as Denmark, more than 6% of children are born with assisted reproductive techniques (ARTs). There is a suggestion that children conceived using ARTs might show a higher prevalence of genetic and epigenetic anomalies. This raises the question of complete molecular characterization of sperm that will be eventually used for ARTs. Our understanding of the molecular landscape of the sperm is likely to increase dramatically in the coming future with the advent of new technologies that permit high throughput and detailed molecular analysis. OMICS involving the exploration of genetic, epigenetic, transcriptomic and proteomic modifications and their interaction with each other is fast becoming a tool of choice to understand and interpret complex biological phenomenon and may be used to understand key molecular events involved in the development of the normal male germ cell lineages and their pathological counterparts. A combination of these approaches together with strict diagnostic criteria will increase the likelihood of success in understanding male infertility and use of ARTs.

Dr. Anu Bashamboo
Dr. Ken McElreavey
Unit of Human Developmental Genetics
Institut Pasteur, Paris
France

1

Obstructive and Non-Obstructive Azoospermia

Antonio Luigi Pastore[1,2*], Giovanni Palleschi[1,2], Luigi Silvestri[1],
Antonino Leto[1] and Antonio Carbone[1,2]
[1]*Sapienza University of Rome, Faculty of Pharmacy and Medicine,
Department of Medico-Surgical Sciences and Biotechnologies,
Urology Unit, S. Maria Goretti Hospital Latina*
[2]*Uroresearch Association®, Latina
Italy*

1. Introduction

Azoospermia is defined as the complete absence of spermatozoa upon examination of the semen [including capillary tube centrifugation (CTC), strictly confirmed by the absence of spermatozoa issued in urine after ejaculation]. The presence of rare spermatozoa (<500.000/ml) in seminal fluid after centrifugation is called "cryptozoospermia". The complete absence of spermatozoa should be confirmed with repeat testing after a long time, because many external factors (e.g., febrile episodes and some therapies) may cause transient azoospermia. Azoospermia is present in approximately 1% of all men, and in approximately 15% of infertile men. Azoospermia may result from a lack of spermatozoa production in the testes (secretory or Non-Obstructive Azoospermia, NOA), or from an inability of produced spermatozoa to reach the emitted semen (excretory or Obstructive Azoospermia, OA); however, in clinical practice both components are sometimes present in a single patient (mixed genesis azoospermia).The initial diagnosis of azoospermia is made when no spermatozoa can be detected on high-powered microscopic examination of centrifuged seminal fluid on at least two occasions. *The World Health Organization (WHO) Laboratory Manual for the Examination of Human Semen and Semen-Cervical Mucus Interactions* recommends that the seminal fluid be centrifuged for 15 minutes, preferably at a centrifugation speed of ≥3000 × *g*.

The evaluation of a patient with azoospermia is performed to determine the etiology of the patient's condition. The numerous etiologies for azoospermia fall into three principal categories: pre-testicular, testicular, and post-testicular.

1. pre-testicular azoospermia affects approximately 2% of men with azoospermia, and is due to a hypothalamic or pituitary abnormality diagnosed with hypogonadotropic hypogonadism;
2. testicular failure or non-obstructive azoospermia is estimated to affect from 49% to 93% of azoospermic men. While the term testicular failure would seem to indicate a complete absence of spermatogenesis, men with testicular failure actually have either

* Corresponding Author

reduced spermatogenesis [hypospermatogenesis], maturation arrest at an early or late stage of spermatogenesis, or a complete failure of spermatogenesis (noted with Sertoli-cell only syndrome);

3. post-testicular obstruction or retrograde ejaculation are estimated to affect from 7% to 51% of azoospermic men. In these cases, spermatogenesis is normal even though the semen lacks spermatozoa.

Diagnosis

The minimum initial evaluation of an azoospermic patient should include a complete medical history, physical examination, and hormone level measurements. Relevant history should investigate prior fertility; childhood illnesses such as orchitis or cryptorchidism; genital trauma or prior pelvic/inguinal surgery; infections; gonadotoxin exposure, such as prior radiation therapy/chemotherapy and current medical therapy; and a familial history of birth defects, mental retardation, reproductive failure, or cystic fibrosis. Physical examination includes: testis size and consistency; consistency of the epididymides; secondary sex characteristics; presence and consistency of the vasa deferentia; presence of a varicocele; and masses upon digital rectal examination. The initial hormonal evaluation should include measurement of serum testosterone (T) and follicle stimulating hormone (FSH) levels.

History and initial investigations for men with azoospermia

Cryptorchidism: the bilateral form is almost always associated with azoospermia and irreversible gonadal secretory dysfunction. The age at which surgical intervention is practiced and subsequent gonadal development may sometimes affect the prognosis. In addition, not infrequently, germinal malformations are also associated with atrophy of the epydidimus and sometimes with iatrogenic damage to the vas deferens. In unilateral cryptorchidism, azoospermia is less frequent; azoospermia in a patient with unilateral cryptorchidism is likely the result of concurrent secretory dysfunction (dysgenesis) or other pathology of the contralateral testis.

Reduced volume of ejaculate: occurs progressively in the post-inflammatory obstruction of the ejaculatory ducts (ED), with a concomitant reduction of seminal fructose and lowering of pH. Ejaculate volume is normally reduced in cases of vas deferens agenesis or in the presence of large seminal cysts (Müllerian or Wolffian). The same phenomenon is present in primary hypogonadism. Partial retrograde ejaculation is present in patients with systemic neuropathy (e.g., juvenile diabetes and multiple sclerosis), and is a possible outcome of endoscopic urological surgery for bladder neck sclerosis.

Urological symptoms and signs: the clinician must always pay close attention to symptoms, even prior symptoms that may previously have had no apparent significance, such as episodes of hemospermia, burning urination, urinary frequency, and urethral catheterization after surgery. All of these symptoms should raise the suspicion that the proximal or distal seminal tract may be obstructed (Silber, 1981). The presence of hypospadias may be associated with urinary abnormalities, hypogonadism, cryptorchidism, and the presence of residues in the Müllerian duct of the prostate (utricular cysts). These cysts can be responsible for extrinsic compression of the ED.

Surgery: Inguinal hernioplasty interventions (often performed during infancy) may have damaged the tubes, and then create a condition of seminal tract obstruction. Resection of the funicular vessels may result in hypotrophy of the gonad.

Family history: Clinicians should be attentive to the concomitant presence of infertility in the patient's male relatives (as a result of chromosomal abnormalities, genetic conditions, tuberculosis, etc.). Scrotal traumas are often responsible for complete or incomplete epididymis obstruction, as well as trophic changes of the gonad.

Prior chemotherapy and radiotherapy: Drug and radiation treatments for tumors usually cause irreversible damage to spermatogenesis. Even high-dose hormone therapy; antibiotic therapy with tetracyclines, nitrofurans, and sulfasalazine; or other drug therapies often temporarily alter spermatogenesis.

Chronic obstructive pulmonary diseases are frequently associated with obstruction of the epididymis (11-21%). This condition is often the result of primary ciliary dyskinesia (also known as Kartagener Syndrome) or cystic fibrosis, the latter often characterized by agenesis of the distal epididymis, vas deferens, and seminal vesicles. The most common cause of congenital bilateral absence of the vas deferens (CBAVD) is a mutation of the cystic fibrosis trans-membrane conductance regulator (CFTR) gene. Almost all males with clinical cystic fibrosis have CBAVD, and approximately 70% of men with CBAVD and no clinical evidence of cystic fibrosis have an identifiable abnormality of the CFTR gene.

The CFTR gene is extremely large and known mutations in the gene are extremely numerous. Clinical laboratories typically test for the 30–50 most common mutations found in patients with clinical cystic fibrosis. However, the mutations associated with CBAVD may be different. Because over 1,300 different mutations have been identified in this gene, this type of limited analysis is only informative if a mutation is found. A negative test result only indicates that the CBAVD patient does not have the most common mutations causing cystic fibrosis. Testing for abnormalities in the CFTR should include, at minimum, a panel of common point mutations and the 5T allele. There is currently no consensus on the minimum number of mutations that should be tested.

Bilateral testicular atrophy may be caused by either primary or secondary testicular failure. Elevated serum FSH associated with either normal or low serum testosterone is consistent with primary testicular failure. All patients with these findings should be offered genetic testing for chromosomal abnormalities and Y-chromosome microdeletions. Low serum FSH associated with bilaterally small testes and low serum testosterone is consistent with hypogonadotropic hypogonadism (secondary testicular failure). These patients usually also have low serum luteinizing hormone (LH) levels. Hypogonadotropic hypogonadism can be caused by hypothalamic disorders (e.g., functioning and non-functioning pituitary tumors). Therefore, these patients should undergo further evaluation, including serum prolactin measurement and imaging of the pituitary gland.

When the vasa deferentia and testes are palpably normal, semen volume and serum FSH are key factors in determining the etiology of azoospermia. Azoospermic patients with normal ejaculate volume may have reproductive system obstruction or spermatogenesis abnormalities. Azoospermic patients with low semen volume and normal-sized testes may have ejaculatory dysfunction or ejaculatory duct obstruction (EDO).

Normal semen volume

The serum FSH level of a patient with normal semen volume is a critical factor with which to establish whether a diagnostic testicular biopsy is needed to investigate spermatogenesis. Although a diagnostic testicular biopsy will determine whether spermatogenesis is impaired, it does not provide accurate prognostic information regarding whether or not sperm will be found on future sperm retrieval attempts for patients with NOA. Therefore, a testicular biopsy is not necessary to establish the diagnosis or to provide clinically useful prognostic information for patients with consistent clinical findings for the diagnosis of NOA (e.g., testicular atrophy or markedly elevated FSH). Conversely, patients who have a normal serum FSH should undergo a diagnostic testicular biopsy, because normal or borderline elevated serum FSH levels may suggest either obstruction or abnormal spermatogenesis. If the testicular biopsy is normal, an obstruction in the reproductive system must be found. Most men with OA, palpable vasa deferentia, and no history of iatrogenic vasal injury present with bilateral epididymal obstruction. Epididymal obstruction can be identified only by surgical exploration. Vasography may be utilized to determine whether there is an obstruction in the vas deferens or ED.

Reduced semen volume

Low ejaculate volume (< 1.0 ml) that is not caused by hypogonadism or CBAVD may be caused by ejaculatory dysfunction, but is most likely caused by EDO. Ejaculatory dysfunction rarely causes low ejaculate volume with azoospermia, although it is a well-known cause of aspermia or low ejaculate volume with oligozoospermia. Additional seminal parameters that may be helpful in determining the presence of EDO are seminal pH and fructose, since the seminal vesicle secretions are alkaline and contain fructose. EDO is detected by transrectal ultrasonography (TRUS). The finding of midline cysts, dilated ED, and/or dilated seminal vesicles (>1.5 cm in antero-posterior diameter) on TRUS is suggestive, but not diagnostic, of EDO. Therefore, seminal vesicle aspiration (SVA) and seminal vesiculography may be performed under TRUS guidance to make a more definitive diagnosis of EDO. The presence of large numbers of sperm in the seminal vesicle of an azoospermic patient is highly suggestive of EDO. Seminal vesiculography performed contemporary with SVA can localize the site of obstruction. EDO is detected by TRUS, and is usually accompanied by dilation of the seminal vesicles (typically >1.5 cm).

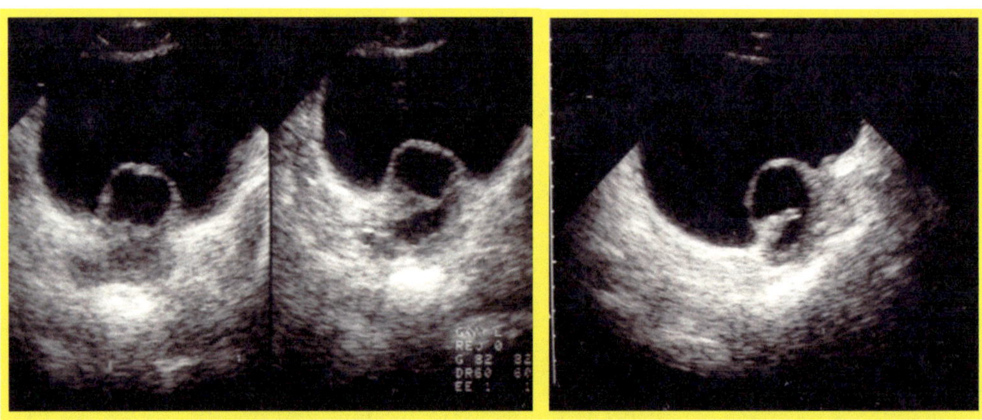

Fig. 1. Ultarsound Investigation: Intraprostatic cyst with ejaculatory duct obstruction

Genetic investigations for men with azoospermia

All men with hypogonadotropic hypogonadism should be referred for genetics counseling, as almost all of the congenital abnormalities of the hypothalamus are due to a genetic alteration.

If a genetic alteration is identified, then genetic counseling is suggested (Level of evidence 2, Grade B recommendation). In addition to mutations in the CFTR gene that give rise to CBAVD, genetic factors may play a role in NOA. The two most common categories of genetic factors are chromosomal abnormalities resulting in impaired testicular function, and Y-chromosome microdeletions leading to isolated spermatogenic impairment.

Chromosomal abnormalities account for approximately 6% of all male infertility, and the prevalence increases with increased spermatogenic impairment (severe oligospermia and NOA).

Approximately 13% of men with NOA or severe oligospermia may have an underlying Y-chromosome microdeletion. Y chromosome microdeletions responsible for infertility – azoospermia factor (AZF) regions a, b, or c – are detected using sequence-tagged sites (STS) and polymerase chain reaction (PCR) analysis. Y chromosome microdeletions carry both prognostic significance for finding sperm, and consequences for offspring if these sperm are utilized. Although successful testicular sperm extraction has not been reported in infertile men with large deletions involving AZFa or AZFb regions, the total number of reports is limited. However, up to 80% of men with AZFc deletions may have retrievable sperm for intracytoplasmic sperm injection (ICSI).

Treatments for azoospermia

Obstructive azoospermia

Instrumental and surgical treatments designed to restore natural fertility

1. Microsurgical recanalization of the proximal seminal tract
a. Obstruction of the epididymis: epididymal tubal vasostomy (vasoepididymostomy)
b. Obstruction of the vas deferens: vasovasostomy
2. Recanalization of the distal seminal tract
a. Transurethral resection of the ejaculatory ducts (TURED)
b. Transrectal ultrasound-guided by unblocking (TRUC)
c. Seminal tract washout treatment
3. Surgical or instrumental sperm collection for artificial reproductive treatment
- Testis
    a. Testicular sperm extraction (TESE)
    b. Testicular sperm aspiration (TESA)
    c. Testicular fine needle aspiration (TEFNA)
- Epididymis
    a. Microsurgical epididymal sperm aspiration (MESA)
    b. Percutaneous epididymal sperm aspiration (PESA)
    c. Epididymal sperm extraction (ESE)
- Vas deferens and distal seminal tract
a. Microscopic vasal sperm aspiration (MVSA)

b. Distal seminal tract aspiration (DISTA)
c. Transrectal ultrasound-guided aspiration of sperm from intraprostatic cysts communicating with the ED
d. Seminal tract washout designed to recover sperm for in vitro fertilization (IVF)

Secretory azoospermia

a. Medical treatment
b. The varicocele in azoospermia
c. Surgical removal of sperm from the testicle or instrument for artificial insemination
    1. Testicular sperm extraction (TESE)
    2. Testicular sperm aspiration (TESA) and Testicular fine needle aspiration (TEFNA)

Retrograde ejaculation

a. Pharmacotherapy
b. Recovery of sperm from the urine as an aid to artificial insemination

Anejaculation

a. Etiologic treatments
b. Treatment aimed to recover sperm for assisted reproductive technology (ART)
    1. Vibratory ED massage
    2. Electroejaculation
    3. Seminal tract washout designed to recover sperm for IVF or cryopreservation of testicular sperm

Obstructive azoospermia

The aim of treating obstructive azoospermia is to restore the patency of the seminal tract and spontaneous fertility. Treatment choice depends on the localization and characteristics of the obstructing lesion. When it is not possible to restore the patency of the seminal tract, the next step is to proceed to surgical sperm recovery (to be used fresh or after cryopreservation for ART).

2. Microsurgery: Reconstruction of the proximal seminal tract

The correct implementation and results of microsurgical reconstruction of the proximal seminal tract depend upon the use of special instruments (surgical microscope), non-reactive suture materials, and the technical skill of the operator. The surgical microscope is essential to evaluate the quantity and quality of sperm during seminal fluid aspiration. This determination dictates the choice of reconstructive surgery.

Surgery is indicated in the following cases:

- Azoospermia confirmed by at least two recent seminal examinations
- Preservation of spermatogenesis on at least one side
- Absence of retrograde ejaculation
- Absence of seminal tract infection

The reconstruction of the seminal tract is still subject to its proximal distal patency, which is demonstrated in the phase immediately preceding reconstructive surgery through cannulation of the deferent (butterfly needle 23-25 Gauge) and injection of at least 10 ml of saline solution.

Epididymal obstructions: Vasoepididymostomy

Vasoepididymostomy is performed to treat congenital, infectious, post-vasectomy or idiopathic obstruction of the epididymis. The rate of restoration of patency varies between 60% and 87%, and spontaneous pregnancies vary between 10% and 43%.5-8 Accuracy of microsurgical technique affects the outcome of reconstructive procedures on the male reproductive system. The best results are achieved by surgeons with training and ongoing experience in microsurgery. To maximize successful outcomes, surgeons performing vasectomy reversal should be comfortable with anastomoses involving extremely small luminal diameters, and must be competent with both vasovasostomy and vasoepididymostomy, because the latter may be unexpectedly necessary in many cases.

Before vasoepididymostomy, or when anastomosis is not feasible, sperm aspiration and cryopreservation should be performed for future use for ICSI, in case of failure of the anastomosis. In some cases, the reappearance of sperm in the seminal liquid happens more than one year after surgery. Stricture of the anastomosis has been observed after some time, at rates varying between 10% and 21%. The absence of sperm in the epididymal tubule or the presence of diffuse fibrosis of the organ are two negative prognostic factors that indicate the presence of a secretory testicular pathology. The presence of ultrasound abnormalities of the distal seminal tract have recently been reported as adverse prognostic factors for the success rates of recanalization. Vasoepididymostomy in patients with obstruction secondary to vasectomy is more advantageous in terms of costs compared with MESA with ICSI pregnancies.

Technical notes

The epididymis is opened where there is a clear tubular dilation due to the obstacle; however, the opening should be as caudal as possible. The liquid that issues from the epididymis is immediately examined to assess the presence and motility of sperm. If the determination is negative, a more proximal tubule will be opened. If the goal is to make an end-to-end vasostomy, after transverse incision of the epididymis tunica vaginalis, the section of the seminal tubules containing sperm should be chosen to perform the anastomosis with the deferent to reduce the possibility of developing strictures in the future. A latero-terminal vasostomy appears to avoid this eventuality without additional effort. Under optical magnification of the field (40×) (the center of a window previously prepared in the tunica vaginalis of the epididymis), a loop is opened longitudinally and the tubulus is anastomosed to deferent with two stitches (8-0 Prolene). To prevent leakage of seminal fluid and the resulting formation of granulomas, the stitches should be as superficial as possible and at the end it is recommended that fibrin glue be placed on the anastomosis.

Obstructions of the vas deferens: Vasovasostomy

The obstruction of the vas deferens that results from vasectomy or, more rarely, from an incorrect vesiculodeferentography, can usually be successfully treated. By contrast, in

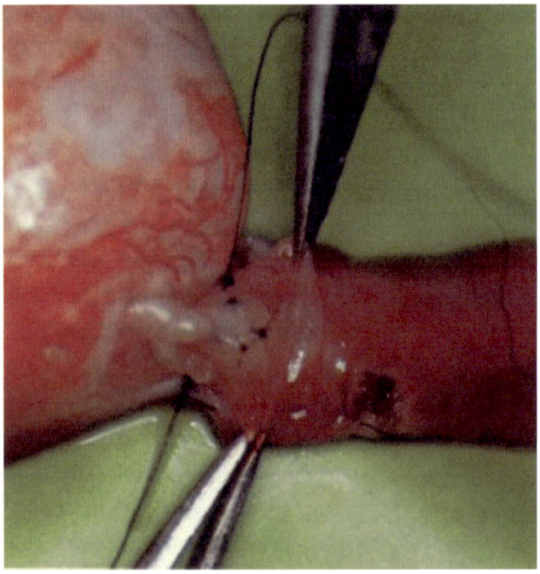

Fig. 2. Vasoepididymostomy

lesions of the distal vas deferens, usually resulting in bilateral herniorrhaphy, the stumps of the vas deferens are often poorly identified in the context of scar tissue. It is therefore necessary to resort to a wide mobilization of the stumps to perform both proximal and distal anastomosis. The outer diameter of the duct remains constant as a result of obstruction, while the inner testicular slope expands approximately 2-4 times. Distal stump sclerosis may progress to scarring. Factors that will influence the success of the anastomosis are:

- The use of a surgical microscope
- The quality of the tissues involved in the anastomosis
- The presence and characteristics of the fluid that is released from the proximal stump of the ductus
- Distal patency of the seminal vesicle
- The duration of obstruction

The recanalization rates extrapolated from the main series (a total of 2385 cases treated) vary between 86% and 93%, while the cumulative spontaneous pregnancy rates range between 52% and 82%. The duration of the obstruction appreciably affect the success rate of vasovasostomy. When the interval between obstruction and recanalization is shorter than 3 years, patency and spontaneous pregnancies are obtained, respectively, in 97% and 76% of cases, compared with 88% and 53% when the interval is between 3 and 8 years, and 71% and 30% when the interval is between 9 and 14 years. Deferential distal obstructions are often incorrigible. In these cases, the aspiration of sperm from the proximal deferential stump may be used or, if there is a concomitant epididymal obstruction, MESA or TESE may be employed (see related chapters).

Technical Notes

Reconstruction of the deferent can be performed in "double layer" or "single layer". In two-layer vasovasostomy, the mucous layer and inner muscle of the two stumps are sutured with 6 sutures (preferably non-absorbable or slow resorption 9/0-10/0); then, the outer muscular and serosal layers are secured with 6 sutures 8/0-9/0, interspersed with the first. However, the sutures pass through the wall of the deferent at ≥6 points, possibly full-thickness.

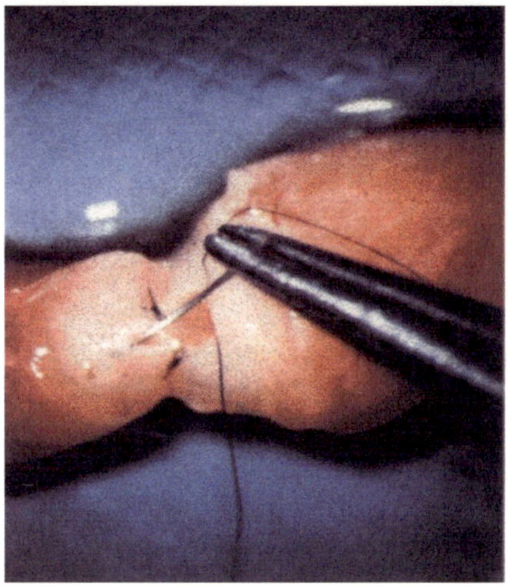

Fig. 3. Vaso-vasostomia

3. Recanalization of the distal seminal tract

Transurethral resection of the ejaculatory ducts (TURED)

Transurethral resection of the ejaculatory ducts (TURED) was proposed in 1973 by Farley and Barnes for the resolution of (EDO). Since then, several studies have documented its effectiveness. The term also includes the endoscopic resection of the ED obstructing prostatic cysts, even if improperly, because in this case the ED are not properly resected, but only the anterior wall of the cyst, making it widely communicate with the prostatic urethra. The indications for TURED are represented by a complete or incomplete congenital or acquired obstruction of the distal seminal tract, caused by atresia, strictures, or scarring; or in the presence of gallstones of ED; or subsequent prostatic cysts, whether or not they communicate with the seminal tract. Only issues relating to the use of TURED in cases of azoospermia will be taken into account.

Until a few years ago, TURED was the only therapeutic option in cases of obstruction of ED. Recently, successful sperm retrieval techniques for assisted reproduction (e.g., ICSI) and the introduction of new techniques (ultrasound-guided sclerotherapy of prostatic cysts, Seminal Tract Wash-out) have reduced its use. Nevertheless, TURED must still be considered an effective therapeutic method that allows patients to obtain natural pregnancies in a significant percentage of cases of obstructive azoospermia. A recent review of 164 cases reported in the literature documented a recanalization rate of 36% and a pregnancy rate of 26%. Regarding cystic obstruction of the ED, TURED could be used in the seminal cysts communicating with the seminal tract. In the presence of non-communicating cysts (Müllerian or median), transrectal ultrasound-guided or percutaneous sclerotherapy are first indicated, and only in case of their failure should TURED be performed.

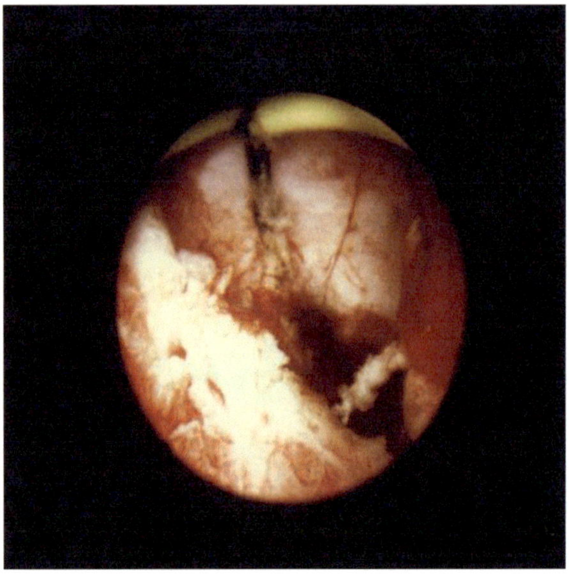

Fig. 4. TURED

Transrectal ultrasonically guided aspiration (TRUCA) of the seminal distal tract

Transrectal ultrasonically guided cyst aspiration (TRUCA) is a minimally invasive technique, suitable to evacuate intraprostatic cysts that are making an extrinsic compression on the ED. The above are of Müllerian cysts that do not communicate with the ED and do not contain sperm. The aspiration of the cyst temporarily or permanently restores normal patency of the ED. This procedure is used as an alternative to endoscopic transurethral incision of the Müllerian cysts.

Technical notes

A transrectal probe of 6.5-7.5 MHz biplanar is used to perform this technique, with a 20-22 G Chiba needle guide connected to a 5 ml syringe for suction. The treatment is conducted with the patient placed on his left side, after oral antibiotic coverage The aspiration is performed with after the patient had abstained from sex from 4 to 5 days to determine the chemical-physical characteristics of the aspirated fluid and the presence of sperm. Shortly after aspiration, the patient is requested to provide a semen sample for analysis. Immediately after, the clinician should recheck the cyst to assess its possible immediate filling (in this case, the cyst is communicating with the seminal tract, and therefore should not be inflexible). For sclerotherapy, an antibiotic (tetracycline) is instilled into the cyst at a rate of one-tenth of the previously aspirated volume. This procedure allows recovery of patency of the distal seminal tract in 75% of patients.

Seminal tract washout therapy aims to restore the patency of the ejaculatory ducts

Seminal Tract Washout (STW) therapy is indicated in azoospermic patients in whom an ultrasound of the distal seminal tract (controlled before and after ejaculation) documents obstruction of the orifices of the ED.1 This framework is characterized by an expansion of products that are associated with dilation of the seminal vesicles throughout their course,

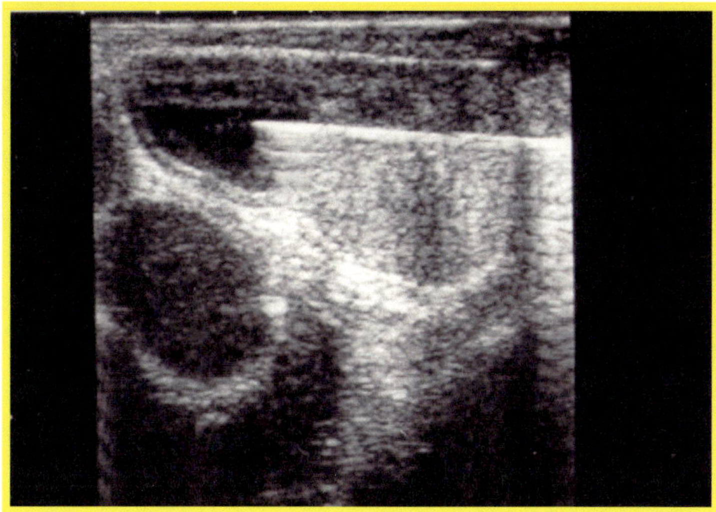

Fig. 5. TRUCA

possibly with seminal calcifications within them. STW is not indicated in patients with a transrectal ultrasound examination that clearly shows a post-inflammatory obstruction of the ED. The STW runs with the same methods described for the STW designed to retrieve sperm for use in assisted reproduction. The unblocking of the orifice of the ED does not rule out the option of recovering and cryopreserving the sperm present in the seminal tract obstruction.

4. Surgical or instrumental sperm collection for artificial insemination

Testicular Sperm Extraction (TESE)

TESE is the extraction of sperm from testicular parenchymal fragments obtained from single or multiple surgical biopsies. TESE was initially introduced by Silber et al. in 1995, as a method of sperm retrieval for ICSI in cases of azoospermia.

TESE is one of several options for sperm retrieval in cases of OA, with directions more or less similar to other techniques. As a testicular removal, it has the advantage over epididymal sperm extraction (ESE) of not obstructing the patency of the epididymis tubule. This advantage can be especially important in cases of potentially reconstructible proximal obstructions (which remain the only curative option in reconstructive surgery), particularly those involving cases of distal ejaculation or anejaculation. Compared with epididymal microsurgical sperm aspiration (MESA), TESE permits the recovery of sperm, and is definitely easier because it does not require the use of a surgical microscope. TESE could be considered the ideal solution to retrieve sperm in those rare cases in which obstructive MESA fails, during the same surgical procedure. TESE is slightly more invasive and complex than the percutaneous techniques; however, in comparison TESE allows the recovery of a more appropriate number of sperm (almost always enough to freeze and use in subsequent cycles of ICSI). Several authors have proposed using TESE directly with cryopreservation in the course of diagnostic testicular biopsy.

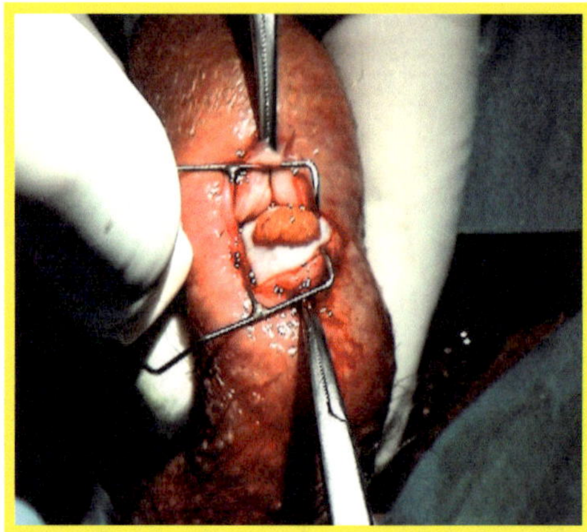

(a)

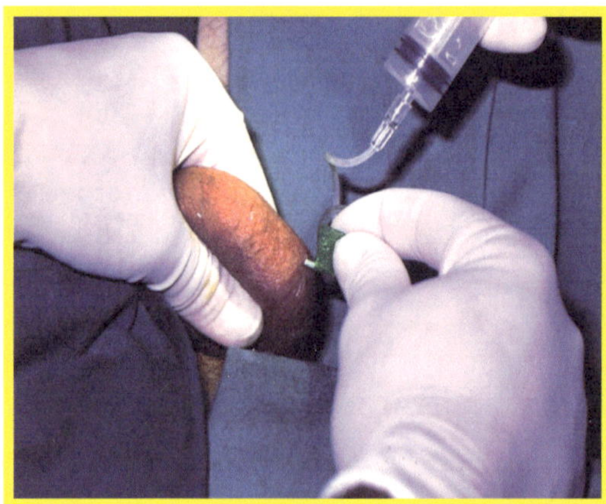

(b)

Fig. 6. (a) TESE, (b) TESA

Epididymal Microsurgical Sperm Aspiration (MESA)

MESA was the first sperm retrieval technique used for ART (Silber, 1987). While it was initially associated with IVF, since 1994 MESA has usually been associated with ICSI, even though the use of IVF may still be justified when sperm of good quality and quantity is recovered. MESA allows better recovery in terms of quantity and quality of sperm. Thanks to microsurgical techniques, it is possible to minimize blood contamination and choose the tubules with the best features for good sperm recovery.13 The chances of sperm retrieval with MESA are >95%, and it is almost always possible to freeze a sufficient number of sperm for any subsequent cycles of ICSI. Therefore, the male partner is usually subjected to a single intervention. The disadvantages of MESA arise because it is a complex technique that requires a manual microsurgical, as well as the availability of an operating microscope and proper instrumentation. The time and costs of MESA intervention are therefore higher than other techniques. MESA is now performed under local anesthesia with the patient's immediate resignation. Normally it is sufficient to intervention only in cases of unilateral and insufficient sperm retrieval.

Technical notes

Traditional technique: General anesthesia, or local infiltration of the umbilical cord and the scrotal skin with any anesthesia care or sedation. A median scrotal incision is made with the opening of the tunica vaginalis and externalization of the testis. Under 20-30× magnification, a slot is removed from the head of the epididymis tunica albuginea and hemostasis is ensured with a bipolar forceps jeweler. The clinician then opens the tubule with microscissors and aspirates the liquid with a 22 or 23 G cannula mounted on an insulin syringe. Slight pressure on the testis and epididymis promotes the release of sperm. The extraction is continued with several syringes until leakage occurs, or until the biologist who monitors the sample finds it sufficient for freezing. Closure of the tubule with a 10/0 stitch is optional. In the variant proposed by Schlegel, instead of opening the tubule with microscissors, the tubule is pricked with a specially prepared, sharp glass micropipette connected to a suction system. This alternative saves time spent searching for the area with better sperm quality and minimizes blood contamination.

Mini-MESA: In this variation of the technique, an incision is made approximately 1 cm from the window as a diagnostic testicular biopsy. Instead of exteriorizing the testicle, only the head of the epididymis is dislocated from the incision and secured with a stitch on the edge of the same. The technique then continues in the same way as the traditional technique, using a surgical microscope for subsequent phases of sperm aspiration from the epididymal tubules. Advantages of this alternative technique include the lack of externalization of the testis, reduction of pain experienced by the patient, and a minimized possibility of postoperative surgical adhesions.

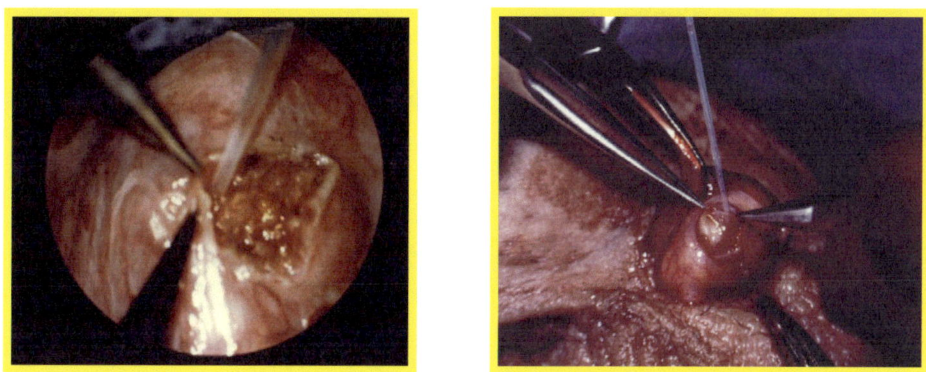

(a) (b)

Fig. 7. (a) MESA, (b) Mini MESA

Epididymal Percutaneous Sperm Aspiration (PESA)

Introduced by Craft in 1995, PESA represented the first "economic" alternative to MESA in patients with OA. Like TESA, PESA has the advantages of being easily implemented, economical, and minimally invasive. The main limitation of PESA is its lower efficacy compared with MESA sperm retrieval. In several studies, PESA seems to allow sperm recovery in approximately 60-70% of OA cases, compared with a 90-95% sperm recovery rate by MESA. The lower sperm recovery rate of PESA is presumably a consequence of the particular anatomic situation of the tubules of the head of the epididymis, which, when obstructed, are not uniformly dilated and do not contain the same amount or quality of sperm. If in the course of MESA is possible to drive on the intake and more dilated tubules with more chance of recovering motile sperm, PESA may just sting tubules without sperm or with sperm of poorer quality. Because PESA results in aspirated sperm of lower quantity and poorer quality, the possibility of freezing sperm for subsequent ICSI cycles is significantly lower with PESA than with MESA. By contrast, compared with TESA, PESA may allow better sperm retrieval, with less contamination from blood or other parenchymal cells. However, PESA involves an increased risk of scrotal hematoma than TESA, caused by the greater vascularity of the area of the head of the epididymis. PESA represents the technique of choice in cases of obstruction or congenital or acquired spermatocele in the epididymis. In this situation, PESA allows easy retrieval of a large amount of sperm with minimal invasiveness, and can be performed without any anesthesia.

Technical Notes

Regarding the need for anesthesia, the same considerations apply to PESA as to TESA. When aspirating, it is best to use a butterfly needle (21 or 22 G) connected to a 20-ml or 50-ml syringe. Aspiration should be applied to only the head of the epididymis, not to the body or tail. The clinician should immobilize the head of the epididymis by holding it between thumb and forefinger, and insert the needle into it. With the syringe, and always under slight suction, advance or retract the needle millimeter-wise until a small amount of clear liquid is observed in the connecting pipe. Continue suction until the flow stops. In most cases, this technique will result in a small quantity of well-aspirated sperm. The aspirated fluid is then diluted in culture medium and examined for sperm. If no sperm is recovered, the clinician should proceed to other aspirations, trying to puncture different parts of the head of the epididymis. It may help to exert pressure on the head of the epididymis for a few minutes, and to keep a bag of ice on the scrotum to minimize the risk of bleeding.

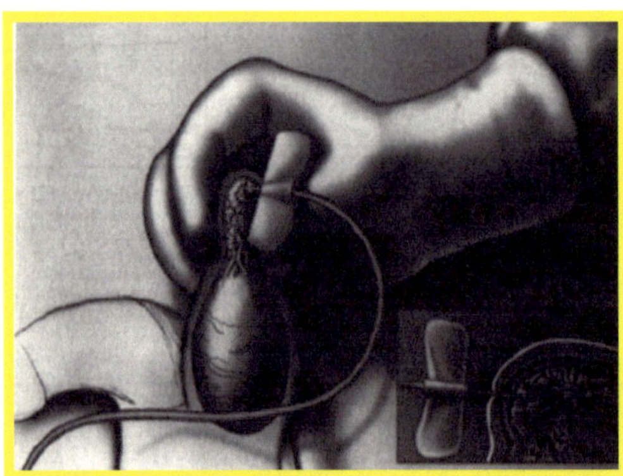

Fig. 8. PESA

5. Epididymis

Epididymal Sperm Extraction (ESE)

ESE is the surgical removal (no need for microsurgical techniques) of more or less substantial portions of the head of the epididymis for sperm extraction. ESE was described for the first time by Kim, although it had already been used sporadically by many clinicians. The extraction technique is identical to TESE. ESE has the advantage of being very fast, does not require the use of a surgical microscope, often provides excellent recoveries that are almost always sufficient to freeze sperm, and is associated with fertilization and pregnancy rates similar to those associated with other techniques. Its main disadvantages are that it is more invasive; the removal or parts of the epididymis is less repeatable (to be performed only in intractable situations of obstruction, such as CBAVD or congenital bilateral agenesis of the vasa deferentia); a higher risk of vascular damage to the testis; and increased blood contamination of the fragment to be treated. ESE is a viable option, and is therefore often used in the course of MESA, when it is not possible to retrieve sperm microaspirates from any of the epididymal sites.

Technical Notes

ESE can be performed under regional anesthesia or sedation. A medial scrotal incision is made, through which the testicle (or simply the head of the epididymis) is exteriorized. With scissors, the surgeon separates it from the testis to approximately 5 mm, dissecting some of the efferent vessels. The surgeon then uses scissors or a scalpel to cut a portion of the epididymis, and the entire head is immersed in a cell culture dish. Next, the biologist will perform the fragmentation of the piece first with scissors or scalpel and then slides with two sterile insulin needles.

Surgical or instrumental collection of sperm for assisted fertilization:
The vas deferens and distal seminal tract

Microscopic Vasal Sperm Aspiration (MVSA)

MVSA consists of the microsurgical aspiration of sperm from the lumen of the deferent. It is indicated in cases of distal deferential obstruction without any possibility of surgical reconstruction (e.g., iatrogenic damage from pelvic surgery or hernioplasty); cases of EDO; cases in which TURED or other techniques cannot be used to harvest sperm (e.g., DISTA); in cases of retrograde ejaculation with insufficient sperm retrieval from the post-orgasm urine; in cases of anejaculation due to different causes; or when vibrostimulation or electroejaculation fail. Finally, MVSA is indicated in selected cases of necrozoospermia or pronounced oligoastenozoospermia in the presence of structural or functional disorders of the emptying of the distal seminal tract that result in prolonged stagnation of the sperm. In these patients, sperm can be obtained from the deferent with good motility and vitality. The recovery of sperm cells that almost always exhibit very good motility makes it possible to opt for less invasive ART techniques (e.g., IVF, intrauterine insemination), as well as freezing. The main disadvantage of MVSA is that the procedure must be performed using microsurgical technique, which is essential for the closure of the rubble of the deferent because of the risk of iatrogenic obstruction.

Technical Notes

MVSA is performed under local anesthesia by infiltration of the scrotal skin. A small incision is made in the scrotum to isolate the deferent and exteriorize it through the surgical access. The vas deferens is cut with a scalpel at the level of a straight portion. With a 23 or 24 G cannula mounted on an insulin syringe or other suction system,3 it is then possible to proceed to the suction of seminal liquid from the lumen of the proximal stump of the deferent. The lumen must be closed with a microsurgical suture (Nylon 10/0), preferably in a double layer (2-3 and 5-6 inside-out stitches).

Distal Seminal Tract Aspiration (DISTA)

Designed as a diagnostic technique, DISTA was subsequently proposed as a treatment to support ART, particularly in cases of azoospermia secondary to an EDO. DISTA involves ultrasound-guided transperineal or transrectal fine needle aspiration of the liquid contained in the seminal vesicles, ED, or cysts of the seminal carrefour in patients with an obstruction of the seminal distal end, thereby achieving sperm retrieval for ART.

The advantage of this technique is that it is minimally invasive compared with TURED; DISTA can be performed under local anesthesia and is easily repeatable. Furthermore, DISTA does not present any of the complications that may arise after TURED, such as the contamination of semen and the reflux of urine into the seminal tract due to the alteration of the antireflux mechanism of the ED. Compared with the techniques used to retrieve sperm from the more proximal seminal tract (deferens: MVSA; epididymis: MESA-PESA; the testis: TESE-TESA), DISTA has the advantages of avoiding the risk of secondary iatrogenic obstructions in these locations; of being quicker and simpler to perform; of being less costly compared with MVSA, MESA, and TESE; and of allowing sperm retrieval that is usually better than TESA, TESE, or PESA. DISTA almost always results in semen that can be frozen for future use in simple ART techniques.

Its disadvantages include the persistent need of an ART technique and its dependence on the availability of an ultrasound machine, as well as even the possibility (albeit negligible) of ascending infections of the seminal tract.

The primary indication for DISTA is cystic duct obstruction (where TURED is not indicated because of high risk); its secondary indication is prostatic cysts communicating with the seminal tract, or intraprostatic cysts in the ED with no obstructions.

Technical Notes

It is advisable to ejaculate the patient immediately before the procedure to increase the number of spermatozoa present in the distal seminal tract. The patient is placed in the lithotomic position or right lateral decubitus. After the administration of systemic antibiotics and enemas (in the case of transrectal puncture), the procedure requires a (preferably linear) transrectal ultrasound probe. The transperineal puncture is performed with local anesthesia. A 20-22 G Chiba type needle is guided by ultrasound to reach the dilated tract (seminal vesicle, ED, prostatic cyst communicating). The liquid content is then aspirated and sent to the laboratory for search and treatment of spermatozoa (swim-up, Percoll, mini-Percoll) to be used for ART.

Transrectal ultrasonically guided sperm cyst aspiration (TRUSCA) can be used to retrieve sperm from Müllerian cysts or the urogenital sinus communicating with one or both ED.

The semen from the aspirated cysts may be suitable for cryopreservation and for subsequent use in ICSI. It may be useful to repeat the procedure a few hours later and immediately after an ejaculation, to increase the likelihood of getting recent sperm flow at the suction site.

Seminal Tract Washout designed to recover sperm for assisted fertilization

Seminal Tract Washout (STW) is an anterograde seminal tract cleaning that pushes spermatozoa from the tails of the epididymis into the bladder, recovering the latter spermatozoa from the bladder by catheterization. The spermatozoa are then cryopreserved or used fresh for ART.

STW is a minimally invasive surgical procedure, applicable in azoospermic (or cryptozoospermic) patients with functional impairment of emptying of the distal seminal tract or a congenital or acquired incomplete anatomic obstruction of the ED. Even in patients with neurogenic anejaculation (an outcome of spinal cord injury of traumatic or iatrogenic origin, juvenile diabetes, or retroperitoneal lymph node dissection for unilateral testicular cancer) and in those with psychogenic anejaculation, sperm retrieval for IVF is satisfactory.

Technical Notes

STW is performed in the outpatient clinic. After the insertion of a Foley Ch 16-18 catheter into the bladder, T6 medium or Ham's F10 is used to wash the bladder and bring the pH to values appropriate to the maintenance of spermatozoa. Twenty milliliters of the same medium are left inside the bladder. Under local funicular anesthesia, the vas deferens is exteriorized with an Allis clamp and loaded between two vascular tapes to insert a 9.5 mm, 25 G butterfly needle.

A 2.5 ml syringe is needed to fill in anterograde direction 20 ml of T6 medium or Ham's F10 for each side. The liquid is immediately recovered from the bladder through the previously inserted catheter and centrifuged (10 min, 600 *g*), and the pellet is treated with the mini-Percoll technique. The obtained sperm can be used for artificial insemination in vivo or in vitro, or cryopreserved and subsequently used for ICSI.

The full-term pregnancy rates of assisted reproductive technologyART with sperm retrieved using STW are high,4 and comparable to those obtained with testicular sperm from obstructive azoospermic subjects.

STW is simple and inexpensive, and does not require microsurgical sutures or paramedical personnel. Compared with TESE and TEFNA, STW allows recovery of a much higher number of sperm, and obtains biological preparations suitable for assisted reproduction techniques in vivo, often without ICSI.

STW is as invasive as a single sample pulp with TESE, and certainly less invasive than multiple TESE withdrawals. It does not require the opening of the tunica vaginalis, the externalization of the gonad, or the suture of the albuginea, and therefore does not carry a risk of bleeding.

6. References

Bhasin S. Approach to the infertile man. J Clin Endocrinol Metab. 2007;92(6):1995-2004.

Campbell AJ, Irvine DS. Male infertility and intracytoplasmic sperm injection (ICSI). Br Med Bull. 2000;56(3):616-29.

Choe JH, Kim JW, Lee JS, Seo JT. Routine screening for classical azoospermia factor deletions of the Y chromosome in azoospermic patients with Klinefelter syndrome. Asian J Androl. 2007 Nov;9(6):815-20. PubMed PMID: 17968468.

Colpi GM, Negri L, Scroppo FI, Grugnetti C, Patrizio P. Seminal Tract Washout: a new diagnostic tool in complicated cases of male infertility. J Androl 15 (Supplement):17S-22S, 1994.

Dixit R, Dixit K, Jindal S, Shah KV. An unusual presentation of immotile-cilia syndrome with azoospermia: Case report and literature review. Lung India. 2009;26(4):142-5. PubMed PMID: 20532000; PubMed Central PMCID: PMC2876703.

Donkol RH. Imaging in male-factor obstructive infertility. World J Radiol 2010;2(5):172-9.

Donoso P, Tournaye H, Devroey P. Which is the best sperm retrieval technique for non-obstructive azoospermia? A systematic review. Hum Reprod Update. 2007 Nov-Dec;13(6):539-49.

Esteves SC, Agarwal A. Novel concepts in male infertility. Int Braz J Urol.2011;37(1):5-15.

Everaert K, De Croo I, Kerckhaert W, Dekuyper P, Dhont M, Van der Elst J, De Sutter P, Comhaire F, Mahmoud A, Lumen N. Long term effects of micro-surgical testicular sperm extraction on androgen status in patients with non obstructive azoospermia. BMC Urol. 2006 Mar 20;6:9.

Ezeh UI. Beyond the clinical classification of azoospermia: opinion. Hum Reprod. 2000 Nov;15(11):2356-9.

Foresta C, Moro E, Ferlin A. Y chromosome microdeletions and alterations of spermatogenesis. Endocr Rev. 2001 Apr;22(2):226-39.

Fullerton G, Hamilton M, Maheshwari A. Should non-mosaic Klinefelter syndrome men be labelled as infertile in 2009? Hum Reprod. 2010 Mar;25(3):588-97.

Garg T, LaRosa C, Strawn E, Robb P, Sandlow JI. Outcomes after testicular aspiration and testicular tissue cryopreservation for obstructive azoospermia and ejaculatory dysfunction. J Urol. 2008 Dec;180(6):2577-80.

Gerris J. Methods of semen collection not based on masturbation or surgical sperm retrieval. Hum Reprod Update. 1999 May-Jun;5(3):211-5.

Ho KL, Wong MH, Tam PC. Microsurgical vasoepididymostomy for obstructive azoospermia. Hong Kong Med J. 2009 Dec;15(6):452-7.

Ichijo S, Sigg C, Nagasawa M, Sirawa Y. Vasoseminal vesiculography before and after ejaculation. Urol. Intern 36:35, 1981

Jarow JP. Seminal vesicle aspiration of fertile men. J Urol 156(3):1005-1007, 1997.

Jarzabek K, Zbucka M, Pepiński W, Szamatowicz J, Domitrz J, Janica J, Wołczyński S, Szamatowicz M. Cystic fibrosis as a cause of infertility. Reprod Biol. 2004;4(2):119-29.

Jee SH, Hong YK. One-layer vasovasostomy: microsurgical versus loupe-assisted. Fertil Steril. 2010 Nov;94(6):2308-11.

Kamal A, Fahmy I, Mansour R, Serour G, Aboulghar M, Ramos L, Kremer J. Does the outcome of ICSI in cases of obstructive azoospermia depend on the origin of the retrieved spermatozoa or the cause of obstruction? A comparative analysis. Fertil Steril. 2010 Nov;94(6):2135-40.

La Marca A, Sighinolfi G, Radi D, Argento C, Baraldi E, Artenisio AC, Stabile G, Volpe A. Anti-Mullerian hormone (AMH) as a predictive marker in assisted reproductive technology (ART). Hum Reprod Update. 2010 Mar-Apr;16(2):113-30.

Lee R, Li PS, Goldstein M, Tanrikut C, Schattman G, Schlegel PN. A decision analysis of treatments for obstructive azoospermia. Hum Reprod. 2008 Sep;23(9):2043-9.

Lee R, Li PS, Schlegel PN, Goldstein M. Reassessing reconstruction in the management of obstructive azoospermia: reconstruction or sperm acquisition? Urol Clin North Am. 2008; 35(2):289-301

Marmar JL. The emergence of specialized procedures for the acquisition, processing, and cryopreservation of epididymal and testicular sperm in connection with intracytoplasmic sperm injection. J Androl. 1998 Sep-Oct;19(5):517-26.

McLachlan RI, O'Bryan MK. Clinical Review#: State of the art for genetic testing of infertile men. J Clin Endocrinol Metab. 2010 Mar;95(3):1013-24.

Merchant R, Gandhi G, Allahbadia GN. In vitro fertilization/intracytoplasmic sperm injection for male infertility. Indian J Urol. 2011;27(1):121-32.

Moon MH, Kim SH, Cho JY, Seo JT, Chun YK. Scrotal US for evaluation of infertile men with azoospermia. Radiology. 2006 Apr;239(1):168-73.

Navarro-Costa P, Gonçalves J, Plancha CE. The AZFc region of the Y chromosome: at the crossroads between genetic diversity and male infertility. Hum Reprod Update. 2010 Sep-Oct;16(5):525-42.

Navarro-Costa P, Plancha CE, Gonçalves J. Genetic dissection of the AZF regions of the human Y chromosome: thriller or filler for male (in)fertility? J Biomed Biotechnol. 2010;2010:936569.

Paz G, Gamzu R, Yavetz H. Diagnosis of nonobstructive azoospermia: the laboratory perspective. J Androl. 2003 Mar-Apr;24(2):167-9.

Poongothai J, Gopenath TS, Manonayaki S. Genetics of human male infertility. Singapore Med J. 2009 Apr;50(4):336-47.

Practice Committee of American Society for Reproductive Medicine in collaboration with Society for Male Reproduction and Urology. The management of infertility due to obstructive azoospermia. Fertil Steril. 2008 Nov;90(5 Suppl):S121-4.

Practice Committee of American Society for Reproductive Medicine. Sperm retrieval for obstructive azoospermia. Fertil Steril. 2008 Nov;90(5 Suppl):S213-8. Review.

Sadeghi-Nejad H, Farrokhi F. Genetics of azoospermia: current knowledge, clinical implications, and future directions. Part I. Urol J. 2006 Fall;3(4):193-203.

Sadeghi-Nejad H, Farrokhi F. Genetics of azoospermia: current knowledge, clinical implications, and future directions. Part II: Y chromosome microdeletions. Urol J. 2007 Fall;4(4):192-206

Schlegel PN, Girardi SK. Clinical review 87: In vitro fertilization for male factor infertility. J Clin Endocrinol Metab. 1997 Mar;82(3):709-16.

Semião-Francisco L, Braga DP, Figueira Rde C, Madaschi C, Pasqualotto FF, Iaconelli A Jr, Borges E Jr. Assisted reproductive technology outcomes in azoospermic men: 10 years of experience with surgical sperm retrieval. Aging Male. 2010 Mar;13(1):44-50.

Sertić J, Cvitković P, Myers A, Saiki RK, Stavljenić Rukavina A. Genetic markers of male infertility: Y chromosome microdeletions and cystic fibrosis transmembrane conductance gene mutations. Croat Med J. 2001 Aug;42(4):416-20.

Shah R. Surgical sperm retrieval: Techniques and their indications. Indian J Urol. 2011; 27(1):102-9.

Sharif K. Reclassification of azoospermia: the time has come? Hum Reprod 2000 Feb;15(2):237-8.

Shridharani A, Sandlow JI. Vasectomy reversal versus IVF with sperm retrieval: which is better? Curr Opin Urol. 2010 Nov;20(6):503-9.

Tanrikut C, Goldstein M. Obstructive azoospermia: a microsurgical success story. Semin Reprod Med. 2009 Mar;27(2):159-64.

Tournaye H. Update on surgical sperm recovery--the European view. Hum Fertil (Camb). 2010 Dec;13(4):242-6.

Van Peperstraten A, Proctor ML, Johnson NP, Philipson G. Techniques for surgical retrieval of sperm prior to intra-cytoplasmic sperm injection (ICSI) for azoospermia. Cochrane Database Syst Rev. 2008 Apr 16;(2):CD002807

Visser L, Westerveld GH, Korver CM, van Daalen SK, Hovingh SE, Rozen S, van der Veen F, Repping S. Y chromosome gr/gr deletions are a risk factor for low semen quality. Hum Reprod. 2009 Oct;24(10):2667-73. Epub 2009 Jul 14. PubMed PMID: 19602516.

Woldringh GH, Besselink DE, Tillema AH, Hendriks JC, Kremer JA. Karyotyping, congenital anomalies and follow-up of children after intracytoplasmic sperm injection with non-ejaculated sperm: a systematic review. Hum Reprod Update. 2010Jan-Feb;16(1):12-9.

Wood S, Sephton V, Searle T, Thomas K, Schnauffer K, Troup S, Kingsland C, Lewis-Jones I. Effect on clinical outcome of the interval between collection of epididymal and testicular spermatozoa and intracytoplasmic sperm injection in obstructive azoospermia. J Androl. 2003 Jan-Feb;24(1):67-72.

Yamaguchi K, Ishikawa T, Nakano Y, Kondo Y, Shiotani M, Fujisawa M. Rapidly progressing, late-onset obstructive azoospermia linked to herniorrhaphy with mesh. Fertil Steril. 2008;90(5):2018.e5-7.

Zielenski J. Genotype and phenotype in cystic fibrosis. Respiration. 2000;67(2):117-33.

2

Gene Mutations Associated with Male Infertility

Kamila Kusz-Zamelczyk, Barbara Ginter-Matuszewska,
Marcin Sajek and Jadwiga Jaruzelska
*Institute of Human Genetics Polish Academy of Sciences,
Poland*

1. Introduction

Infertility is a complex medical problem for several reasons. It is very frequent, since about 15% of couples worldwide fail to conceive, the male factor being involved in roughly 50% of cases. Secondly, the background of male infertility seems extremely heterogeneous including many environmental causes. Thirdly, in as many as 30% of individuals, the origin of infertility remains unknown (Poongothai et al., 2009). Chromosomal aberrations involving an abnormal number or structure of sex chromosomes or autosomes are found in approximately 5% of infertile men (for review see Ferlin et al., 2007). These aberrations often result in congenital syndromes, male infertility being one of their numerous features. Among them, Klinefelter syndrome is relatively common. It is caused by the presence of an extra X chromosome, 47,XXY. Another example is the 46,XX male syndrome. In a majority of cases, it results from translocation of a Y chromosome segment, containing the *SRY* gene, on the X chromosome. Structural aberrations of autosomes are much more frequent in males with isolated infertility than in the general population. For instance, Robertsonian translocation is 9-fold more frequent in infertile patients than in the general population. The most common Robertsonian translocation associated with male infertility is the one originating from chromosomes 13 and 14. Also reciprocal translocations are more frequent (4-10-fold) in infertile than in fertile males (for review see O'Flyn O'Brien et al., 2010). In the recent years much attention has been paid to mutations causing male infertility. These mutations were identified in genes known to be responsible for male germ cell development or, for other male reproductive processes. Thousands of genes in these categories are expressed in human testes and any of them can potentially cause infertility when mutated. This circumstance makes studies on genetic causes of male infertility extremely complex. Therefore, the generation of about 400 mouse models of male infertility in recent years has been very helpful to select the best human candidates for mutation screening in infertile men. These models represent defects at different steps of sperm cell development (Matzuk & Lamb, 2008). In fact, several hundred mutations have been identified in men suffering reproductive defects and by analogy with the mouse model, these mutations might affect human male reproduction. Also, state of the art technologies, such as genome-wide scanning, currently provide an enormous amount of new mutation records. Unexpectedly, this large amount of data on genetic variation contrasts with a very low number of reports describing well documented causative male infertility mutations. This is due to multiple obstacles in collecting additional necessary data. One of the major difficulties is collection of DNA samples from some family members of the proband. This is hampered by the fact that in many instances infertility remains a very personal issue of the couple. This problem makes the study of inheritance patterns difficult. Secondly, the frequency of the mutated alleles is usually very low. Thirdly, the negative mutational effect is not obvious in many cases. The use of specific functional tests is necessary in such situations but often very difficult to establish. Therefore, simple testing for infertility causing mutations is so far limited to Y-chromosome microdeletions testing using commercially available PCR-based kits (for review see O'Flynn O'Brien et al., 2010). Studies on the gene content of the target AZF (Azoospermia Factor) region on the Y revealed few genes which encode nucleic acid binding proteins (for review see Navarro-Costa et al., 2010a). One of the first cloned and also the best studied among them is the *DAZ* (Deleted in Azoospermia) gene which contains an RNA-binding domain (Reijo et al., 1995). Studies of this gene in humans and in several model organisms from the fly to the mouse revealed that DAZ binds the 3'untranslated region (3'UTR) of specific mRNAs to regulate translation in germ cells (Fox et al., 2005). Later on, several other RNA-binding proteins cooperating with DAZ in 3'UTR mediated translational regulation in human male germ cells have been cloned and their status in infertile males was investigated. At the present time, even more attention has been given to the structure of 3'UTRs which are targets for several types of small regulatory RNAs (srRNAs). Importantly, these targets may not be properly recognized when mutated. This issue opens a new field in the research on male infertility and the underlying genetic causes.

2. Autosomal single-gene mutations causing non-syndromic male infertility

A small number of well documented cases of autosomal gene mutations causing non-syndromic male infertility are reviewed below. Several of theses genes cause a distinct spermatozoa defect in the semen of the patients when mutated. These autosomal gene mutations were identified in course of a candidate gene mutation screening strategy or by the genome-wide scanning approach.

2.1 *AURKC* gene mutations in macrozoospermia

The genome-wide microsatellite scanning was performed in 10 infertile males suffering from macrozoospermia and originating from North Africa. Identification of a homozygous frame-shift mutation c.114delC in *AURKC* (Aurora Kinase C) gene in all 10 patients provided a strong support for its causative effect and the macrozoospermia phenotype (Dieterich et al., 2007). This finding was reinforced by further studies showing that 100% (66 individuals) of infertile macrozoospermic men originating from North Africa carried an *AURKC* gene mutation in both alleles. Moreover, the majority of them were c.114delC homozygotes (Dieterich et al., 2007, 2009; Kerch et al., 2011). The remaining patients were c.114delC/c.436-2A→G or c.114delC/p.Cys229Tyr compound heterozygotes (Ben Khelifa et al.; 2011, Dieterich et al., 2009). Importantly, no homozygotes were found in the several control groups of fertile men (Dieterich et al., 2007, Kerch et al., 2011). Pedigree analysis in two families revealed that all homozygous males were infertile whereas homozygous females and heterozygous males were fertile (Dieterich et al., 2007, 2009). This indicates a recessive inheritance model for *AURKC* mutation transmission with the infertility phenotype restricted to men. The c.114delC mutation introduces a frameshift p.Leu49TrpfsX22 resulting in premature stop codon. Indeed, a premature translational termination yielding a truncated protein lacking the kinase domain was demonstrated using a functional test (Dieterich et al., 2007). Spermatozoa of homozygous patients were all tetraploid indicating a cytokinesis arrest at the first meiotic division (Dieterich et al., 2009). Accordingly, the mutated *AURKC* gene has been associated with macrozoospermia characterized by a large-headed multiflagellar polyploid sperm. Also, mouse males characterized by *Aurkc* gene disruption presented with 20% of the sperm cells with characteristic macrozoospermic large heads (Kimmins et al., 2007). Consistent with this phenotype, this kinase was shown to localize at the centrosome suggesting a role in cell division (Kimura et al., 1999). Interestingly, although the *AURKC* gene mutations are deleterious only in male patients, Aurora Kinase C is highly expressed in both male (Bernard et al., 1998) and female gonads (Yan et al., 2005). These data indicate that, for couples with male infertility caused by *AURKC* gene mutation, the ISCI approach should not be encouraged.

2.2 *SPATA16* and *DPY19L2* gene mutations in globozoospermia

In course of infertility related genome-wide scan, *SPATA16* (spermatogenesis-associated 16) gene a mutation was identified in a consanguineous Ashkenazi Jewish family including three brothers suffering from globozoospermia. The same homozygous c.848G→A mutation of *SPATA16* gene was identified in all affected brothers. Since, both parents as well as two unaffected brothers were heterozygous and a healthy brother was a wild-type homozygote, an autosomal recessive inheritance of *SPATA16* gene mutation has been certified. Moreover, this mutation was absent in control group of fertile males. The functional analysis demonstrated that c.848G→A mutation altered the *SPATA16* pre-mRNA splicing process causing protein truncation. Namely, it disrupted the tetratricopeptide repeat (TRP) functional domain which is responsible for peptide-peptide interaction. The SPATA16 protein is specifically expressed in human testis and localizes to the Golgi apparatus (Xu et al., 2003). Accordingly, the mouse homologue localizes to the proacrosomic vesicles which at the spermatid stage are transported to the acrosome (Lu et al., 2006). While these data strongly suggested that *SPATA16* mutation caused globozoospermia, no causative *SPATA16* mutation was identified in additional 29 patients with the same phenotype (Dam et al., 2007).

Later on, two independent genome-wide scans of globozoospermic patients revealed a *DPY19L2* gene mutation underlying this phenotype. In the first study this mutation was found in a Jordanian consanguineous family including 10 siblings. In this family, four among five brothers suffering from complete globozoospermia, as well as three fertile brothers underwent the analysis. In all four analyzed infertile brothers a homozygous large ~200 kb deletion was identified. The only gene this deletion encompassed was the *DPY19L2*. Moreover, all fertile brothers were wild-type homozygotes at that *locus* (Koscinski et al., 2011). The second scan was performed on 20 patients mostly of the North African origin, suffering a complete globozoospermia. Also in this study a homozygous *DPY19L2* gene deletion was found in 15 out of 20 infertile men (Harbuz et al., 2011). Finally, a search for such *DPY19L2* deletions was performed on a third group of 28 globozoospermic patients. In this search, homozygous deletions were identified in 4 out of 28 infertile men. Differences of the deletion breakpoints identified in this group, suggested recurrent mutational events (Koscinski et al., 2011). A nonallelic homozygous recombination is the most probable bases for this mutational event, given that the *DPY19L2* gene is surrounded by two low copy repeats (Harbuz et al., 2011; Koscinski et al., 2011). The *DPY19L2* locus represents a copy number variant (CNV), since duplications as well as heterozygous deletions were found with frequency 1:76 and 1:222, respectively, in the large almost 5 thousands group of healthy individuals. However, no homozygous *DPY19L2* gene deletion was observed in this group of people (Koscinski et al., 2011). The persuasive pedigree analysis, a high frequency of homozygous deletion encompassing *DPY19L2* gene in globozoospermic patients as well as the lack of homozygous deletions in the control group, altogether indicate that this gene is a globozoospermia factor essential for the sperm head elongation and acrosome forming. As expected, the *DPY19L2* gene is predominantly expressed in testis (Harbuz et al., 2011). The *C.elegans* homologue is involved in the cell polarity as it was shown in the human sperm cells (Honigberg et al., 2000).

2.3 *DNAI1*, *DNAH5* and *DNAH11* asthenozoospermia associated genes

Mutation screening of three dynein encoding genes *DNAI1*, *DNAH5* and *DNAH11*, was performed in a group of 91 asthenozoospermic Italian patients of Caucasian origin, including familial cases. A causative mutation was identified in each of these genes. One of them, a p.Arg663Cys amino acid substitution of *DNAI1* was found in two infertile brothers and two other unrelated patients. The p.Glu2666Asp mutation of the *DNAH5* gene, however, was present in only one man. Finally, the p.Ile3040Val nonsynonymous mutation of the *DNAH11* gene was identified in two first cousins and in one unrelated patient. In both familial cases, mutations were inherited from the mothers indicating an autosomal dominant pattern of dynein gene transmission with the infertility phenotype restricted to men. None of the three mutations were identified in the control group of 200 fertile men. The three mutations targeted the highly conserved amino acid sites and, moreover, were localized either within or near the functional dynein domain (Zuccarello et al., 2008). Taken together, the presence of familial asthenozoospermia cases associated with two dynein gene mutations, their location at highly conserved amino acid positions, as well as lack of all three dynein gene mutations in the control group, indicate that these mutations can be considered as asthenozoospermia causative mutations. The *DNAI1*, *DNAH5* and *DNAH11* genes were found to be expressed in testis and trachea (Bartoloni et al., 2002; Bush & Ferkol, 2006; Guichard et al., 2001; Hornef et al., 2006; Kispert et al., 2003; Noone et al., 2002; Olbrich et al., 2002; Pennarun et al., 1999; Schwabe et al., 2008; Zariwala et al., 2001, 2006, as cited in Zuccarello et al., 2008). The encoded proteins, axonemal dynein intermediate chain 1, axonemal dynein heavy chain 5 and axonemal dynein heavy chain 11 respectively, belong to the axonemal dynein cluster present in cilia and sperm tails. It was known that the presence of mutations in both alleles in a single dynein gene cause primary ciliary dyskinesia and Kartagener Syndrome which are usually associated with asthenozoospermia (for review see Escudier et al., 2009). Notably, this study shows that mutations in dynein encoding genes present in only one allele cause a non syndromic, male infertility phenotype.

2.4 *CATSPER1* gene mutations in oligo-astheno-theratozoospermia

The *CATSPER1(Cation channel sperm-associated protein 1)* gene was selected for mutation analysis after allelic homozygosity screening in two consanguineous Iranian families with familial cases of non-syndromic male infertility. Oligozoospermia, no motile sperm or sperm with lowered motility, but also increased counts of sperm with abnormal morphology were observed in the patients. In the first family, the homozygous insertion c.539-540insT was found in two infertile brothers, whereas two other fertile brothers as well as the parents were heterozygous. In the second family, a different homozygous mutation, an insertion c.948-949insATGGC, was found in the infertile proband and his sister, the latter with unknown fertility status. None of these mutations were present in the control group of 579 fertile Italian men. Both mutations were frame shifts mutations resulting in premature stop codons, p.Lys180LysfsX9 and p.Asp317MetfsX18, respectively, producing a truncated protein lacking six transmembrane domains as well as the P loop (Avenarius et al., 2009). Therefore, in all probability, the CATSPER1 channel activity was abolished in homozygous patients. The *CATSPER1* gene was associated with oligo-astheno-theratozoospermia compound semen abnormality. The *CATSPER1* gene encodes the first of the four sperm-specific CATSPER voltage-gated calcium channels. Its mouse homologue is specifically expressed in the plasma membrane of the sperm tail element known as the principal piece (Ren et al., 2001) and it is required for calcium mediated hyperactivation of sperm motility (Carlson et al., 2003).

2.5 *NR5A1* (*SF-1*) azoospermia or oligozoospermia associated gene

Recently it has been shown, that mutations of *NR5A1* (nuclear receptor 5A1) gene, also known as *SF-1* (steroidogenic factor 1), may cause a non-syndromic spermatogenic failure. Mutation screening of the *NR5A1* gene in 315 mixed ancestry patients with azoospermia or oligozoospermia revealed 6 heterozygous mutations, 2 among them present in one allele, in 7 infertile men. A deleterious allele carrying a double mutation p.Gly123Ala/p.Pro129Leu was identified in three patients of 31, 37 and 42 years of age. While the youngest among them had a progressive loss of sperm cell concentration and quality, the two oldest patients suffered azoospermia. This may indicate that this double mutation at the heterozygous status causes a progressive degradation of sperm cells. The other four mutations, p.Pro311Leu, p.Arg191Cys, p.Gly121Ser and p.Asp238Asn, were identified in single patients and were associated with azoospermia or severe oligozoospermia phenotype. None of these mutations were observed in over 700 fertile or normozoospermic men from the mixed origin population nor in almost 1400 samples from numerous other worldwide populations (Bashamboo et al., 2010). Functional tests for the *NR5A1* mutations demonstrated that all of them abolished transactivation ability of SF-1 (Bashamboo et al., 2010, Laurenco et al., 2009). Although family pedigrees of the probands were not studied, the lack of these mutations in the vast control groups as well as the clear results of the functional tests altogether indicate that these *NR5A1* gene mutations are causative for infertility. The *NR5A1* gene encodes a transcriptional regulator playing a key role in many aspects of adrenal and reproductive development. The previously identified heterozygous mutations of this gene were associated with a wide spectrum of phenotypes including anorchia, gonadal dysgenesis 46,XY, genital ambiguity, micropenis, and cryptorchidism, as well as ovarian failure (for review see Lin & Achermann, 2008, Schimmer & White, 2010). It has been postulated that mutations which induce a more severe functional failure of the NR5A1 factor are associated with severe phenotypes while milder ones are associated with non syndromic infertility (Lin & Achermann, 2008).

3. The Y-chromosome and azoospermia factor region (AZF)

In 1976, a cytogenetic study performed on blood lymphocytes in a group of 1170 infertile men with azoospermia, revealed deletions of the long Y-chromosome arm (Yq) in six of them (Tiepolo & Zuffardi, 1976). This indicated the presence of a gene on the Yq, initially called AZF for AZoospermia Factor, the lack of which have caused azoospermia phenotype. This initial finding has been followed by many reports describing smaller internal deletions within Yq. The deletion overlapping region has been named the azoospermia factor (AZF) region. Tremendous technological progress related to the Human Genome Project provided powerful molecular tools such as short Sequence Tagged Sites (STSs) to accurately delimit and precisely map single AZF deletions. This approach enabled identification of a large number of microdeletions in infertile men, mapping to different sites within AZF region. According to initial findings, specific phenotypes of spermatogenic failure were associated with distinct microdeletion locations within the AZF region. These associations served to designate three AZF subregions: AZFa, AZFb and AZFc (Figure 1) (Vogt et al., 1996). In the meantime, over 20 genes involved in spermatogenesis were identified in the AZF region (for review see Navarro-Costa et al., 2010a). Therefore, an attempt was made by many researchers to address whether there were correlations between definite infertility phenotypes and specific deleted AZF genes. The identification of such correlations could be beneficial for male infertility genetic diagnosis, as well as for Intra Cytoplasmic Sperm Injection (ICSI) prediction outcomes in infertile couples with male infertility factors.

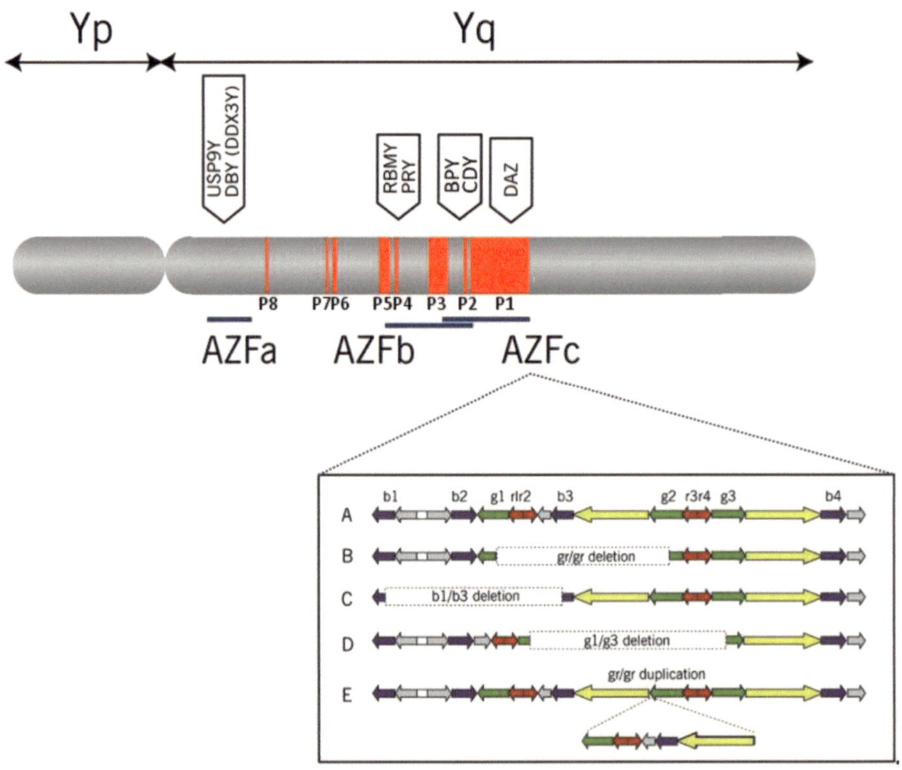

Fig. 1. The structure of AZF subregions and associated genes on the Y-chromosome. A, the ampliconic sequences mapped in the AZFc region, named after colors: blue (b), green (g), red (r), grey and yellow. B-D, the common types of subdeletions (gr/gr, b1/b3, g1/g3). E, a duplication (gr/gr) on the AZFc region. Genes representative of each subregion are indicated between two Y-chromosome schemes (modified O'Flynn O'Brien et al., 2010).

3.1 AZFa

This region is the most proximal AZF subregion. One of the genes it encodes is a single copy *DBY* gene, also called *DDX3Y*, with a corresponding copy on the X-chromosome. *DBY* encodes a Y-linked DEAD box RNA helicase of unknown function. Although this gene is ubiquitously transcribed, which is a hallmark of the Y-chromosome genes with a X-chromosome counterpart, DBY protein expression is limited to the premeiotic spermatogonia (Ditton et al., 2004). In 13 men with maturation arrest and 3 men with hypospermatogenesis, reduced levels of *DBY* transcripts in the testis was detected, while the other examined AZF genes were transcribed at the normal level (Lardone et al., 2007). This finding pointed out the importance of DBY for male reproduction. Furthermore, *DBY* gene deletions have been identified in 3 men with Sertoli Cell-Only Syndrome (SCOS), which is characterized by a lack of germ cells. However, these deletions removed both, the *DBY* as well as the closely mapping *USP9Y* gene (Sargent et al., 1999). For that reason, in this group of patients, the SCOS phenotype could not be assigned specifically to *DBY* gene. The second AZFa gene, *USP9Y*, encodes the Y-linked ubiquitin specific peptidase 9. It is the only gene reported as an isolated deleted gene of AZF region associated with infertility. It has been later shown, however, that a loss or partial deletion of *USP9Y* gene may cause variable phenotypes from azoospermia (Sun et al., 1999), through oligozoospermia (Brown et al., 1998) up to subfertility (Krausz et al., 2006). It seems that the phenotype associated with the *USP9Y* gene defects varies according to the specific carriers or some other factors which are still unknown. Moreover, a dysfunctional *USP9Y* gene was reported to be passed to the next generation in one family (Luddi et al., 2009). Thus, it seems that the *DBY* gene plays a more crucial role in male reproduction than the *USP9Y* gene.

3.2 AZFb

The *RBMY* gene was the first candidate gene from the AZFb subregion, proposed to be involved in spermatogenesis (Ma et al., 1993). One of the six copies of this gene located on the Y chromosome, *RBMY1*, encodes a Y-linked RNA binding motif protein, which is a testis-specific splicing factor expressed in the nuclei of male germ cells (for review see Vogt, 2005). One man manifesting azoospermia and the maturation arrest phenotype, reduction of *RBMY1* expression was demonstrated. Given that an AZFc deletion was also present, the significance of the *RBMY1* expression reduction could not be assessed (Lavery et al., 2007). However, severe spermatogenic failure and SCOS or hypospermatogenesis was also reported in men carrying microdeletions removing various genes of AZFb area, excluding the *RBMY* gene (Ferlin et al., 2003). This might suggest that some additional AZFb genes contribute to a similar histological and clinical infertility phenotype when deleted. The strongest candidate is a family of *PRY* genes which are involved in the regulation of apoptosis during the spermatogenic process (Stouffs et at., 2004). Furthermore, spermatogenesis was completely arrested before or at the meiosis stage, when both genes were removed (Vogt et al., 1996). This suggests that, in the AZFb region, the *RBMY* and *PRY* genes are crucial for the male reproduction.

3.3 AZFc

This subregion encodes several protein-coding gene families, including three copies of *BPY* and two copies of the *CDY* gene. However, the functions of the *BPY* and *CDY* genes are not known yet (Kuroda-Kawaguchi et al., 2001). This subregion encodes four copies of the *DAZ* (Deleted in AZoospermia) gene, one of the first cloned AZF genes, encoding a germ cell-specific RNA binding protein (Reijo et al., 1995). Deletions of *DAZ2*, *DAZ3*, or *DAZ4* were identified in infertile patients but also in fertile men. In the latter case they were considered familial variants transmitted from father to son (Vogt et al., 1996; Saxena et al., 2000; Fernandes et al., 2002, 2004). Only, *DAZ1/DAZ2* double deletions were reported to be restricted to infertile men (Fernandes et al., 2006). It suggests that expression of *DAZ1* is crucial for spermatogenesis (Fernandes et al., 2002), although a case of one fertile man carrying a *DAZ1* deletion has been reported (Machev et al., 2004).

It has been recently demonstrated that genes related to the AZFb and AZFc subregions are located in so-called "amplicons". They represent subregions containing a series of inversely repeated units organized in eight palindromes, P8-P1, as ordered from the most proximal up to the most terminal towards the centromere (Figure 1). A peculiarity of amplicons compared to other AZF regions is their high density of the Y-chromosome genes with testis predominant expression (Kuroda-Kawaguchi et al., 2001; Skaletsky et al., 2003). Moreover, it has been shown that AZFb plus the AZFc subregion contain large segments of duplicated sequence with the proximal end of the AZFc overlapping with the distal end of AZFb (Figure 1) (Repping et al., 2002). Although complete AZFc deletions, removing 3.5 Mb between the b2/b4 amplicons, are most commonly found, a number of smaller, partial AZFc subdeletions have also been identified (Figure 1B-D) (for review see Navarro-Costa et al., 2010b). These partial deletions were associated with variable semen phenotypes, ranging from normospermic to azoospermic. This phenotypic diversity has been suggested to be a consequence of different origins, that undergo differential evolution over generations within distinct ethnic groups, reflecting specific environmental pressures (Bateson et al., 2004). This was observed in the cases of the most frequent deletions of the AZFc region, the gr/gr subdeletions (Figure 1B). Gr/gr subdeletions removing a 1.6 Mb fragment of AZFc region were identified as risk factors for spermatogenic failure in several studies, while in others such an association was not found (for review see Navarro-Costa et al., 2010b). Surprisingly, an analysis of the Han Chinese population revealed that a duplication of the gr/gr region (Figure 1E) may be deleterious for fertility (Lin et al.; 2007). Given that, the gr/gr deletions can be passed from father to son, the gr/gr deletion results in subfertility rather than in complete infertility (Poongothai et al., 2009). This picture appears even more complex due to some other studies indicating no association between spermatogenesis and the genes in the AZFc region (Saut et al., 2002).

3.4 Genotype-phenotype correlations in infertile males carrying AZF region microdeletions

Microdeletions of AZFa subregion are relatively rare. They are responsible for infertility in 1% of men with NonObstructive Azoospermia (NOA). In the majority of cases, patients with the AZFa deletions lack germ cells in seminiferous tubules or show the presence of germ cells only in the minority of tubules. Therefore, it is assumed that AZFa microdeletions correlate with SCOS phenotype (for review see Sadeghi-Nejad & Farrokhi, 2007). Microdeletions in AZFb are responsible for infertility in 1-2% of men with NOA. However, in contrast to AZFa, patients carrying AZFb deletions present with variable phenotypes. Namely, in about half of such cases, a maturation arrest phenotype at the stage of primary spermatocytes was found (for review see Vogt, 2005). Moreover, patients carrying large

AZFb deletions are azoospermic whereas those harboring smaller AZFb deletions present with a range of infertile phenotypes, including severe or even mild oligozoospermia. The most common aberrations, however, which occur in AZF are multiple gene deletions encompassing both, AZFb and AZFc subregions, resulting in a wide range of infertility phenotypes (for review see Navarro-Costa et al., 2010a). Also AZFc deletions are responsible for a variety of phenotypes ranging from azoospermia to severe oligozoospermia. In addition, AZFc deletions are the most frequently identified microdeletions in patients with NOA. They are responsible for up to 12% of azoospermia and 6% of severe oligozoospermia cases (Kuroda-Kawaguchi et al., 2001).

Today the Y chromosome microdeletions are the most frequently known genetic cause of severe spermatogenic impairment. Therefore, it is important for men suffering azoospermia or severe oligozoospermia to undergo tests for AZF microdeletions. Importantly, the only molecular genetic tests which are routinely performed to identify the cause of male infertility are those for microdeletion identification within the AZF region. These tests are PCR-based, find the most commonly deleted STSs and are commercially available. They are of great importance for both, a correct diagnosis, as well as for genetic counseling. Knowledge about the type of AZF deletion may help the clinician to select patients for, and to determine the best type of, Artificial Reproductive Technology (ART). It is known that sometimes such men can still father children with help of ART, including ICSI. Moreover, the combination of ICSI with testicular sperm recovery offers even azoospermic men the possibility of fathering their own genetic children. However, men carrying AZFc microdeletions must realize that their male offspring will almost certainly be subfertile (for review see Poongothai et al., 2009).

4. 3'UTR-mediated translational regulation and male infertility

Identification of *DAZ*, the first AZFc gene causing male infertility, stimulated much research on its role in human germ cell development as well as in model organisms such as flies, worms, frogs and the mouse. Nowadays, *DAZ* is the best studied among other so far weakly assessed AZF genes. Four Y-chromosome copies of *DAZ* arose most likely by amplification of the original autosomal *DAZL* (*DAZ*-Like) gene (Saxena et al., 1996). The DAZ protein family which emerged from this genomic reshuffling is thought to control meiosis and maintenance of germ cells (Reynolds et al., 2005). The DAZ proteins contain an RNA-binding domain suggesting involvement in RNA regulation (Saxena et al., 1996). In particular, DAZ was later shown to bind another highly conserved RNA-binding protein, PUMILIO2 (Moore et al., 2003). This protein was earlier identified as a translational repressor in body patterning and germ cell development of the fly (Wharton et al., 1998). Interaction with PUMILIO2 highlights involvement of DAZ in a type translational regulation mediated by the 3'UTR, which is crucial in many developmental processes, including that of germ cells. This regulation involves recognition of specific nucleotide motifs within 3'UTRs by definite complexes of RNA-binding proteins. By this means, specific mRNAs are stimulated for translation or are directed towards P-bodies, cytoplasmic storage and degradation centres (for review see Kishore et al., 2010). Therefore, one can imagine that elimination of PUMILIO2-binding partner caused by *DAZ* gene deletions may bring about translational deregulation of specific mRNAs in the male germ cells resulting in male infertility. An unsuccessful attempt has been made to identify *PUMILIO2* gene mutations that potentially could disable DAZ-PUMILIO2 interaction, causing infertility phenotypes similar to those found with DAZ deletions (Kusz et al., 2006). Two other PUMILIO2-binding, male germ cell specific, highly conserved RNA-binding proteins, NANOS2 and NANOS3, were not found to be dysfunctional in genetic screens for mutations in a series of infertile males (Kusz et al., 2009a; Kusz et al., 2009b). Inactivation of both genes (Nanos2 and Nanos3) cause male infertility in the mouse (Tsuda et al., 2003).

The GEMIN3, a miRNA biogenesis factor (Mourelatos et al., 2002) has recently been found to bind PUMILIO2 and NANOS1 proteins within the chromatoid body, a structure analogous to P-bodies of somatic cells (Ginter-Matuszewska et al., 2011). This finding strongly suggests participation of miRNAs in 3'UTR mediated translational regulation in partnership with these proteins in human male germ cells. Many recently identified potential PUMILIO2 mRNA targets contain several predicted miRNA binding sites (Galgano et al., 2008). Moreover, various microRNAs as well as other small regulatory RNAs are expressed in human male germ cells and they seem to be active in spermatogenesis (He et al., 2009). Their biogenesis and involvement in male infertility is summarized bellow.

5. Small regulatory RNAs in reproduction and male infertility

There is a growing body of data indicating that one of the most important class of regulatory noncoding RNAs discovered in recent years, the small regulatory RNAs (srRNAs), play a major role in human spermatogenesis and may contribute to male infertility. Most of these RNAs are involved in RNA interference (RNAi), a phenomenon which usually leads to gene silencing. The length of srRNAs ranges between 20-30 nt. srRNAs contain 5' phosphate and 3'-OH groups which can be modified. All of them are loaded into specific effector complexes named RNA Induced Silencing Complexes (RISCs) to silence specific RNA targets (for review see Czech & Hannon, 2011). There are three major classes of srRNAs: microRNAs (miRNAs), short interfering RNAs (siRNAs) and PIWI interacting RNAs (piRNAs).

5.1 miRNAs

The first miRNA was discovered in *C. elegans*, when it was found that the *lin-4* gene, known for its role in early larval development timing, encodes two short RNAs, one ~22 nt and the second one ~61 nt. The longer molecule, which folds into a stem-loop structure, turned out to be a precursor of the shorter one. Interestingly, both molecules were complementary to multiple sites present in 3' UnTranslated region (3'UTR) of the *lin-14* mRNA. This enables *lin-4* RNAs to bind the *lin-14* 3'-UTR, which results in translational repression of *lin-14* mRNA (Lee et al., 1993). Seven years later, a second 22 nt regulatory *let-7* miRNA encoded in l*et-7* gene was identified. This miRNA promotes later larval development timing in the *C. elegans* (Reinhart et al., 2000). Soon after, *let-7* homologues, as well as a large number of other miRNAs, were discovered in the fly, many other animal groups and the human genome (for review see Bartel, 2004). Among over one thousand miRNAs identified in humans, some are ubiquitous whereas some other are tissue specific, e.g., are only expressed in testis (e.g. Bentwich et al., 2005).

The primary miRNA precursors known as pri-miRNAs are transcribed usually by RNA polymerase II, or in some cases RNA polymerase III. All known human pri-miRNAs contain a 5′cap structure and a 3′polyA tail (Cai et al., 2004). These miRNA precursors are cleaved by an RNase III named Drosha, resulting in 60-80 nt pre-miRNA molecules containing a hairpin loop with two 3′ overhanging nucleotides. The human Drosha enzyme contains four distinct domains: catalytic, double-stranded RNA binding, proline-rich, and serine and arginine-rich domains. Drosha is a component of a 500 kDa miRNA processing complex. Another crucial component interacting with Drosha and necessary for pre-miRNA processing in humans is the DGCR8 protein (DiGeorge syndrome critical region gene 8) (Gregory et al., 2004)

The next step in miRNA biogenesis is the export of pre-miRNA from the nucleus to the cytoplasm. This process is mediated by Exportin 5 protein, a member of cariopherin family. The loading of cargo on Exportin 5 requires binding of the phosphorylated Ran-GTP, a member of GTPases family. Hydrolysis of Ran-GTP to Ran-GDP causes cargo release. Binding of Exportin 5 to pre-miRNA requires the presence of a minihelix motif with a stem built of fourteen base pairs at the 5' end and 3-8 overhanging nucleotides at the 3' end (for review see Kim, 2004). Once in the cytoplasm, pre-miRNAs are cleaved by Dicer, a type of RNase III which cuts the last base pair of the stem-loop. The double stranded cleavage product contains 5' phosphate and two 3′ overhanging nucleotides. To perform this activity in humans, Dicer cooperates with TRPB and PACT proteins (Kok et al., 2007).

After this maturation step, the miRNA-miRNA* duplex (miRNA-guide strand and miRNA*-passenger strand) are loaded into the RISC complex which contains Argonaute (AGO) protein, a member of Argonaute superfamily. Among human ARGONAUTE proteins (AGO1-4) only AGO2 has slicer activity (Parker & Barford, 2006; Wang et al., 2009). Generally the miRNA strand characterized by a less thermodynamically stable 5' end of the miRNA duplex is selected as the guide strand within miRISC complex (Schwarz et al., 2003). It has been proposed that the passenger strand is removed in the cleavage-independent manner by unwinding (Kawamata et al., 2009; Yoda et al. 2010). The guide strand is responsible for miRISC specific mRNA recognition. The miRISC binds to recognition sequences located within 3′UTR of mRNA complementary to the guide strand, although this complementarity is usually not complete. This binding induces translational repression or, rarely, stimulation through a mechanism which is not fully understood (for review see Bartel, 2009; Huntzinger & Izzauralde, 2011). Four alternative ways of translational repression have been proposed: inhibition at the translation initiation or elongation, co-transcriptional protein degradation or premature translational termination. Intensive studies are in progress to decipher this intricate, miRNA mediated, posttranscriptional silencing mechanism (for review see Djuranovic et al., 2011; Huntzinger & Izzauralde, 2011). Meanwhile, it has been demonstrated that single nucleotide polymorphisms (SNPs) identified at various miRNA binding sites in 3′UTRs of specific mRNAs may cause diseases, including human male infertility.

The miRNA expression profile analysis using miRCURY™ LNA microarray platform was performed in testis samples originating from 3 patients diagnosed with non-obstructive azoospermia (NOA). These profiles were compared with profiles from testis samples of two fertile individuals who underwent orchiectomy due to prostate carcinoma. By this approach a total of 173 miRNAs were selected to be differentially expressed in NOA patients compared to fertile controls. 19 of them were upregulated whereas 154 downregulated (Lian et al., 2009). Among 154 downregulated miRNAs, at least 12 (7.8%) were found to be testis specific in the mouse (Ro et al., 2007). The results obtained by microarray analysis were confirmed by real time RT-PCR, on a selected group of four miRNAs: *miR-302a, miR-491-3p, miR-520d-3p* and *miR-383*. The first two *miR-302a, miR-491-3p* were upregulated, while *miR-520d-3p* and *miR-383* were downregulated in NOA patients. Additionally, downregulation of *miR-383* in these patients was confirmed by *in situ* hybridization. Interestingly, specific expression profiles were found to be correlated with miRNA genomic cluster localization. While chromosomes 14, 19 and X appeared to encode a significant number (62) of downregulated miRNA genes from this study, the majority of upregulated miRNA genes mapped to chromosome 17. For example, the expression of 12 out of 13 members of a miRNA cluster on human chromosome 14q32.31 were downregulated in infertile men, with only one, the *miR-654-5p*, upregulated. An opposite bias was found in two miRNA gene clusters located on chromosome 19q13.42. However, in one of these clusters only two miRNAs, *mir-371* and *mir-372* were downregulated, the *mir-373-5p* of the same cluster being upregulated. The second cluster contains 13 nonconserved downregulated miRNAs. A bioinformatic analysis was performed to select for potential targets of these differentially expressed miRNAs. The identified potential target genes, *TIMP3*, *SOX9* and *GAD45G* (Lian et al., 2009), had been previously shown to be upregulated in testis of infertile patients (Rockett et al., 2004). The *TIMP3* gene, is a potential target for downregulated *miR-1, miR-181a, miR-221* and *miR-9**. This gene is involved in testis development and differentiation (Zeng et al, 1998). The second target encoding a well described transcription factor *SOX9*, is probably regulated by *mir-145* (Lian et al., 2009) and is required for testis determination and development but also for spermatogenesis (Schumacher et al, 2008). Finally, the third target gene encoding GAD45G, an apoptosis inducer and cell growth inhibitor in response to stress shock (Ying et al., 2005), is also a potential target of *miR-383* (Lian et al., 2009). It is expected that expression of those three target genes might significantly contribute to male infertility. In addition, several members of the *mir-17-92* and *mir-371,2,3* clusters which are downregulated in NOA patients testicular tissue, are considered potential novel oncogenes due to their participation in the development of human testicular germ cell tumors (TGCTs). For example, the mir-17-92 cluster, which is rarely expressed in NOA patients, is highly expressed in the carcinoma in situ (CIS) testis tumor. These miRNAs act as apoptosis inhibitors by means of translational downregulation of E2F transcription factor 1(E2F1) in CIS cells. Therefore, the lowered expression of these miRNAs observed in NOA patients may contribute to increased apoptosis in the gonadal tissue (Lin et al., 1999, Novotny et al., 2007 Voorhoeve et al., 2006). Molecular consequences of *miR-383* downregulation were further investigated. Consistent with the miRNA microarray results the expression of *miR-383* was significantly decreased in testicular specimens of the patients with maturation arrest (MA). In addition, real-time PCR results also revealed a significant downregulation of miR-383 expression in testes obtained from NOA patients compared with normal controls, as previously reported (Lian et al., 2009). This downregulation may be exclusive for MA patients, as *miR-383* was not altered in infertile patients with hypospermatogenesis (HA). Regulation of *miR-383* expression takes place mainly at the transcription level, although additional layers of post-transcriptional regulation exist. The testicular embryonal carcinoma cell line (NT2) which shows overexpression of *miR-383* manifests with significantly decelerated cell proliferation, G1 cell cycle arrest and apoptosis stimulation. Inhibition of endogenous *miR-383* expression resulted in a significant stimulation of proliferation, a decrease of cell number in the G1 phase, and suppression of basal levels of apoptosis. Interferon regulatory factor-1 (IRF1) was predicted and experimentally verified as being the *miR-383* target gene. Since the effects of IRF1 silencing in NT2 cells were very similar to the ones caused by *miR-383* overexpression, this may suggest a promitogenic role of *miR-383* in NT2 cells. This effect is opposite to that found in most other cell lines from other tissues (for review see Kroger et al., 2002). The negative correlation between *miR-383* and IRF1 expression was confirmed *in vivo* in the mouse testes. It was further investigated since IRF1 regulates a set of genes involved in apoptosis, cell cycle and DNA repair. The mRNA and protein expression level of the cell cycle *Cyclin D1, CDK2* and *p21* genes was positively correlated with IRF1 levels in NT2 cells. Moreover, silencing of Cyclin D1 resulted in inhibition of proliferation due to arrest at the G1 phase. Silencing of Cyclin D1 caused a dramatic enhancement of the *miR-383* effects. Meanwhile, silencing of p21 caused partial inhibition of *miR-383*-induced G1-phase arrest. It was reported that Cyclin D and p21 in complex with CDK4 are required for phosphorylated retinoblastoma protein (pRb)-mediated G1/S transition. This phosphorylation was inhibited by *miR-383* which also repressed CDK4 expression by the proteasome-dependent pathway. Immunostaining of cyclin D1, p21, CDK2, CDK4 and phosphorylated pRb (P-pRb) in testis tissue of MA patients revealed higher expression of all these proteins in some seminiferous tubules. However, in the MA patients studied, enhanced nuclear staining for P-pRb was the only finding present in all of them. These results indicate that dysregulation of the *miR-383*-mediated pRb pathways might contribute to spermatogenic failure in MA patients. Interestingly, a loss of pRb expression is often associated with occurrence of testis germ cell tumor (TGCT). The existence of the widespread expression of P-pRb in the testes of MA patients indicates a status of "physiological absence of pRb" in infertile men. TGCTs were reported to occur three times more frequently in infertile than fertile man. Therefore, activated P-pRb expression caused by *miR-383* downregulation could be associated with a higher frequency of TGCTs (Lian et al., 2010).

In a recent bioinformatic study of 140 mRNAs involved in mammalian spermatogenesis (database founded), 21 human mRNAs carried, in total, 39 SNPs which occurred in the predicted miRNA-binding sites. Six among those SNPs were demonstrated to induce a significant change of Gibbs binding free energy value at a rate higher than 5.27 kJ/mol. This alteration indicated a possible disabling of miRNA interaction. These potentially causative six SNPs were located in the 3'UTRs of five mRNAs encoding CYP19, Serpina5, CGA, CPEB1 and CPEB2 spermatogenic proteins. As the next step, a total number of 494 patients manifesting with azoospermia or severe oligozoospermia and 357 fertile males were tested for these 6 SNPs. One of them, a mutant allele rs2303846 identified in *CPEB1* gene, was correlated with infertility. Also the mutant allele rs6631 (A→T transversion) of the *CGA* gene was found to be associated with idiopathic male infertility. The following miRNAs were predicted to bind the site containing the rs6631 SNP in *CGA*: *miR-610, miR-34c-5p* and *miR-1302*. While the *miR-1302* was predicted to bind more stably the rs6631-A allele than rs6631-T, a reverse correlation was found for *miR-610* and *miR-34c-5p*. To confirm these predictions, dual-luciferase reporter assays were performed in human HEK293T cells. At the beginning, these cells were tested for expression of these three miRNAs. As the next step, the cells were transfected with constructs containing a luciferase reporter cDNA in fusion with the modified *CGA* 3'UTR representing rs6631-A or rs6631-T alleles, or with a deleted miRNA binding site. The *miR-1302* was found to negatively regulate *CGA* expression given that rs6631 related A→T substitution disrupted the repression by 26% (H. Zhang et al.,

2011). Possibly the resulting *CGA* overexpression is the direct cause of idiopathic male infertility. The *CGA* gene encodes the α-subunit of glycoprotein hormones, such as thyrotropin (the pituitary TSH), lutropin (LH), follitropin (FSH), and the placental chorion gonadotropin (human chorionic gonadotropin, hCG). These hormones play important roles in thyroid and in gonadal development and function (Baenziger & Green, 1988). Heterodimerization of α- and β-subunits is a critical event for their function (Bieche et al., 2002). Disruption of CGA expression causes a lack of biologically active FSH, LH and TSH hormones and results in hypogonadism. The α-subunit alone has some growth factor activity and it can induce lactotrope differentiation and the subsequent secretion of prolactin (PRL) (Begeot et al., 1984; Blithe et al., 1991; Lapthorn et al., 1994; Kendall et al., 1995). While CGA and PRL are known to play important roles in gonadal development, one can assume that overexpression of CGA may elevate the risk of male infertility (H. Zhang et al., 2011).

In a separate study on human 5 day embryos (blastocyst stage) originating from fertile donors, or from male factor infertility couples, 12 miRNAs (*RNU48, let-7a, let-7b, let-7c, let-7g, miR-19a, miR-19b, miR-21, miR-24, miR-34b, miR-92,* and *miR*-93) were selected because of their expression at that developmental stage. Interestingly, a significant decrease in expression of *let-7a* and *miR-24* was observed in blastocysts derived from couples with a male factor infertility compared to fertile donors. This decrease was associated with significantly altered expression of two genes. One of these genes encodes a decay promoting factor, KHSRP, while the second one encodes a transcription factor, NFAT5. The corresponding mRNAs were predicted targets for *miR-24*. While the decrease of *miR-24* in male infertility factor blastocysts was correlated with a significant increase of KHSRP expression, the expression of NFAT5 was decreased. The gene ontology (GO) biological processes annotation for the *let-7a* and *miR-24* targets revealed involvement in cell growth and maintenance, transcription and protein metabolism. The GO molecular function annotation indicates signal transducer and nucleic acid binding activity (McCallie et al., 2010). In addition, lowered or lack of expression of *let-7a* and *miR-24* was previously found to be associated with several types of human neoplasia. Malignant melanoma, gastric carcinoma, lymphoma and chronic lymphatic leukemia were associated with a lack of *let-7a* expression (Marton et al., 2008; Muller & Bosserhoff, 2008; Sampson et al., 2007; H. H. Zhang et al., 2007). Likewise, *miR-24* was shown to be responsible for downregulation of a tumor suppressor gene *p16* in cervical carcinoma cells a decreased level of *miR-24* caused increase of *p16* expression resulting in replicative senescence (Lal et al., 2008). These findings may suggest a possible role for embryonic miRNAs in etiology of human male infertility and several cancers (McCallie et al., 2010).

5.2 siRNAs

The siRNAs were first discovered in plants (Hamilton & Baulcombe, 1999). Although, in the animal kingdom, biogenesis of siRNA is best understood in *D. melanogaster,* this process seems to be very similar in mammals. siRNAs are derived from long dsRNAs. These long precursors are processed to siRNA duplexes by Dicer 2 (DCR2) (Lee et al., 2004). In mammals, Dicer is also responsible for siRNA and miRNA processing (for review see Jaskiewicz & Filipowicz, 2008). The siRNAs are processed from single stranded transcripts that can form long hairpins or dsRNAs derived from paired single stranded molecules. The siRNA duplexes are incorporated into RISC (siRISC). During siRISC assembly, the passenger strand of siRNA is cleaved by the AGO protein which has a slicer activity (AGO2 in human) (for review see Czech and Hannon, 2011). The mature siRISC binds complementary mRNA to form an effector complex. The siRNA guides AGO2 to catalyze cleavage of the target mRNA at a site that is ~10 nt distant from the 5' of siRNA. After AGO2 cleavage, the target mRNA is degraded and the RISC is recycled to cleave the next mRNA target molecules (Elbashir, et al., 2001; Liu. et al., 2004; Meister et al., 2004; Song et al., 2004). The siRNA mechanism functions in mammalian reproduction, since endogenous siRNAs were found to be in abundant in mouse oocytes, ES cells and spermatogenic cells (Babiarz et al., 2008; Song et al., 2011 Tam et al., 2008; Watanabe et al., 2008). Involvement of siRNA phenomena in male human infertility is a matter of future studies.

5.3 piRNAs

Piwi-interacting RNAs (piRNAs) are a class of small regulatory RNAs of the 24-30 nt. These srRNAs differ from miRNAs and siRNAs in that they are not produced by Dicer enzymes and do not require formation of a stable double-stranded RNA intermediates for their biogenesis (for review see Simonelig, 2011). piRNAs also vary from other srRNAs in that they were described primarily in gonads in many animal species from *Drosophila* to mammals. The principal role of piRNAs is to protect the genome against transposable elements (TEs) which represent as much as 45% of human DNA and which are known to move and replicate within the genome (Lander et al. 2001). Derepression of transposable elements (TEs), occurring through epigenetic reprogramming of the mammalian embryonic germline, requires the existence of an efficient mechanism coordinating the piwi/piRNA pathway and the *de novo* DNA methylation machinery. Accumulating evidence indicates that piRNA-binding, mammalian piwi homologues such as Miwi, Miwi2, and Mili proteins, are required for the germline maintenance and spermatogenesis in *Drosophila* and the mouse (Thomson & Lin, 2009). This view is supported by the fact that piRNAs are expressed in mouse male germ cells, particularly in pachytene spermatocytes and round spermatids (Klattenhoff & Theurkauf, 2008). Deficiency of Mili and Miwi2 leads to arrest of gametogenesis and complete sterility in males (Aravin et al., 2007; Carmell et al., 2007; Kuramochi-Miyagawa et al. 2008). Thus, it is likely that Mili and Miwi2 partners, the piRNAs, are potentially involved in regulating the meiotic and postmeiotic processes of male germ cell development, as they do in the fly. There are hundreds of thousands if not millions of individual piRNA genes which are transcribed from piRNA clusters from several, up to 200, kilobases in length. Each cluster contain multiple sequences that generate piRNAs. Moreover, in a number of clusters transcription occurs in both directions. It is currently unclear how primary piRNA are produced from piRNA clusters. They are not produced by Dicer enzymes and do not require formation of stable double-stranded RNA intermediates (Vagin et al., 2006). There are two alternative and distinct pathways of piRNA biogenesis. The first one is primary piRNA biogenesis and the second one is the so called "ping-pong amplification loop" pathway. These pathways are conserved in many animal species (Houwing et al., 2008; Kawaoka et al. 2009; Lau et al. 2006; Robine et al. 2009). In the mouse pro-spermatogonia, the primary piRNAs are produced through primary processing which generates an initial pool of piRNAs that target many TEs. Thereafter they are amplified through the ping-pong pathway, which requires slicer activity of Mili and Miwi2 proteins. In the ping-pong cycle, piRNA molecules that target active TE elements are highly amplified (for review see Siomi et al. 2011). In mouse spermatocytes, primary piRNA biogenesis is the only process that generates piRNA, whereas in pre-meiotic spermatogonia, specific sequences generated by the primary pathway are amplified in the ping-pong cycle. In the mouse, Mili and Miwi2 function in the ping-pong cycle (Aravin et al., 2007). The piRISC complexes loaded by piRNA silence complementary RNA targets. Silencing occurs by cleavage and also through some chromatin effects (Nishida et al.; 2007; for review see Thomson & Lin, 2009). Deficiency of piwi proteins in flies, but also in mice, leads to the lack of primary piRNA, although it is unlikely that piwi-proteins are directly involved in primary piRNA processing. Finally, the piRNA pathway phenomenon opens a new fascinating field for exploration of potential roles of piRNAs in human germ cell development, infertility and the origin of TGCTs.

Therefore, to get more insight into the potential contribution of the piRNA pathway in human male infertility, the genetic variation of several piwi homologues, HIWI, HILI, HIWI3 and HIWI2, was studied in 490 patients with idiopathic azoospermia or oligozoospermia and in 468 fertile males from a Chinese Han population. Among 9 SNPs identified in the patients, 2 exhibited a significant association with the risk of oligozoospermia under a dominant model (variant containing versus homozygous wild-type genotype). Although the biological effects of one of these SNPs, a T->C transition (rs508485) in *HIWI2* 3'UTR was not clear, individuals carrying this transition in at least one allele, had a significantly increased risk of oligozoospermia. In contrast, individuals carrying a non-synonymous rs11703684 Val471Ile mutation in the *HIWI3* gene exhibited a borderline significantly reduced oligozoospermia risk compared with individuals with the wild-type genotype. After classification according the age or smoking status, a protective effect of the Val471Ile mutation on spermatogenesis was more obvious in non-smokers. Interestingly, the Val471Ile mutation was located within the PIWI functional domain which is crucial for RNA-mediated silencing in germ cells. While the function of HIWI3 protein in human spermatogenesis remains unclear, these finding may suggest a significant role of the piwi homologue in spermatogenesis. Altogether, the genetic variations identified in this study are more likely to be associated with oligozoospermia rather than azoospermia (Gu et al., 2010). Certainly, more studies are needed in various worldwide populations to properly assess the contribution of the piRNA pathway to defects in human male infertility.

6. Future directions

A tremendous technological advance in screening for male infertility causing mutations has been made in the recent years, enabling the collection of a large amount of data. Paradoxally, the latest advances in understanding posttranscriptional mechanisms of gene expression regulation in germ cells has revealed that a search for male infertility causing defects is even more complex than it had been expected several years ago. It is clear nowadays, that a gene can be disrupted not only by a mutation occurring within the open reading frame or promoter of a specific gene, but also within it's 3'UTR. This region seems to be rich in signals necessary for proper expression. First of all, it contains recognition signals for specific RNA-binding proteins. This seems particularly important in the light of a recent hypothesis that mRNAs that encode functionally related proteins are coordinately regulated during development and form the so-called posttranscriptional RNA regulons, involving specific complexes of RNA-binding proteins (Keene, 2007). One can imagine that point mutations targeting these specific nucleotide motifs in 3'UTR may disrupt protein recognition causing a severe mRNA deregulation. This notion is further compounded by the presence in 3′UTRs of small regulatory RNA recognition sites, including those for miRNAs. As summarized in this chapter, there is a high probability that male infertility can be induced by point mutations within miRNA recognition sites. It has been recently demonstrated that a single nucleotide point mutation within the recognition site for a specific microRNA caused Crohn disease (Brest et al., 2010). Involvement of miRNAs in male infertility has been poorly assessed so far but may be quite complex. It is known that miRNAs can function in a combinatorial manner, given that an mRNA molecule may contain recognition sites for several miRNAs. On the other hand, each miRNA may repress up to hundreds of mRNAs. According to a recent, competing endogenous RNAs (ceRNA) hypothesis, mRNAs, transcribed pseudogenes, and long noncoding RNAs cooperate using miRNA recognition sites. These form large-scale regulatory networks across the transcriptome (Salmena et al., 2011). Dissection of these basic processes is certainly very important for a better understanding of germ cell development and male infertility.

7. Acknowledgments

We thank Dr Robert P Erickson for critical reading of the manuscript. This work was supported by a grant from Ministry of Science and Higher Education no. N N401 318439 to JJ.

8. References

Aravin, A.A.; Sachidanandam, R.; Girard, A.; Fejes-Toth, K. & Hannon, G.J. (2007). Developmentally regulated piRNA clusters implicate MILI in transposon control. *Science*, Vol.316, No.5825, (May 2007), pp. 744-747, ISSN 0036-8075

Avenarius, M.R.; Hildebrand, M.S.; Zhang, Y.; Meyer, N.C.; Smith, L.L.; Kahrizi, K.; Najmabadi, H. & Smith, R.J. (2009). Human male infertility caused by mutations in the CATSPER1 channel protein. *American Journal of Human Genetics*, Vol.84, No.4, (April 2009), pp. 505-510, ISSN 0002-9297

Babiarz, J.E.; Ruby, J.G.; Wang, Y.; Bartel, D.P. & Blelloch, R. (2008). Mouse ES cells express endogenous shRNAs, siRNAs, and other Microprocessor-independent, Dicer-dependent small RNAs. *Genes & Development*, Vol.22, No.20, (October 2008), pp. 2773-2785, ISSN 0890-9369

Baenziger, J.U. & Green, E.D. (1988). Pituitary glycoprotein hormone oligosaccharides: structure, synthesis and function of the asparagine-linked oligosaccharides on lutropin, follitropin and thyrotropin. *Biochimica et Biophysica Acta*, Vol.947, No.2, (June 1988), pp. 287-306, ISSN 0006-3002

Bartel D.P. (2004). MicroRNAs: genomics, biogenesis, mechanism, and function. *Cell*, Vol.116, No.2 (January 2004), pp. 281-297, ISSN 0092-8674

Bartel D.P. (2009). MicroRNAs: Target Recognition and Regulatory Functions. *Cell*, Vol.136, No.2, (January 2009), pp. 216-233, ISSN 0092-8674

Bashamboo, A.; Ferraz-de-Souza, B.; Lourenço, D.; Lin, L.; Serbie, N.J.; Montjean, D.; Bignon-Topalovic, J.; Mandelbaum, J.; Siffroi, J.P.; Christin-Maitre, S.; Radhakrishna, U.; Rouba, H.; Ravel, C.; Seeler, J.; Achermann, J.C. & McElreavey K. (2010). Human male infertility associated with mutations in NR5A1 encoding steroidogenic factor 1. *American Journal of Human Genetics,* Vol.87, No.4, (October 2010), pp. 505-512, ISSN 0002-9297

Bateson, P.; Barker, D.; Clutton-Brock, T.; Deb, D.; D'Udine, B.; Foley, R.A.; Gluckman, P.; Godfrey, K.; Kirkwood, T.; Lahr, M.M.; McNamara, J.; Metcalfe, N.B.; Monaghan, P.; Spencer, H.G. & Sultan, S.E. (2004). Developmental plasticity and human health. *Nature,* Vol.430, No.6998, (July 2004), pp. 419–421, ISSN 0369-6243

Begeot, M.; Hemming, F.; DuBois, P.; Combarnous, Y.; DuBois, M. & Aubert, M. (1984). Induction of pituitary lactotrope differentiation by luteinizing hormone asubunit. *Science,* Vol.226, No.4674, (November 1984), pp. 566-568, ISSN 0036-8075

Ben Khelifa, M.; Zouari, R.; Harbuz, R.; Halouani, L.; Arnoult, C.; Lunardi, J. & Ray, P.F. (2011). A new AURKC mutation causing macrozoospermia: implications for human spermatogenesis and clinical diagnosis. *Molecular Human Reproduction,* Epub ahead of print, (August 2011), ISSN 1360-9947

Bentwich, I.; Avniel, A.; Karov, Y.; Aharonov, R.; Gilad, S.; Barad, O.; Barzilai, A.; Einat, P.; Einav, U.; Meiri, E.; Sharon, E.; Spector, Y. & Bentwich, Z. (2005). Identification of hundreds of conserved and nonconserved human microRNAs. *Nature Genetics,* Vol.37, No.7, (July 2005), pp. 766-770, ISSN 1061-4036

Bernard, M.; Sanseau, P.; Henry, C.; Couturier, A. & Prigent, C. (1998). Cloning of STK13, a third human protein kinase related to Drosophila aurora and budding yeast Ipl1 that maps on chromosome 19q13.3-ter. *Genomics,* Vol.53, No.3, (November 1998), pp. 406-409, ISSN 0888-7543

Bieche, I.; Latil, A.; Parfait, B.; Vidaud, D.; Laurendeau, I.; Lidereau, R.; Cussenot, O. & Vidaud, M. (2002). CGA gene (coding for the a subunit of glycoprotein hormones) overexpression in ERa- positive prostate tumors. *European Urology,* Vol.41, No.3, (March 2002), pp. 335-341, ISSN 0302-2838

Blithe, D.L.; Richards, R.G. & Skarulis, M.C. (1991). Free alpha molecules from pregnancy stimulate secretion of prolactin from human decidual cells: a novel function for free alpha in pregnancy. *Endocrinology,* Vol.129, No.4, (October 1991), pp. 2257-2259, ISSN 0013-7227

Brest, P.; Lapaquette, P.; Souidi, M.; Lebrigand, K.; Cesaro, A.; Vouret-Craviari, V.; Mari, B.; Barbry, P.; Mosnier, J.F.; Hébuterne, X.; Harel-Bellan, A.; Mograbi, B.; Darfeuille-Michaud, A. & Hofman, P. (2011). A synonymous variant in IRGM alters a binding site for miR-196 and causes deregulation of IRGM-dependent xenophagy in Crohn's disease. *Nature Genetics,* Vol.43, No.3, (March 2011), pp. 242-245, ISSN 1061-4036

Brown, G.M.; Furlong, R.A.; Sargent, C.A.; Erickson, R.P.; Longepied, G.; Mitchell, M.; Jones, M.H.; Hargreave, T.B.; Cooke, H.J. & Affara, N.A. (1998). Characterisation of the coding sequence and fine mapping of the human DFFRY gene and comparative expression analysis and mapping to the Sxrb interval of the mouse Y chromosome of the Dffry gene. *Human Molecular Genetics,* Vol.7, No.1, (January 1998), pp. 97–107, ISSN 0964-6906

Cai, X.; Hagedorn, C. & Cullen, B. (2004). Human microRNAs are processed from capped, polyadenylated transcripts that can also function as mRNAs. *RNA,* Vol.10, No.12, (December 2004), pp. 1957-1966, ISSN 1355-8382

Carlson, A.E.; Westenbroek, R.E.; Quill, T.; Ren, D.; Clapham, D.E.; Hille, B.; Garbers D.L. & Babcock, D.F. (2003). CatSper1 required for evoked Ca2+ entry and control of flagellar function in sperm. *Proceedings of the National Academy of Sciences of the United States of America,* Vol.100, No.25, (December 2003), pp. 14864-14868, ISSN ISSN 0027-8424

Carmell, M.A.; Girard, A.; van de Kant, H.J.; Bourc'his, D.; Bestor, T.H.; de Rooij, D.G. & Hannon, G.J. (2007). MIWI2 is essential for spermatogenesis and repression of transposons in the mouse male germline. *Developmental Cell,* Vol.12, No.4, (April 2007), pp. 503-514, ISSN 1534-5807

Czech, B. & Hannon G. (2011). Small RNA sorting: matchmaking for Argonautes. *Nature Reviews. Genetics,* Vol.12, No.1, (January 2011), pp. 19-31, ISSN 1471-0056

Dam, A.H.; Koscinski, I.; Kremer, J.A.; Moutou, C.; Jaeger, A.S.; Oudakker, A.R.; Tournaye, H.; Charlet, N.; Lagier-Tourenne, C.; van Bokhoven, H. & Viville, S. (2007). Homozygous mutation in SPATA16 is associated with male infertility in human globozoospermia. *American Journal of Human Genetics,* Vol.81, No.4, (October 2007), pp. 813-820, ISSN 0002-9297

Dieterich, K.; Soto Rifo, R.; Faure, A.K.; Hennebicq, S.; Ben Amar, B.; Zahi, M.; Perrin, J.; Martinez, D.; Sèle, B.; Jouk, P.S.; Ohlmann, T.; Rousseaux, S.; Lunardi, J. & Ray, P.F. (2007). Homozygous mutation of AURKC yields large-headed polyploid spermatozoa and causes male infertility. *Nature Genetics,* Vol.39, No.5, (May 2007), pp. 661-665, ISSN 1061-4036

Dieterich, K.; Zouari, R.; Harbuz, R.; Vialard, F.; Martinez, D.; Bellayou, H.; Prisant, N.; Zoghmar, A.; Guichaoua, M.R.; Koscinski, I.; Kharouf, M.; Noruzinia, M.; Nadifi, S.; Sefiani, A.; Lornage, J.; Zahi, M.; Viville, S.; Sèle, B.; Jouk, P.S.; Jacob, M.C.; Escalier, D.; Nikas, Y.; Hennebicq, S.; Lunardi, J. & Ray, P.F. (2009). The Aurora Kinase C c.144delC mutation causes meiosis I arrest in men and is frequent in the North African population. *Human Molecular Genetics,* Vol.18, No.7, (April 2009), pp. 1301-1309, ISSN 0964-6906

Ditton, H.J.; Zimmer, J.; Kamp, C.; Rajpert-De Meyts, E. & Vogt, P.H. (2004). The AZFa gene DBY (DDX3Y) is widely transcribed but the protein is limited to the male germ cells by translation control. *Human Molecular Genetics,* Vol.13, No.19, (October 2004), pp. 2333–2341, ISSN 0964-6906

Djuranovic, S.; Nahvi, A. & Green, R. (2011). A Parsimonious model for Gene Regulation by miRNAs. *Science,* Vol.331, No.6017, (February 2011), pp. 550-553, ISSN 0036-8075

El Kerch, F.; Lamzouri, A.; Laarabi, F.Z.; Zahi, M.; Ben Amar, B. & Sefiani, A. (2011). Confirmation of the high prevalence in Morocco of the homozygous mutation c.144delC in the aurora kinase C gene (AURKC) in the teratozoospermia with large-headed spermatozoa. *Journal de Gynécologie Obstétrique et Biologie de la Reproduction,* Vol.40, No.5, (Jun 2011), pp. 329-333, ISSN 0368-2315

Elbashir, S.M.; Martinez, J.; Patkaniowska, A.; Lendeckel, W. & Tuschl, T. (2001). Functional anatomy of siRNAs for mediating efficient RNAi in Drosophila melanogaster embryo lysate. *The EMBO Journal,* Vol.20, No.23, (December 2001), pp. 6877-6888, ISSN 0261-4189

Escudier, E.; Duquesnoy, P.; Papon, J.F. & Amselem, S. (2009). Ciliary defects and genetics of primary ciliary dyskinesia. *Paediatric Respiratory Reviews,* Vol.10, No.2, (Jun 2009), pp. 51-54, ISSN 1526-0542

Ferlin, A.; Moro, E.; Rossi, A.; Dallapiccola, B. & Foresta, C. (2003). The human Y chromosome's azoospermia factor b (AZFb) region: sequence, structure, and deletion analysis in infertile men. *Journal of Medical Genetics*, Vol.40, No.1, (January 2003), pp. 18–24, ISSN 0022-2593

Ferlin, A.; Raicu, F.; Gatta, V.; Zuccarello, D.; Palka, G.; Foresta, C. (2007). Male infertility: role of genetic background. *Reproductive biomedicine online,* Vol.14, No.6, (Jun 2007), pp. 734-745, ISSN 1472-6483

Fernandes, A.T.; Fernandes, S.; Gonçalves, R.; Sá, R.; Costa, P.; Rosa, A.; Ferrás, C.; Sousa, M.; Brehm, A. & Barros, A. (2006). DAZ gene copies: evidence of Y chromosome evolution. *Molecular Human Reproduction,* Vol.12, No.8, (August 2006), pp. 519–523, ISSN 1360-9947

Fernandes, S.; Huellen, K.; Gonçalves, J.; Dukal, H.; Zeisler, J.; Rajpert De Meyts, E.; Skakkebaek, N.E.; Habermann, B.; Krause, W.; Sousa, M.; Bartos, A. & Vogt, P.H. (2002). High frequency of DAZ1/DAZ2 gene deletions in patients with severe oligozoospermia. *Molecular Human Reproduction,* Vol.8, No.3, (March 2002), pp. 286–298, ISSN 1360-9947

Fernandes, S.; Paracchini, S.; Meyer, L.H.; Floridia, G.; Tyler-Smith, C. & Vogt P.H. (2004). A large AZFc deletion removes DAZ3/DAZ4 and nearby genes from men in Y haplogroup N. *American Journal of Human Genetics,* Vol.74, No.1, (January 2004), pp. 180–187, ISSN 0002-9297

Fox, M.; Urano, J. & Reijo Pera, R.A. (2005). Identification and characterization of RNA sequences to which human PUMILIO-2 (PUM2) and deleted in Azoospermia-like (DAZL) bind. *Genomics,* Vol.85, No.1, (January 2005), pp. 92-105, ISSN 0888-7543

Galgano, A.; Forrer, M.; Jaskiewicz, L.; Kanitz, A.; Zavolan, M. & Gerber, A.P. (2008). Comparative analysis of mRNA targets for human PUF-family proteins suggests extensive interaction with the miRNA regulatory system. *PLoS One,* Vol.3, No.9, (September 2008), pp. e3164, ESSN 1932-6203

Ginter-Matuszewska, B.; Kusz, K.; Spik, A.; Grzeszkowiak, D.; Rembiszewska, A.; Kupryjanczyk, J. & Jaruzelska, J. (2011). NANOS1 and PUMILIO2 bind microRNA biogenesis factor GEMIN3, within chromatoid body in human germ cells. *Histochemistry and Cell Biology,* Vol.136, No.3, (September 2011), pp. 279-287, ISSN 0948-6143

Gregory, R.; Yan, K.; Amuthan, G.; Chendrimada, T.; Doratotaj, B.; Cooch, N. & Shiekhattar, D. (2004). The Microprocessor complex mediates the genesis of microRNAs. *Nature,* Vol.432, No.7014, (November 2004), pp. 235-240, ISSN 0028-0836

Gu, A.; Ji, G.; Shi, X.; Long, Y.; Xia, Y.; Song, L.; Wang, S. & Wang, X. (2010). Genetic variants in Piwi-interacting RNA pathway genes confer susceptibility to spermatogenic failure in a Chinese population. *Human Reproduction,* Vol.25, No.12, (December 2010), pp. 2955-2961, ISSN 0268-1161

Hamilton, A.J. & Baulcombe, D.C. (1999). A species of small antisense RNA in posttranscriptional gene silencing in plants. *Science,* Vol.286, No.5441, (October 1999), pp. 950-952, ISSN 0036-8075

Harbuz, R.; Zouari, R.; Pierre, V.; Ben Khelifa, M.; Kharouf, M.; Coutton, C.; Merdassi, G.; Abada, F.; Escoffier, J.; Nikas, Y.; Vialard, F.; Koscinski, I.; Triki, C.; Sermondade, N.; Schweitzer, T.; Zhioua, A.; Zhioua, F.; Latrous, H.; Halouani, L.; Ouafi, M.; Makni, M.; Jouk, P.S.; Sèle, B.; Hennebicq, S.; Satre, V.; Viville, S.; Arnoult, C.; Lunardi, J. & Ray, P.F. (2011). A recurrent deletion of DPY19L2 causes infertility in man by blocking sperm head elongation and acrosome formation. *American Journal of Human Genetics,* Vol.88, No.3, (March 2011), pp. 351-361, ISSN 0002-9297

He, Z.; Kokkinaki, M.; Pant, D.; Gallicano, G.I. & Dym, M. (2009). Small RNA molecules in the regulation of spermatogenesis. *Reproduction.* Vol.137, No.6, (June 2009), pp. 901-911, ISSN 1470-1626

Honigberg, L. & Kenyon C. (2000). Establishment of left/right asymmetry in neuroblast migration by UNC-40/DCC, UNC-73/Trio and DPY-19 proteins in C. elegans. *Development,* Vol.127, No.21, (November 2000), pp. 4655-4668, ISSN 1011-6370

Houwing, S.; Berezikov, E. & Ketting, R.F. (2008). Zili is required for germ cell differentiation and meiosis in zebrafish. *The EMBO Journal,* Vol.27, No.20, (October 2008), pp. 2702-2711, ISSN 0261-4189

Huntzinger, E. & Izzauralde, E. (2011). Gene silencing by microRNAs: contributions of translational repression and mRNA decay. *Nature Reviews. Genetics,* Vol.12, No.2, (February 2011), pp. 99-110, ISSN 1471-0056

Jaskiewicz, L. & Filipowicz, W. (2008). Role of Dicer in posttranscriptional RNA silencing. *Current Topics in Microbiology and Immunology,* Vol.320, pp. 77-97, ISSN 0070-217X

Kawamata, T.; Seitz, H. & Tomari, Y. (2009). Structural determinants of miRNAs for RISC loading and slicer-independent unwinding. *Nature Structural & Molecular Biology,* Vol.16, No.9, (September 2009), pp. 953-960, ISSN 1545-9993

Kawaoka, S.; Hayashi, N.; Suzuki, Y.; Abe, H.; Sugano, S.; Tomari, Y.; Shimada, T. & Katsuma, S. (2009). The Bombyx ovary-derived cell line endogenously expresses PIWI/PIWI-interacting RNA complexes. *RNA,* Vol.15, No.7, (July 2009), pp. 1258-1264, ISSN 1355-8382

Keene, J.D. (2007). RNA regulons: coordination of post-transcriptional events. *Nature Reviews Genetics,* Vol.8, No.7, (July 2007), pp. 533-543, ISSN 1471-0056

Kendall, S.K.; Samuelson, L.C.; Saunders, T.L.; Wood, R.I. & Camper, S.A. (1995). Targeted disruption of the pituitary glycoprotein hormone alpha-subunit produces hypogonadal and hypothyroid mice. *Genes & Development,* Vol.9, No.16, (August 1995), pp. 2007-1019, ISSN 0890-9369

Kim, V. (2004). MicroRNA precursors in motion: exportin-5 mediates their nuclear export. *Trends in Cell Biology,* Vol.14, No.4, (April 2004), pp. 156-159, ISSN 0962-8924

Kimmins, S.; Crosio, C.; Kotaja, N.; Hirayama, J.; Monaco, L.; Höög, C.; van Duin, M.; Gossen, J.A. & Sassone-Corsi, P. (2007). Differential functions of the Aurora-B and Aurora-C kinases in mammalian spermatogenesis. *Molecular Endocrinology,* Vol.21, No.3, (March 2007), pp. 726-739, ISSN 0952-5041

Kimura, M. ; Matsuda, Y., Yoshioka, T & Okano, Y. (1999). Cell cycle-dependent expression and centrosome localization of a third human aurora/Ipl1-related protein kinase, AIK3. *Journal of Biological Chemistry,* Vol.12, No.274, (March 1999), pp. 7334-7340, ISSN 0021-9258

Kishore, S.; Luber, S. & Zavolan, M. (2010). Deciphering the role of RNA-binding proteins in the post-transcriptional control of gene expression. *Briefings in Functional Genomics,* Vol.9, No.5-6, (December 2010), pp. 391-404, ISSN 2041-2649

Klattenhoff, C. & Theurkauf, W. (2008). Biogenesis and germline functions of piRNAs. *Development,* Vol.135, No.1, (January 2008), pp. 5-9, ISSN 1011-6370

Kok, K.H.; Ng, M.H.J.; Ching, Y.P. & Jin, D.Y. (2007). Human TRBP and PACT directly interact with each other and associate with dicer to facilitate the production of small interfering RNA. *The Journal of Biological Chemistry*, Vol.282, No.24, (June 2007), pp. 17649–17657, ISSN 0021-9258

Koscinski, I.; Elinati, E.; Fossard, C.; Redin, C.; Muller, J.; Velez de la Calle, J.; Schmitt, F.; Ben Khelifa, M.; Ray, P.F.; Kilani, Z.; Barratt, C.L. & Viville, S. (2011). DPY19L2 deletion as a major cause of globozoospermia. *American Journal of Human Genetics*, Vol.88, No.3, (March 2011), pp. 344-350, ISSN 0002-9297

Krausz, C.; Degl'Innocenti, S.; Nuti, F.; Morelli, A.; Felici, F.; Sansone, M.; Varriale, G. & Forti, G. (2006). Natural transmission of USP9Y gene mutations: a new perspective on the role of AZFa genes in male fertility. *Human Molecular Genetics*, Vol.15, No.18, (September 2006), pp. 2673–2681, ISSN 0964-6906

Kroger, A.; Koster, M.; Schroeder, K.; Hauser, H. & Mueller, P.P. (2002). Activities of IRF-1. *Journal of Interferon & Cytokine Research The Official Journal of the International Society for Interferon and Cytokine Research*, Vol.22, No.1, (January 2002), pp. 455-461, ISSN 1079-9907

Kuramochi-Miyagawa, S.; Watanabe, T.; Gotoh, K.; Totoki, Y.; Toyoda, A.; Ikawa, M.; Asada, N.; Kojima, K.; Yamaguchi, Y.; Ijiri, T.W.; Hata, K.; Li, E.; Matsuda, Y.; Kimura, T.; Okabe, M.; Sasaki, Y.; Sasaki, H. & Nakano, T. (2008). DNA methylation of retrotransposon genes is regulated by Piwi family members MILI and MIWI2 in murine fetal testes. *Genes & development*, Vol.22, No.7, (April 2008), pp. 908-917, ISSN 0890-9369

Kuroda-Kawaguchi, T.; Skaletsky, H.; Brown, L.G.; Minx, P.J.; Cordum, H.S.; Waterston, R.H.; Wilson, R.K.; Silber, S.; Oates, R.; Rozen, S. & Page D.C. (2001). The AZFc region of the Y chromosome features massive palindromes and uniform recurrent deletions in infertile men. *Nature Genetics*, Vol.29, No.3, (November 2001), pp. 279–286, ISSN 1061-4036

Kusz, K.; Ginter-Matuszewska, B.; Ziolkowska, K.; Spik, A.; Bierla, J.; Jedrzejczak, P.; Latos-Bielenska, A.; Pawelczyk, L. & Jaruzelska, J. (2007). Polymorphisms of the human PUMILIO2 gene and male sterility. *Molecular Reproduction and Development*, Vol.74, No.6, (June 2007), pp. 795-799, ISSN 1040-452X

Kusz, K.; Tomczyk, L.; Sajek, M.; Spik, A.; Latos-Bielenska, A.; Jedrzejczak, P.; Pawelczyk, L. & Jaruzelska, J. (2009a). The highly conserved NANOS2 protein: testis-specific expression and significance for the human male reproduction. *Molecular Human Reproduction*, Vol.15, No.3, (March 2009), pp. 165-171, ISSN 1360-9947

Kusz, K.; Tomczyk, L.; Spik, A.; Latos-Bielenska, A.; Jedrzejczak, P.; Pawelczyk, L. & Jaruzelska, J. (2009b). NANOS3 gene mutations in men with isolated sterility phenotype. *Molecular Reproduction and Development*, Vol.76, No.9, (September 2009), pp. 804, ISSN 1040-452X

Lal, A.; Kim, H.H.; Abdelmohsen, K.; Kuwano, Y.; Pullmann, R. Jr; Srikantan, S.; Subrahmanyam, R.; Martindale, J.L.; Yang, X.; Ahmed, F.; Navarro, F.; Dykxhoorn, D.; Lieberman, J. & Gorospe, M. (2008). p16(INK4a) translation suppressed by miR-24. *PLoS One*, Vol.3, No.3, (March 2008), pp. e1864, ESSN 1932-6203

Lander, E.S.; Linton, L.M.; Birren, B.; Nusbaum, C.; Zody, M.C.; Baldwin, J.; Devon, K.; Dewar, K.; Doyle, M.; FitzHugh, W.; Funke, R.; Gage, D.; Harris, K.; Heaford, A.; Howland, J.; Kann, L.; Lehoczky, J.; LeVine, R.; McEwan, P.; McKernan, K.;

Meldrim, J.; Mesirov, J.P.; Miranda, C.; Morris, W.; Naylor, J.; Raymond, C.; Rosetti, M.; Santos, R.; Sheridan, A.; Sougnez, C.; Stange-Thomann, N.; Stojanovic, N.; Subramanian, A.; Wyman, D.; Rogers, J.; Sulston, J.; Ainscough, R.; Beck, S.; Bentley, D.; Burton, J.; Clee, C.; Carter, N.; Coulson, A.; Deadman, R.; Deloukas, P.; Dunham, A.; Dunham, I.; Durbin, R.; French, L.; Grafham, D.; Gregory, S.; Hubbard, T.; Humphray, S.; Hunt, A.; Jones, M.; Lloyd, C.; McMurray, A.; Matthews, L.; Mercer, S.; Milne, S.; Mullikin, J.C.; Mungall, A.; Plumb, R.; Ross, M.; Shownkeen, R.; Sims, S.; Waterston, R.H.; Wilson, R.K.; Hillier, L.W.; McPherson, J.D.; Marra, M.A.; Mardis, E.R.; Fulton, L.A.; Chinwalla, A.T.; Pepin, K.H.; Gish, W.R.; Chissoe, S.L.; Wendl, M.C.; Delehaunty, K.D.; Miner, T.L.; Delehaunty, A.; Kramer, J.B.; Cook, L.L.; Fulton, R.S.; Johnson, D.L.; Minx, P.J.; Clifton, S.W.; Hawkins, T.; Branscomb, E.; Predki, P.; Richardson, P.; Wenning, S.; Slezak, T.; Doggett, N.; Cheng, J.F.; Olsen, A.; Lucas, S.; Elkin, C.; Uberbacher, E.; Frazier, M.; Gibbs, R.A.; Muzny, D.M.; Scherer, S.E.; Bouck, J.B.; Sodergren, E.J.; Worley, K.C.; Rives, C.M.; Gorrell, J.H.; Metzker, M.L.; Naylor, S.L.; Kucherlapati, R.S.; Nelson, D.L.; Weinstock, G.M.; Sakaki, Y.; Fujiyama, A.; Hattori, M.; Yada, T.; Toyoda, A.; Itoh, T.; Kawagoe, C.; Watanabe, H.; Totoki, Y.; Taylor, T.; Weissenbach, J.; Heilig, R.; Saurin, W.; Artiguenave, F.; Brottier, P.; Bruls, T.; Pelletier, E.; Robert, C.; Wincker, P.; Smith, D.R.; Doucette-Stamm, L.; Rubenfield, M.; Weinstock, K.; Lee, H.M.; Dubois, J.; Rosenthal, A.; Platzer, M.; Nyakatura, G.; Taudien, S.; Rump, A.; Yang, H.; Yu, J.; Wang, J.; Huang, G.; Gu, J.; Hood, L.; Rowen, L.; Madan, A.; Qin, S.; Davis, R.W.; Federspiel, N.A.; Abola, A.P.; Proctor, M.J.; Myers, R.M.; Schmutz, J.; Dickson, M.; Grimwood, J.; Cox, D.R.; Olson, M.V.; Kaul, R.; Raymond, C.; Shimizu, N.; Kawasaki, K.; Minoshima, S.; Evans, G.A.; Athanasiou, M.; Schultz, R.; Roe, B.A.; Chen, F.; Pan, H.; Ramser, J.; Lehrach, H.; Reinhardt, R.; McCombie, W.R.; de la Bastide, M.; Dedhia, N.; Blöcker, H.; Hornischer, K.; Nordsiek, G.; Agarwala, R.; Aravind, L.; Bailey, J.A.; Bateman, A.; Batzoglou, S.; Birney, E.; Bork, P.; Brown, D.G.; Burge, C.B.; Cerutti, L.; Chen, H.C.; Church, D.; Clamp, M.; Copley, R.R.; Doerks, T.; Eddy, S.R.; Eichler, E.E.; Furey, T.S.; Galagan, J.; Gilbert, J.G.; Harmon, C.; Hayashizaki, Y.; Haussler, D.; Hermjakob, H.; Hokamp, K.; Jang, W.; Johnson, L.S.; Jones, T.A.; Kasif, S.; Kaspryzk, A.; Kennedy, S.; Kent, W.J.; Kitts, P.; Koonin, E.V.; Korf, I.; Kulp, D.; Lancet, D.; Lowe, T.M.; McLysaght, A.; Mikkelsen, T.; Moran, J.V.; Mulder, N.; Pollara, V.J.; Ponting, C.P.; Schuler, G.; Schultz, J.; Slater, G.; Smit, A.F.; Stupka, E.; Szustakowski, J.; Thierry-Mieg, D.; Thierry-Mieg, J.; Wagner, L.; Wallis, J.; Wheeler, R.; Williams, A.; Wolf, YI.; Wolfe, K.H.; Yang, S.P.; Yeh, R.F.; Collins, F.; Guyer, M.S.; Peterson, J.; Felsenfeld, A.; Wetterstrand, K.A.; Patrinos, A.; Morgan, M.J.; de Jong, P.; Catanese, J.J.; Osoegawa, K.; Shizuya, H.; Choi, S. & Chen, Y.J. (2001). Initial sequencing and analysis of the human genome. *Nature*, Vol.409, No.6822, (February 2001), pp. 860-921, ISSN 0028- 0836

Lapthorn, A.J.; Harris, D.C.; Littlejohn, A.; Lustbader, J.W.; Canfield, R.E.; Machin, K.J.; Morgan, F.J. & Isaacs, N.W. (1994). Crystal structure of human chorionic gonadotropin. *Nature*, Vol.369, No.6480, (June 1994), pp. 455-461, ISSN 0028-0836

Lardone, M.C.; Parodi, D.A.; Valdevenito, R.; Ebensperger, M.; Piottante, A.; Madariaga, M.; Smith, R.; Pommer, R.; Zambrano, N. & Castro, A. (2007). Quantification of DDX3Y, RBMY1, DAZ and TSPY mRNAs in testes of patients with severe impairment of spermatogenesis. *Molecular Human Reproduction,* Vol.13, No.10, (October 2007), pp. 705–712, ISSN 1360-9947

Lau, N.C.; Seto, A.G.; Kim, J.; Kuramochi-Miyagawa, S.; Nakano, T.; Bartel, D.P. & Kingston, R.E. (2006). Characterization of the piRNA complex from rat testes. *Science*, Vol.313, No.5785, (July 2006), pp. 363-367, ISSN 0036- 8075

Lavery, R.; Glennon, M.; Houghton, J.; Nolan, A.; Egan, D. & Maher, M. (2007). Investigation of DAZ and RBMY1 gene expression in human testis by quantitative real-time PCR. *Archives of Andrology,* Vol.53, No.2, (March-April 2007), pp. 71–73, ISSN 0148-5016

Lee, R.C.; Feinbaum, R.L. & Ambros, V. (1993). The C. elegans heterochronic gene lin-4 encodes small RNAs with antisense complementarity to lin-14. *Cell,* Vol.75, No.5, (December 1993), pp. 843-854, ISSN 0092-8674

Lee, Y.S.; Nakahara, K.; Pham, J.W.; Kim, K.; He, Z.; Sontheimer, E.J. & Carthew, R.W. (2004). Distinct roles for Drosophila Dicer-1 and Dicer-2 in the siRNA/miRNA silencing pathways. *Cell,* Vol.117, No.1, (April 2004), pp. 69-81, ISSN 0092-8674

Lian, J.; Tian, H.; Liu, L.; Zhang, X.S.; Li, W.Q.; Deng, Y.M.; Yao, G.D.; Yin, M.M. & Sun, F. (2010). Downregulation of microRNA-383 is associated with male infertility and promotes testicular embryonal carcinoma cell proliferation by targeting IRF1. *Cell Death & Disease,* Vol.1, (November 2010), pp. e94, ESSN 2041-4889

Lian, J.; Zhang, X.; Tian, H.; Liang, N.; Wang, Y.; Liang, C.; Li, X. & Sun, F. (2009). Altered microRNA expression in patients with non-obstructive azoospermia. *Reproductive Biology and Endocrinology,* Vol.7, (February 2009), pp. 13, ESSN 1477-7827

Lin, L. & Achermann J.C. (2008). Steroidogenic factor-1 (SF-1, Ad4BP, NR5A1) and disorders of testis development. *Sexual Development,* Vol.2, No.4-5, (November 2008), pp. 200-209, ISSN 1661-5425

Lin, Y.W.; Hsu, L.C.; Kuo, P.L.; Huang, W.J.; Chiang, H.S.; Yeh, S.D.; Hsu, T.Y.; Yu, Y.H.; Hsiao, K.N.; Cantor, R.M. & Yen, P.H. (2007). Partial duplication at AZFc on the Y chromosome is a risk factor for impaired spermatogenesis in Han Chinese in Taiwan. *Human Mutation,* Vol.28, No.5, (May 2007), pp. 486–494, ISSN 1059-7794

Liu, J.; Carmell, M.A.; Rivas, F.V.; Marsden, C.G.; Thomson, J.M.; Song, J.J.; Hammond, S.M.; Joshua-Tor, L. & Hannon, G.J. (2004). Argonaute2 is the catalytic engine of mammalian RNAi. *Science,* Vol.305, No.5689, (September 2004), pp. 1437-1441, ISSN 0036-8075

Lourenço, D.; Brauner, R.; Lin, L.; De Perdigo, A.; Weryha, G.; Muresan, M.; Boudjenah, R.; Guerra-Junior, G.; Maciel-Guerra, A.T.; Achermann, J.C.; McElreavey, K. & Bashamboo, A. (2009). Mutations in NR5A1 associated with ovarian insufficiency. *New England Journal of Medicine,* Vol.360, No.12, (March 2009), pp.1200-1210, ISSN 0028-4793

Lu, L.; Lin, M.; Xu, M.; Zhou, Z.M. & Sha, J.H. (2006). Gene functional research using polyethylenimine-mediated in vivo gene transfection into mouse spermatogenic cells. *Asian Journal of Andrology,* Vol.8, No.1, (January 2006), pp. 53-59, ISSN 1008-682X

Luddi, A.; Margollicci, M.; Gambera, L.; Serafini, F.; Cioni, M.; De Leo, V.; Balestri, P. & Piomboni, P. (2009). Spermatogenesis in a man with complete deletion of USP9Y.

The New England Journal of Medicine, Vol.360, No.9, (February 2009), pp. 881–885, ISSN 0028-4793

Ma, K.; Inglis, J.D.; Sharkey, A.; Bickmore, W.A.; Hill, R.E.; Prosser, E.J.; Speed, R.M.; Thomson, E.J.; Jobling, M.; Taylor, K.; Wolfe, J.; Cooke, H.J.; Hargreave, T.B. & Chandley, A.C. (1993). A Y chromosome gene family with RNA-binding protein homology: candidates for the azoospermia factor AZF controlling human spermatogenesis. *Cell,* Vol.75, No.7, (December 1993), pp. 1287–1295, ISSN 0092-8674

Machev, N.; Saut, N.; Longepied, G.; Terriou, P.; Navarro, A.; Levy, N.; Guichaoua, M.; Metzler-Guillemain, C.; Collignon, P.; Frances, A.M.; Belougne, J.; Clemente, E.; Chiaroni, J.; Chevillard, C.; Durand, C.; Ducourneau, A.; Pech, N.; McElreavey, K.; Mattei, M.G. & Mitchell, M.J. (2004). Sequence family variant loss from the AZFc interval of the human Y chromosome, but not gene copy loss, is strongly associated with male infertility. *Journal of Medical Genetics,* Vol.41, No.11, (November 2004), pp. 814-825, ISSN 0022-2593

Marton, S.; Garcia, M.R.; Robello, C.; Persson, H.; Trajtenberg, F.; Pritsch, O.; Rovira, C.; Naya, H.; Dighiero, G. & Cayota, A. (2008). Small RNAs analysis in CLL reveals a deregulation of miRNA expression and novel miRNA candidates of putative relevance in CLL pathogenesis. *Leukemia Official Journal of the Leukemia Society of America, Leukemia Research Fund, U.K,* Vol.20, No.2, (February 2008), pp. 330-338, ISSN 0887-6924

Matzuk, M.M. & Lamb, D.J. (2008). The biology of infertility: research advances and clinical challenges. *Nature Medicine,* Vol.14, No.11 (November 2008), pp. 1197-1213, ISSN 1078-8956

McCallie, B.; Schoolcraft, W.B. & Katz-Jaffe, M.G. (2010). Aberration of blastocyst microRNA expression is associated with human infertility. *Fertility and Sterility,* Vol.93, No.7, (May 2010), pp. 2374-2382, ISSN 0015-0282

Meister, G.; Landthaler, M.; Patkaniowska, A.; Dorsett, Y.; Teng, G. & Tuschl, T. (2004). Human Argonaute2 mediates RNA cleavage targeted by miRNAs and siRNAs. *Molecular Cell,* Vol.15, No.2, (July 2004), pp. 185-197, ISSN 1097-2765

Moore, F.L.; Jaruzelska, J.; Fox, M.S.; Urano, J.; Firpo, M.T.; Turek, P.J.; Dorfman, D.M. & Pera, R.A. (2003). Human Pumilio-2 is expressed in embryonic stem cells and germ cells and interacts with DAZ (Deleted in AZoospermia) and DAZ-like proteins. *Proceedings of the National Academy of Sciences of the United States of America,* Vol.100, No.2, (January 2003), pp. 538-543, ISSN 0027-8424

Mourelatos, Z.; Dostie, J.; Paushkin, S.; Sharma, A.; Charroux, B.; Abel, L.; Rappsilber, J.; Mann, M. & Dreyfuss, G. (2002). miRNPs: a novel class of ribonucleoproteins containing numerous microRNAs. *Genes & Development,* Vol.16, No.6, (March 2002), pp. 720-728, ISSN 0890-9369

Muller, D.W. & Bosserhoff, A.K. (2008). Integrin beta 3 expression is regulated by let-7a miRNA in malignant melanoma. *Oncogene,* Vol.27, No.52, (November 2008), pp. 6698-6706, ISSN 0950-9232

Navarro-Costa, P.; Plancha, C.E. & Gonçalves, J. (2010a). Genetic dissection of the AZF regions of the human Y chromosome: thriller or filler for male (in)fertility? *Journal of Biomedicine & Biotechnoogy,* Epub 2010:936569, (June 2010), ISSN 1110-7243

Navarro-Costa, P.; Gonçalves J. & Plancha, C.E. (2010b). The AZFc region of the Y chromosome: at the crossroads between genetic diversity and male infertility. *Human Reproduction Update*, Vol.16, No.5, (September-October 2010), pp. 525-542, ISSN 1355-4786

Nishida, K.M.; Saito, K.; Mori, T.; Kawamura, Y.; Nagami-Okada, T.; Inagaki, S.; Siomi, H. & Siomi, M.C. (2007). Gene silencing mechanisms mediated by Aubergine piRNA complexes in Drosophila male gonad. *RNA*, Vol.13, No.11, (November 2007), pp. 1911-1922, ISSN 1355-8382

Novotny, G.W.; Sonne, S.B.; Nielsen, J.E.; Jonstrup, S.P.; Hansen, M.A.; Skakkebaek, N.E.; Rajpert-De Meyts, E.; Kjems, J. & Leffers, H. (2007). Translational repression of E2F1 mRNA in carcinoma in situ and normal testis correlates with expression of the miR-17-92 cluster. *Cell Death and Differentiation*, Vol.14, No.4, (April 2007), pp. 879-882, ISSN 1350-9047

O'Flynn O'Brien, K.L.; Varghese, A.C. & Agarwal, A. (2010). The genetic causes of male factor infertility: a review. *Fertility and Sterility*, Vol.93, No.1, (January 2010), pp. 1-12, ISSN 0015-0282

Parker, J.S. & Barford, D. (2006). Argonaute: A scaffold for the function of short regulatory RNA. *Trends in Biochemical Sciences*, Vol.31, No.11, (November 2006), pp. 622-630, ISSN 0968-0004

Poongothai, J.; Gopenath, T.S. & Manonayaki, S. (2009). Genetics of human male infertility. *Singapore Medical Journal,* Vol.50, No.4, (April 2009), pp. 336-347, ISSN 0037-5675

Reijo, R.; Lee, T.Y.; Salo, P.; Alagappan, R.; Brown, L.G.; Rosenberg, M.; Rozen, S.; Jaffe, T.; Straus, D.; Hovatta, O.; Chapelle, A.; Silber, S. & Page, D.C. (1995). Diverse spermatogenic defects in humans caused by Y chromosome deletions encompassing a novel RNA-binding protein gene. *Nature Genetics,* Vol.10, No.4, (August 1995), pp. 383–393, ISSN 1061-4036

Reinhart, B.J.; Slack, F.J.; Basson, M.; Bettinger, J.C.; Pasquinelli, A.E.; Rougvie, A.E.; Horvitz, H.R. & Ruvkun, G. (2000). The 21 nucleotide let-7 RNA regulates developmental timing in Caenorhabditis elegans. *Nature*, Vol.403, No.6772, (February 2000), pp. 901-906, ISSN 0028-0836

Ren, D.; Navarro, B.; Perez, G.; Jackson, A.C.; Hsu, S.; Shi, Q.; Tilly, J.L.; & Clapham, D.E. (2001). A sperm ion channel required for sperm motility and male fertility. *Nature,* Vol.413, No.6856, (2001 October), p.603-609, ISSN 0028-0836

Repping, S.; Skaletsky, H.; Lange, J.; Silber, S.; Van Der Veen, F.; Oates, R.D.; Page, D.C. & Rozen, S. (2002). Recombination between palindromes p5 and p1 on the human y chromosome causes massive deletions and spermatogenic failure. *American Journal of Human Genetics,* Vol.71, No.4, (October 2002), pp. 906–922, ISSN 0002-9297

Reynolds, N.; Collier, B.; Maratou, K.; Bingham, V.; Speed, R.M.; Taggart, M.; Semple, C.A.; Gray, K. & Cooke, H.J. (2005). Dazl binds in vivo to specific transcripts and can regulate the pre-meiotic translation of Mvh in germ cells. *Human Molecular Genetics,* Vol.14, No.24, (December 2005), pp. 3899-3909, ISSN 0964-6906

Ro, S.; Park, C.; Sanders, K.M.; McCarrey, J.R. & Yan, W. (2007). Cloning and expression profiling of testis-expressed microRNAs. *Developmental Biology,* Vol.311, No.2, (November 2007), pp. 592-602, ISSN 0012-1606

Robine, N.; Lau, N.C.; Balla, S.; Jin, Z.; Okamura, K.; Kuramochi-Miyagawa, S.; Blower, M.D. & Lai, E.C. (2009). A broadly conserved pathway generates 3'UTR-directed primary piRNAs. *Current Biology*, Vol.19, No.24, (December 2009), pp. 2066-2076, ISSN 0960-9822

Rockett, J.C.; Patrizio, P.; Schmid, J.E.; Hecht, N.B. & Dix, D.J. (2004). Gene expression patterns associated with infertility in humans and rodent models. *Mutation Research*, Vol.549, No.1-2, (May 2004), pp. 225-240, ISSN 0027-5107

Sadeghi-Nejad, H. & Farrokhi, F. (2007). Genetics of azoospermia: current knowledge, clinical implications, and future directions. Part II: Y chromosome microdeletions. *Urology Journal*, Vol.4, No.4, (Fall 2007), pp. 192-206, ISSN 1735-1308

Salmena, L.; Poliseno, L.; Tay, Y.; Kats, L. & Pandolfi, P.P. (2011). A ceRNA Hypothesis: The Rosetta Stone of a Hidden RNA Language? *Cell*, Vol.146, No.3, (August 2011), pp. 353-358, ISSN 0092-8674

Sampson, V.B.; Rong, N.H.; Han, J.; Yang, Q.; Aris, V.; Soteropoulos, P. ; Petrelli, N.J.; Dunn, S.P. & Krueger, L.J. (2007). MicroRNA let-7a down-regulates MYC and reverts MYC-induced growth in Burkitt lymphoma cells. *Cancer Research*, Vol.67, No.20, (October 2007), pp. 9762-9770, ISSN 0008-5 472

Sargent, C.A.; Boucher, C.A.; Kirsch, S.; Brown, G.; Weiss, B.; Trundley, A.; Burgoyne, P.; Saut, N.; Durand, C.; Levy, N.; Terriou, P.; Hargreave, T.; Cooke, H.; Mitchell, M.; Rappold, G.A. & Affara, N.A. (1999). The critical region of overlap defining the AZFa male infertility interval of proximal Yq contains three transcribed sequences. *Journal of Medical Genetics*, Vol.36, No.9, (September 1999), pp. 670-677, ISSN 0022-2593

Saut, N.; Terriou, P.; Navarro, A.; Levy, N. & Mitchell, M.J. The human y chromosome genes bpy2, cdy1 and daz are not essential for sustained fertility. (2000). *Molecular Human Reproduction*, Vol.6, No.9, (September 2000), pp. 789–793, ISSN 1360-9947

Saxena, R.; Brown, L.G.; Hawkins, T.; Alagappan, R.K.; Skaletsky, H.; Reeve, M.P.; Reijo, R.; Rozen, S.; Dinulos, M.B.; Disteche, C.M. & Page, D.C. (1996). The DAZ gene cluster on the human Y chromosome arose from an autosomal gene that was transposed, repeatedly amplified and pruned. *Nature Genetics*, Vol.14, No.3, (November 1996), pp. 292-299, ISSN 1061-4036

Saxena, R.; De Vries, J.W.A.; Repping, S.; Alagappan R.K.; Skaletsky, H.; Brown L.G.; Ma, P.; Chen, E.; Hoovers, J.M.N. & Page, D.C. (2000). Four genes in two clusters found in the AZFc region of the human Y chromosome. *Genomics*, Vol.67, No.3, (August 2000), pp. 256–267, ISSN 0888-7543

Schimmer, B.P. & White, P.C. (2010). Minireview: steroidogenic factor 1: its roles in differentiation, development, and disease. *Molecular Endocrinology*, Vol.24, No.7, (July 2010), pp. 1322-1337, ISSN 0952-5041

Schumacher, V.; Gueler, B.; Looijenga, L.H.; Becker, J.U.; Amann, K.; Engers, R.; Dotsch, J.; Stoop, H.; Schulz, W. & Royer-Pokora, B. (2008). Characteristics of testicular dysgenesis syndrome and decreased expression of SRY and SOX9 in Frasier syndrome. *Molecular Reproduction and Development*, Vol.75, No.9, (September 2008), pp. 1484-1494, ISSN 1040-452X

Schwarz, D.S.; Hutvágner, G.; Du, T.; Xu, Z.; Aronin, N. & Zamore, P.D. (2003). Asymmetry in the assembly of the RNAi enzyme complex. *Cell*, Vol.115, No.2, (October 2003), pp. 199-208, ISSN 0092-8674

Simonelig, M. (2011). Developmental functions of piRNAs and transposable elements: A Drosophila point-of-view. *RNA Biology*, Vol.8, No.5, (September/October 2011), pp. 1-6, ISSN 1547-6286

Siomi, M.C.; Sato, K.; Pezic, D. & Aravin, A.A. (2011). PIWI-interacting small RNAs: the vanguard of genome defence. *Nature Reviews. Molecular Cell Biology*, Vol.12, No.4, (April 2011), pp. 246-258, ISSN 1471-0072

Skaletsky, H.; Kuroda-Kawaguchi, T.; Minx, P.J.; Cordum, H.S.; Hillier, L.; Brown, L.G.; Repping, S.; Pyntikova, T.; Ali, J.; Bieri, T.; Chinwalla, A.; Delehaunty, A.; Delehaunty, K.; Du, H.; Fewell, G.; Fulton, L.; Fulton, R.; Graves, T.; Hou, S.F.; Latrielle, P.; Leonard, S.; Mardis, E.; Maupin, R.; McPherson, J.; Miner, T.; Nash, W.; Nguyen, C.; Ozersky, P.; Pepin, K.; Rock, S.; Rohlfing, T.; Scott, K.; Schultz, B.; Strong, C.; Tin-Wollam, A.; Yang S.P.; Waterston, R.H.; Wilson, R.K.; Rozen, S. & Page, D.C. (2003). The male-specific region of the humanYchromosome is a mosaic of discrete sequence classes. *Nature*, Vol.423, No.6942, (June 2003), pp. 825–837, ISSN 0369-6243

Song, J. J.; Smith, S. K.; Hannon, G. J. & Joshua-Tor, L. (2004). Crystal structure of Argonaute and its implications for RISC slicer activity. *Science*, Vol.305, No.5689, (September 2004), pp. 1434-1437, ISSN 0036-8075

Song, R.; Hennig, G.W.; Wu, Q.; Jose, C.; Zheng, H. & Yan, W. (2011). Male germ cells express abundant endogenous siRNAs. *Proceedings of the National Academy of Sciences of the United States of America*, Vol.108, No.32, (August 2011), pp. 13159-13164, ISSN 0027-8424

Stouffs, K.; Lissens, W.; Verheyen, G.; Van Landuyt, L.; Goossens, A.; Tournaye, H.; Van Steirteghem, A. & Liebaers, I. (2004). Expression pattern of the Y-linked PRY gene suggests a function in apoptosis but not in spemiatogenesis. *Molecular Human Reproduction*, Vol.10, No.1, (January 2004), pp. 15–21, ISSN 1360-9947

Sun, C.; Skaletsky, H.; Birren, B.; Devon, K.; Tang, Z.; Silber, S.; Oates, R. & Page, D.C. (1999). An azoospermic man with a de novo point mutation in the Y chromosomal gene USP9Y. *Nature Genetics*, Vol.23, No.4, (December 1999), pp. 429–432, ISSN 1061-4036

Tam, O.H.; Aravin, A.A.; Stein, P.; Girard, A.; Murchison, E.P.; Cheloufi, S.; Hodges, E.; Anger, M.; Sachidanandam, R.; Schultz, R.M. & Hannon, G.J. (2008). Pseudogene-derived small interfering RNAs regulate gene expression in mouse oocytes. *Nature*, Vol.453, No.7194, (May 2008), pp. 534-538, ISSN 0028-0836

Thomson, T. & Lin, H. (2009). The biogenesis and function of PIWI proteins and piRNAs: progress and prospect. *Annual Review of Cell and Developmental Biology*, Vol.25, pp. 355-376, ISSN 1081-0706

Tiepolo, L. & Zuffardi, O. (1976). Localization of factors controlling spermatogenesis in the nonfluorescent portion of the human Y chromosome long arm. *Human Genetics*, Vol.34, No.2, (October 1976), pp. 119-124, ISSN 0340-6717

Tsuda, M.; Sasaoka, Y.; Kiso, M.; Abe, K.; Haraguchi, S.; Kobayashi, S. & Saga, Y. (2003). Conserved role of nanos proteins in germ cell development. *Science*, Vol.301, No.5637, (August 2003), pp. 1239-1241, ISSN 0036-8075

Vagin, V.V.; Sigova, A.; Li, C.; Seitz, H.; Gvozdev, V. & Zamore, P.D. (2006). A distinct small RNA pathway silences selfish genetic elements in the germline. *Science*, Vol.313, No.5785, (July 2006), pp. 320-324, ISSN 0036-8075

Vogt, P.H. (2005). Azoospermia factor (AZF) in Yq11: towards a molecular understanding of its function for human male fertility and spermatogenesis. *Reproductive Biomedicine Online*, Vol.10, No.1, (January 2005), pp. 81-93, ISSN 1472-6483

Vogt, P.H.; Edelmann, A.; Kirsch, S.; Henegariu, O.; Hirschmann, P.; Kiesewetter, F.; Köhn, F.M.; Schill, W.B.; Farah, S.; Ramos, C.; Hartmann, M.; Hartschuh, W.; Meschede, D.; Behre, H.M.; Castel, A.; Nieschlag, E.; Weidner, W.; Gröne, H.J.; Jung, A.; Engel, W. & Haidl, G. (1996). Human Y chromosome azoospermia factors (AZF) mapped to different subregions in Yq11. *Human Molecular Genetics*, Vol.5, No.7, (July 1996), pp. 933-943, ISSN 0964-6906

Voorhoeve, P.M.; le Sage, C.; Schrier, M.; Gillis, A.J.; Stoop, H.; Nagel, R.; Liu, Y.P.; van Duijse, J.; Drost, J.; Griekspoor, A.; Zlotorynski, E.; Yabuta, N.; De Vita, G.; Nojima, H.; Looijenga, L.H. & Agami, R. (2006). A genetic screen implicates miRNA-372 and miRNA-373 as oncogenes in testicular germ cell tumors. *Cell*, Vol.124, No.6, (March 2006), pp. 1169-1181, ISSN 0092-8674

Wang, Y.; Juranek, S.; Li, H.; Sheng, G.; Wardle, G.S.; Tuschl, T. & Patel, D.J. (2009). Nucleation, propagation and cleavage of target RNAs in Ago silencing complexes. *Nature*, Vol.461, No.7265, (October 2009), pp. 754-761, ISSN 0028-0836

Watanabe, T.; Totoki, Y.; Toyoda, A.; Kaneda, M.; Kuramochi-Miyagawa, S.; Obata, Y.; Chiba, H.; Kohara, Y.; Kono, T.; Nakano, T.; Surani, M.A.; Sakaki, Y. & Sasaki, H. (2008). Endogenous siRNAs from naturally formed dsRNAs regulate transcripts in mouse oocytes. *Nature*, Vol.453, No.7194, (May 2008), pp. 539-543, ISSN 0028-0836

Wharton, R.P.; Sonoda, J.; Lee, T.; Patterson, M. & Murata, Y. (1998). The Pumilio RNA-binding domain is also a translational regulator. *Molecular Cell*, Vol.1, No.6, (May 1998), pp. 863-872, ISSN 1097-2765

Xu, M.; Xiao, J.; Chen, J.; Li, J.; Yin, L.; Zhu, H.; Zhou, Z. & Sha, J. (2003). Identification and characterization of a novel human testis-specific Golgi protein, NYD-SP12. *Molecular Human Reproduction*, Vol.9, No.1, (January 2003), pp. 9-17, ISSN 0268-1161

Yan, X.; Wu, Y.; Li, Q.; Cao, L.; Liu, X.; Saiyin, H. & Yu, L. (2005). Cloning and characterization of a novel human Aurora C splicing variant. *Biochemical and Biophysical Research Communications*, Vol.4, No.328, (March 2005), pp. 353-361, ISSN 0006-291X

Yoda, M.; Kawamata, T.; Paroo, Z.; Ye, X.; Iwasaki, S.; Liu, Q. & Tomari, Y. (2010). ATP-dependent human RISC assembly pathways. *Nature Structural & Molecular Biology*, Vol.17, No.1, (January 2010), pp. 17-23, ISSN 1545- 9993

Zeng, Y.; Rosborough, R.C.; Li, Y.; Gupta, A.R. & Bennett, J. (1998). Temporal and spatial regulation of gene expression mediated by the promoter for the human tissue inhibitor of metalloproteinases- 3 (TIMP-3)-encoding gene. *Developmental Dynamics an Official Publication of the American Association of Anatomists*, Vol.211, No.3, (March 1998), pp. 228-237, ISSN 1058-8388

Zhang, H.; Kolb, F.A.; Brondani, V.; Billy, E. & Filipowicz, W. (2008). Mouse ES cells express endogenous shRNAs, siRNAs, and other Microprocessor-independent, Dicer-dependent small RNAs. *Genes & Development*, Vol.21, No.20, (October 2008), pp. 5875-5885, ISSN 0890-9369

Zhang, H.; Liu, Y.; Su, D.; Yang, Y.; Bai, G.; Tao, D.; Ma, Y. & Zhang, S. (2011). A single nucleotide polymorphism in a miR-1302 binding site in CGA increases the risk of idiopathic male infertility. *Fertility and Sterility*, Vol.96, No.1, (July 2011), pp. 34-39, ISSN 0015-0282

Zhang, H.H.; Wang, X.J.; Li, G.X.; Yang, E. & Yang, N.M. (2007). Detection of let-7a microRNA by real-time PCR in gastric carcinoma. *World Journal of Gastroenterology*, Vol.13, No.20, (May 2007), pp. 2883-2888, ISSN 1007-9327

Zuccarello, D.; Ferlin, A.; Cazzadore, C.; Pepe, A.; Garolla, A.; Moretti, A.; Cordeschi, G.; Francavilla, S. & Foresta, C. (2008). Mutations in dynein genes in patients affected by isolated non-syndromic asthenozoospermia. *Human Reproduction*, Vol.23, No.8, (August 2008), pp. 1957-1962, ISSN 0268-1161

3

Apoptosis, ROS and Calcium Signaling in Human Spermatozoa: Relationship to Infertility

Ignacio Bejarano[1], Javier Espino[1], Sergio D. Paredes[2], Águeda Ortiz[1], Graciela Lozano[1], José Antonio Pariente[1], Ana B. Rodríguez[1]

[1]University of Extremadura, Department of Physiology
[2]Complutense University of Madrid, Department of Physiology (School of Medicine)
Spain

1. Introduction

Apoptosis or programmed cell death is a physiological process involving a finely regulated cascade of biochemical events. The main features of this pathway are the activation of specific proteases such as caspases, the release of pro-apoptotic mitochondrial factors, and finally changes in nuclear morphology and DNA fragmentation. Throughout the apoptotic process, one of the responsible signals for initiating the process of programmed cell death is a sustained and manteined increase in intracellular calcium levels ($[Ca^{2+}]_i$). Experimental evidence suggests that an increase in $[Ca^{2+}]_i$ could be associated with the apoptotic signal. In fact, an overload of $[Ca^{2+}]_i$ due to depletion of intracellular stores or calcium influx from the extracellular medium has been suggested to be a signal that precedes the apoptotic process. Additionally, apoptosis also can be stimulated by oxidizing agents such as hydrogen peroxide and menadione, and inhibited by antioxidants.

Mainly two pathways have been described inducing apoptotic cell death, which differ in how the death signal is transduced. The first is the extrinsic pathway, triggered by binding of extracellular death ligands, such as factor activating ExoS ligand (FasL), to its cell-surface death receptor, such as Fas. Membrane death receptors form a complex known as the death-inducing signaling complex, which recruits procaspase-8 becoming activated caspase-8, and subsequently processes other downstream caspases. The second is the intrinsic pathway, which is mediated by mitochondrial alterations. The protein Bid, a natural substrate of caspase-8, is the nexus between the extrinsic and intrinsic pathway. In response to apoptotic stimuli, several proteins are released from the mitochondrial intermembrane space into the cytoplasm. Such mitochondrial alterations stimulate the generation of reactive oxygen species (ROS), which together with activation of DNAses by caspases and mitochondrial signals, undergo DNA damage.

The apoptotic process has been described in many cell types, including both sperm and intratesticular germ cells from different animal species, including humans. The process is similar to that carried out in somatic cells. Apoptosis may play a major role at causing diseases related to male infertility. Actually, it is known that apoptosis is involved in the genesis of several diseases of the male genital tract as defective spermatogenesis, decreased sperm motility, sperm DNA fragmentation, testicular torsion, varicocele and immunological infertility.

On the other hand, melatonin is known to regulate seasonal and circadian rhythms of mammals, but emerging evidence suggests that melatonin possesses protective effects against free radicals and apoptosis. For this reason, this indolamine appears to be a good candidate to improve sperm quality and protect from oxidative stress. Little is known, however, about the mechanisms that carry out such effects. In this regard, melatonin, which has an uncommonly low toxicity profile, may be used as a powerful free-radical scavenger, and anti-apoptotic agent in ejaculated human spermatozoa to supplement sperm preparation media, therefore increasing success of assisted reproductive techniques. Moreover, characterization of the role of melatonin on apoptosis and oxidative damage in ejaculated human spermatozoa may be helpful to preserve high rates of functional spermatozoa after manipulation for their use in any assisted reproduction program.

2. Apoptosis

Apoptosis is a basic biological principle of programmed cell death that occurs in almost every cell type (Kerr et al., 1972). It is a physiological process initiated by environmental or developmental stimuli, which are in charge of removing redundant cells, and maintains tissue homeostasis in a safe and non-immunogenic manner, whereas necrosis leads to plasma membrane rupture, release of pro-inflammatory intracellular molecules and collateral tissue damage (Kerr et al., 1972). The activation of a genetic program that controls designs and initiates a cascade of events leads the cell forward an organized and noiseless destruction. Apoptosis does not take place randomly, but it is a process with energy requirements, like ATP. Additionally it does not initiate inflammatory response, allowing the elimination of undesirable cells without modifying the architecture and physiology of tissues around. A major component of the apoptotic machinery involves a family of aspartic acid-directed cysteine proteases, called caspases (cysteinyl aspartate-specific proteases), which cleave multiple protein substrates *en masse*, leading to the loss of cellular structure and function and, ultimately, resulting in cell death (Stennicke & Salvesen, 1997). Traditionally, two general apoptotic pathways have been described. The first is the extrinsic pathway, triggered by binding of an extracellular death ligand, such as factor activating ExoS ligand (FasL), to its cell-surface death receptor, such as Fas (Ashkenazi & Dixit, 1998). The second is the intrinsic pathway, which is mediated by mitochondrial alterations. In response to apoptotic stimuli, several proteins are released from the mitochondrial intermembrane space into the cytoplasm (Green & Reed, 1998). Some of the well-characterized proteins include cytochrome *c*, which mediates the activation of caspase-9 (Li et al., 1997), thus triggering a cascade of caspase activation, including caspase-3, that promotes cellular self-destruction.

Reproductive phenomena are also under these regulation events. These include from the development of germ cells (spermatogenesis and oogenesis), follicular development and maturation, to the interaction of gametes with subsequent fertilization and embryo implantation. For instance, in human beings, after twenty weeks of development, females show 7 millions of germ cells, which are decreased to 2 millions of ovocytes in birth and finally 300,000 in the beginning of sexual maturity (Baker, 1963). Further than 90 % of ovocytes in ovary degenerate throughout the reproductive period of life (Hsueh et al., 1994). Theoretically, a normal testicle losses 75 % of spermatozoa due to the degeneration of germ cells throughout the spermatogenesis (Rodríguez et al., 1997). In human reproductive system, cell death can be observed in ovocyte degeneration (Morita & Tilly, 1999), in follicular atresia (Hsueh y cols., 1994), in ovulation (Murdoch, 2000), in the luteolisis (Davis & Rueda, 2002) and in germ cells of testis (Sinha-Hikim & Swerdloff, 1999; Koji, 2001). In males who suffer infertility from unknown origin, increased DNA damage and subsequent fragmentation of oligonucleosome in sperm cells have been reported. The presence of apoptotic signals in spermatozoa has been controversial for long time, especially due to the low transcriptional activity in these cells (Grunewald et al., 2005) and the inability to transfer studies on somatic cells to sperm behavior. Early works denied the existence of apoptosis in human ejaculated spermatozoa (Weil et al., 1998) and others have considered that the presence of endogenous debris in ejaculated spermatozoa indicates incomplete maturation during spermatogenesis (Sakkas et al., 1999a). Nonetheless, the presence and activation of apoptotic signals in human spermatozoa in response to various stimuli, is presently widely accepted (Eley et al., 2005; Barroso et al. 2006; Bejarano et al., 2008; Lozano et al., 2009).

During spermatogenesis, germ cells are in continuous proliferation, being apoptosis the process in charge of maintaining the homeostasis in testis. The hormonal control, both central (exerted by adenohypophysis FSH) and local (exerted by testosterone in Leydig cells), acts as the main mechanism for spermatogenesis regulation, as well as regulating pathway-specific apoptotic genes and proteins rather than proliferation (Ruwanpura et al., 2010). Damages in DNA (intrinsic pathway) and the signal when a ligand binds to specific death membrane receptors (extrinsic pathway) are the major mechanisms to trigger apoptosis in germ cells (Ruwanpura et al., 2010).

The ejaculated sperm deposited in the female reproductive tract must be subjected to a rigorous controlled program of senescence, so that they can activate mechanisms for removal from the cervix and uterine cavity (Aitken & Koppers, 2011). Phosphatidylserine externalization is a typical signal of apoptosis in somatic cells. It is thought that externalized phosphatidylserine in the surface of sperm is a consequence of apoptosis triggered by oxidative stress suffered in the female tract (Lozano et al., 2009). This phenomemon seem to activate the phagocytic cells responsible for senescent spermatozoa elimination (Kurosaka et al., 2003). Thus, leukocyte antigens recognize and phagocytize sperm without an inflammatory reaction. However, phosphatidylserine exposure is not only related to apoptosis in sperm but also is associated with a decreased ability to fertilize (Said et al., 2005). In 2003, De Vries and colleagues published a paper linking the externalization of phosphatidylserine in the training process (De Vries et al., 2003); and in 2005, it was reported the externalization of this phospholipid after induction of acrosome reaction by calcium ionophore A23187 (Martin et al., 2005). Other authors found a reduced capacitation and subsequent acrosome reaction in sperm that had externalized phosphatidylserine (Grunewald et al., 2006).

Signs of apoptosis in mature spermatozoa are found primarily associated with the mitochondrial pathway: activation of initiator caspase-9, disruption of mitochondrial membrane potential, activation of the main executioner caspase-3 and subsequent cellular collapse (Paasch et al., 2004; Bejarano et al., 2008). Experimental evidence points to an apparent exclusive cellular location of active caspase-3 to the mid-piece of spermatozoa (Oehninger et al., 2003). This is consistent with the fact that mitochondria are mainly located in that area, and also consistent with mitochondrial association of caspases-3 decribed by Nicholson (Nicholson, 1999).

Moreover, caspases are a family of cysteinyl aspartic-specific proteases which represent the central component of apoptotic machinery. Caspases are involved in both physiological processes, like spermatogenesis, and andrological pathologies, including varicocele, immunological infertility and reduced sperm fertilizing potential (Said et al., 2004). Besides other apoptotic events, caspase activity has been associated with spermatozoa immaturity, low count, reduced motility (Marchetti et al., 2004), decreased fertilization rates (Grunewald et al., 2008) and loss of plasma membrane integrity, as shown by phosphatidylserine externalization (Paasch et al., 2004).

Another point of connection between apoptosis and sperm capacitation is associated with the cytosolic protease calpain and its natural inhibitor calpastatin. Both proteins are located between the plasma membrane of sperm and the acrosome (Yudin et al., 2000). Calpain is a calcium-dependent protease, involved in sperm capacitation, acrosome reaction and cell fusion, which are essential processes for ovum fertilization. Numerous studies have shown the relationship between calpain and sperm motility and acrosome reaction (Ozaki et al., 2001). Caspase-1, a pro-inflammatory and executioner cystein-protease of apoptosis, is activated in human sperm within the activation cascade of caspases in response to apoptosis stimuli (Paasch et al., 2004). Caspase-1 cleaves directly calpastatin resulting in an increased activity of calpain (Wang et al., 1998). These results together, suggest that apoptotic signals are activated by capacitation and acrosome reaction, and consequently calpain performs an enhancing effect on apoptosis. Other studies showed that inhibition of both caspase-1 and calpain partially suppresses the capacitation process without apoptosis signaling, supporting the relevant role of both proteases for capacitation and fertilization capacity in human sperm. In this line, inhibition of $[Ca^{2+}]_i$ sensor, calmodulin, inhibited events related to capacitation, as well as triggering a strong activation of caspases-9 and -3, with a previous disruption of mitochondrial membrane potential. Thus, these findings suggest that apoptosis and capacitation are inverse processes in human sperm. Although apoptotic spermatozoa are not able to be capacitated, capacitated spermatozoa present inhibition apoptosis signaling (Grunewald et al., 2009b). Therefore a strong dependence of $[Ca^{2+}]_i$ is displayed by both processes apoptosis and capacitation. This is consistent with results showing caspase-3 dependence of calcium signaling (Bejarano et al., 2008).

On the other hand, several studies have shown evidence on the effects of some factors on caspases and their relationship to male infertility. For example, treatment with prolactin, besides causing spermatogonial apoptosis, augments significantly caspase activity in testicular tissue when treated simultaneously with cycloheximide, a well-known pesticide (Yazawa et al., 2000). However, the pancaspase inhibitor z-VAD-fmk inhibits prolactin-induced apoptosis in germ cells, which indicates the essential role of caspases in prolactin-induced apoptosis (Yazawa et al., 2001). But in general, exposure to antiandrogens increases both expression and activity of caspases in a dose-dependent manner, as revealed by experiments carried out with flutamine (Omezzine et al., 2003).

Caspase-8 constitutes a key factor in crosstalk between the two propagation pathways of death signals, especially when activated by external cytokines. Upon activation by external death signals, caspase-8 can directly either activate executioner caspases or truncate the Bcl-2 family member, Bid, into tBid, which, once truncated, translocates from cytosol to mitochondria where it promotes permeability and release of cytochrome *c* (Lee et al., 1999).

2.1 Extrinsic apoptosis

The extrinsic pathway constitutes another main manner to trigger apoptosis by external signals through specific death receptors, called FAS receptors. This pathway has been shown being activated in physiologically and experimentally-induced apoptosis in germinal cells (Shaha, 2007). Fas expression in human testis is related to cellular degeneration within the meiosis process, arresting maturation during the spermatogenesis. Evidence indicates that Fas gene expression is likely involved in the elimination of defective germ cells which have alterations in meiotic maturation (Francavilla et al., 2002). A massive apoptotic wave appears in early stages of normal mature spermatozoa in order to keep the ratio between some germinal cell stages and Sertoli cells. In addition, it has been shown that Sertoli cells express FasL, which lead to the destruction of Fas-positive germ cells, thereby limiting the germ cell population to a number that Sertoli cells can support (Celik-Ozenci et al., 2006). Such events are in agreement with the "abortive apoptosis", theory which proposes that apoptotic processes start in germinal cells but are not completed, and therefore Fas-positive sperm can be found in ejaculated semen. In this regard, in normal sperm, less than 10% of spermatozoa are Fas-positive. However, in oligozoospermic samples and in men whose spermatozoa have poor motility and morphology Fas-positive spermatozoa oscillates between 10-50% (Sakkas et al., 1999a). Although, some authors have reported no evidence of Fas expression in ejaculated sperm, neither non-normozoospermic nor normozoospermic patients (Perticarari et al., 2008), a recent study has confirmed the presence of a low Fas expression, asserting its ability as selected apoptotic marker on cell surface of ejaculated spermatozoa (Soleimani et al., 2010). The triggered apoptosis in germinal cells could be attributed to a molecular mechanism which avoids the transmission of any abnormality to offspring (Koji, 2001).

Northern blottings carried out in mouse testis have shown that this organ represent the main constitutive source of FasL in the organism (Suda et al., 1993). Fas system is involved in the control of immune system and is responsible of autoimmune diseases when it is not functional. Bellgrau and collegues reported that allografts of testes were accepted in mice, unless they were derived from gld mice (non-functional FasL), or were grafted into lpr mice (lack of Fas). They also showed that Sertoli cells were identified as the testicular cells that express FasL and this receptor was therefore proposed to be responsible for immune privilege in the testis (Bellgrau et al., 1995). However, other researchers sustain that the expression or overexpression of FasL induce proinflammatory immune response after allo- and xeno-transplantation (Allison et al., 1997). Additionally, Riccioli and collegues showed that through Fas system cells express FasL on germ cells surface, and not on Sertoli cells as showed by other authors, therefore discarding the theories of maintenance of immunoprivilege and regulation of physiological germ cells apoptosis. Given that FasL is present in germ cell membrane, FasL may represent a self-defence mechanism against lymphocytes present in the female genital tract, as corroborated experimentally (Riccioli et al., 2003). Experimental evidence carried out on mice revealed the presence of FasL on epididymal spermatozoa, suggesting that this system plays a self-protective role of male gametes against immune attacks along the male and female genital tract (Riccioli et al., 2003). Supplementary studies have shed new light about the role of Fas depending on its location. Two different forms of Fas were observed in sperm: Membrane cell bound (mFas) and soluble Fas (sFas) besides of matrilisyn (MMP-7), the methalloprotease which cleaves mFas to sFAS. mFas was found on normozoospermic men and it was absent in sperm cells from pathological donors suggesting that normozoospermic germ cells are equipped with Fas system protection against hostility into human genital tract. On the other hand, germ cells from infertile samples showed matrilysin and sFas, and consequently they are prone to suffer apoptotic process in human genital tract (Riccioli et al., 2005).

Apart from the physiological role of Fas, many external toxicants have been described to cause cell damage where Fas takes an essential part triggering apoptosis. For instance, bisphenol A, a potential endocrine disruptor and testicular toxicant, induces germ cell apoptosis through Fas/FasL and the subsequent activation of the mitochondrial apoptotic pathway (Wang et al., 2010). Zearalenone, which is a non-steroidal estrogenic mycotoxin, causes testicular toxicity through the modulation of Fas/FasL (Jee et al., 2010). Lead-induced apoptosis is involved in the increase of Fas expression (Dong et al., 2009). Intra-peritoneal injection of ethanol in mice also causes a rise in Fas/FasL expression. Moreover, this toxicant causes damage to mitochondria, activating the intrinsic pathway of apoptosis (Jana et al., 2010). In this line many toxicants have been shown to promote apoptosis through Fas pathway, including cocaine (Jia et al., 2008), dexamethasone (Khorsandi et al., 2008), mono-(2-ethylhexyl) phthalate (Chandrasekaran et al., 2005), among others. Additionally, the gonads are very sensitive to exogenous stimuli such as X-rays and heat; these factors seem to be related to infertility in both sexes. Several studies of apoptosis on male infertility establish an association between increased cell death and fertility problems. Actually, an increase in apoptotic germ cells in testis of patients suffering severe oligozoospermia and azoospermia has been reported (Lin et al., 1997).

Li and co-workers reported that BID, a pro-apoptotic Bcl-2 family member, is a specific substrate of caspase-8 in the Fas apoptotic signaling pathway. While non-truncated BID is localized in cytosol, truncated BID (tBID) translocates to mitochondrial outer membrane and thus transduces extracellular apoptotic signals to mitochondria. tBID induces release of cytochrome *c*, loss of mitochondrial membrane potential, cell shrinkage, and nuclear condensation in a caspase-dependent fashion. Thus, BID is a mediator of mitochondrial damage induced by caspase-8 (Li et al., 1998).

2.2 Intrinsic apoptosis

Apart from the extrinsic pathway, intrinsic apoptosis is also involved in both physiological and pathological processes. The anti-apoptotic Bcl-2 family members play a critical role in the intracellular balance, likely hormonally-controlled, determining which cell lives or which one dies (Rodríguez, 1997). As mentioned before, apoptosis is present in the normal human testis involving all classes of germ cells. In this regard, Oldereids reported that there was a preferential expression of Bax, Bcl-xL, Bcl-2, Bad and Bak in germ cell compartments suggesting that these apoptotic proteins are involved in differentiation and maturation through the various stages of human spermatogenesis (Oldereid et al., 2001), under intrinsic apoptosis control. During the male embryo development, primordial germ cells migrate from allantoids, where they are generated to develope gonads, known as gonadal ridge. In this process apoptosis occurs in order to eliminate cells with anomalous migration, which therefore would be cause of physiological anomalies. Redundant primordial germ cells are controlled by the balance of Bcl-xL and Bax proteins, which determine the death or survival process. Thus, in case of cell death, apoptosis is carried out affecting permeability of mitochondria and their subsequent collapse (Rucker et al., 2000).

According to recent studies, hormones control apoptosis in different stages of maturity. Follicle-stimulating hormone (FSH) and testosterone play a role predominantly acting as survival factors. Studies to test the action of testosterone showed that the hormone influence, at least in rodents, is exercised through both pathways, intrinsic and extrinsic, in spermatocytes and spermatids. Studies in gonadotrophin-deficient men suggest that the hormonal control on apoptosis of spermatogonia is exercised through the intrinsic pathway (Rawanpura et al., 2008).

Experimental evidence have shown that mitochondrial membrane potential ($\Delta\Psi_m$) could be used as a trustable tool to determine the sperm quality, given that the $\Delta\Psi_m$ and sperm functions are correlatively related. For instance, studying JC-1 staining, a probe sensitive to $\Delta\Psi_m$, it was observed a relationship with events such as compromise plasma membrane permeability (Troiano et al., 1998), DNA damage (Donelli et al., 2000), motility and *in vitro* fertilization rates (Marchetti et al., 2004) or even presence of phosphatidylserine (Barroso et al., 2006). In all cases, a correlation between sperm quality and $\Delta\Psi_m$ could be found. This suggests that $\Delta\Psi_m$ may be used as a diagnosis of dysfunctional spermatozoa suffering from apoptotic process, low motility, DNA damage or other types of undesirable occurrences. In this way, the rates of pregnancy among barren couples could be easily improved when abnormal sperm is discarded. Interestingly, those spermatozoa showing high $\Delta\Psi_m$ have shown intact functionality of acrosome as well as high motility values and fertilizing capacity (Gallon et al., 2006). Likewise, low $\Delta\Psi_m$ is related to low rates of pregnancy (Marchetti et al., 2004). Together, these results suggest the importance of mitochondrial functionality for fertilizing capacity of human spermatozoa.

The use of chemotherapeutic agents leads to undesirable consequences on sperm functionality, damaging DNA and/or triggering apoptosis affecting mitochondria. For instance, betulinic acid (BA) has been shown to disrupt $\Delta\Psi_m$, activating subsequently caspase-9 and -3. These events of intrinsic programmed cell death have been related to a significant decrease of spermatozoa motility (Dathe et al., 2005), given that they induce apoptosis through mitochondria, the cell energy source necessary for sperm motility or velocity. Pre-incubation of spermatozoa with z-VAD-fmk inhibited only in a partial way the loss of $\Delta\Psi_m$ under BA treatment, which is indicative that BA-induced mitochondrial disruption is independent of caspase activation (Espinoza et al., 2009). Together these results suggest that inducers of the mitochondrial pathway of apoptosis applied in the treatment of cancer affect directly to men fertility. High $\Delta\Psi_m$ has been positively correlated to sperm concentration and negatively to levels of ROS. This is consistent with low rates of *in vitro* fertilization (IVF) (Wang et al., 2003). Controversially, the anticancer agent cisplatin is able to induce caspase-8 and apaf-1, activating caspase-3 and -2 even with caspase-9 blocked. This implies that cisplatin leads to apoptosis independently of mitochondria (Muller et al., 2003).

Hyperthermia is the base for cryptorchidism. Exposure of germ cells at mild heat results in induction of apoptosis. Besides FasL, Bax translocation to mitochondria, caspases-3, -6, -9, -7 activation and cytochrome *c* release have been detected under hyperthermia treatment. However, heat-induced apoptosis in FasL-defective cells was not blocked. These results demonstrate that heat-induced apoptosis occurs via mitochondria (Said et al., 2004).

Alkylating drugs against cancer such as cyclophosphamide (CP) have unwanted results in patients' germ cells, both in seminogram parameters and in causing DNA damage as a consequence. However, it has been described that these unwanted effects could be mitigated by the presence of antioxidants, e.g. astaxanthin, a red carotenoid pigment (Tripathi & Jena, 2008). Genotoxicity of different anti-neoplastic agents, including methotrexate or tamoxifen, induces hazards in both somatic and germ cells, as a consequence of cancer treatment side effects. However, pretreatment with the antioxidant taurine alleviates chromosomal aberrations, and restores GSH levels, increasing the count and motility of spermatozoa and decreasing abnormalities (Allam et al., 2011).

3. ROS generation and oxidative stress

Aerobic organisms are continuously exposed to ROS. The main source of ROS is the electron transport chain within the inner mitochondrial membrane. Apoptosis can also be stimulated by ROS in several cell types (Brookes et al., 2004; Bejarano et al., 2008; Lozano et al., 2009). Aerobic cells are equipped with the necessary antioxidant machinery to scavenge ROS and keep free radicals at homeostatic levels avoiding pathological effects due to oxidative stress. It has been long recognised that ROS may form an important link similar to the second messenger intracellular communication, or even taking part in physiological processes such as "the respiratory burst" in macrophages or neutrophils. Nevertheless, physiological levels of ROS are also required for normal sperm functions including hyperactivation, capacitation and acrosome reaction (Sikka et al., 1995). The amount of scavenging enzymes of spermatozoa is limited as well as their cytoplasm, in which these enzymes are found, making them highly susceptible to ROS damage. Actually, it has been suggested that the damage to the acrosome membrane may not be related to sperm motility (Griveau et al., 1995). Lipid peroxidation caused by oxidative stress conditions during the transport of sperm through the epididymis not only affects the plasma membrane of these cells in close contact with each other during transport, but can also inhibit the acrosome reaction by damaged acrosome membrane with no apparent effect on motility (Oehninger et al., 1995).

When global levels of ROS, overcome the available total antioxidant capacity (TAC) oxidative stress occurs, which results in oxygen and oxygen-derived oxidants. Given that ROS are able to readily permeate membranes, within cells, DNA, proteins and lipids suffer from oxidative damage, leading cells into apoptosis. ROS present in seminal plasma can be originated from several sources, both endogenous and exogenous. The ejaculated semen is made up of different types of cells, including mature and immature spermatozoa, leukocytes and epithelial cells, being leukocytes and immature spermatozoa the major source of ROS (Kothary et al., 2010). Leukocytes, more specifically neutrophils and monocytes, are present in semen, avoiding the presence of pathogens. In line with this, during infection leukocytes produce high amount of ROS (Tremellen et al., 2008). A detrimental activity of superoxide dismutase (SOD) and increased levels of pro-inflammatory interlekin-8 can also be detected (Blake et al., 1987). Semen contains antioxidants that protect germ cells from environmental oxidative hazard. However, antioxidants are removed by assisted reproductive techniques, leaving sperm cells especially vulnerable to oxidative damage. Semen manipulation, like cryopreservation or repeated cycles of centrifugation, has unwanted effects on germ cells. After cryopreservation and thawing or centrifugation, an excess of ROS is detected evoking oxidative stress in germ cells due to lowered intracellular antioxidant levels. As expected, these effects cause irreversible damage to DNA (Agarwal et al., 1994; Kumar et al., 2011). In this regard, the application of antioxidants appears as a tool to protect germ cells from manipulation-induced oxidative damage. Growing studies support the beneficial effect of antioxidants. For example, the exposure of post-thawed spermatozoa showing increased levels of ROS to ascorbate or catalase reduced ROS production and subsequent apoptotic events, such as loss of $\Delta\Psi_m$, PI and Annexin V staining. Moreover, a considerable improvement in sperm parameters was also appreciated (Li et al., 2010). Similar results were obtained with other antioxidants like cystein, taurine, chloropromazine, and treating samples with the antioxidant enzymes SOD and glutathione peroxidease (Paudel et al., 2010; Thuwanut et al., 2010). The use of melatonin, which has an uncommomly low toxicity profile, has been also proposed as a powerful antioxidant and anti-apoptotic agent in ejaculated human spermatozoa (Espino et al., 2010).

Apart from leukocytes, immature spermatozoa are an additional source of ROS. Erroneous spermatogenesis does not allow the regular extrusion of cytoplasm from potential germ cells for maturation process. Thus, these sperm cells contain an excess of cytoplasm and are considered immature (teratozoospermic). The excess activates the NADPH system (Kothary et al., 2010), mainly in mitochondria, resulting in an increase of free radicals. Moreover, mitochondria have been reported to be the main source of ROS in infertile men (Plante et al., 1994). It has been reported a positive tendency between teratozoospermia and ROS production at pathological levels, as well as apoptosis and DNA damage in spermatozoa (Sikka et al., 1995). In this regard, it has been reported that H_2O_2-evoked oxidative stress induces mitochondrial ROS generation affecting mitochondria functionality and activating caspase-9 in human spermatozoa (Espino et al., 2010). Caspase-9 is an initiator protease considered to be involved in the initial steps of mitochondrial apoptosis. The pre-incubation of spermatozoa with the specific inhibitor of caspase-9, z-LEHD-fmk, was able to block H_2O_2-evoked caspase-3 activation (Bejarano et al., 2008). Taken together, these findings strongly suggest that oxidative stress leads cells into apoptosis through the mitochondrial pathway. Evidence suggests that ROS-mediated damage to sperm significantly contributes to 30–80% of pathological cases (Shekarriz et al., 1995; Agarwal et al., 2006).

Natural antioxidants including melatonin are currently acquiring great importance for cell protection against oxidative hazards. Melatonin reduces calcium-evoked ROS generation, as well as caspase-9, what means that melatonin protects mitochondria, blocking the apoptotic process (Espino et al., 2010). Similarly, myo-inositol, the most important form in nature of inositol, a component of vitamin B, has been suggested to have an antioxidant seminal action. Particularly, myo-inositol has shown capacity to ameliorate mitochondrial function of oligo-astheno-theratozoospemic patients. This indicates that the molecule may be used for the treatment against male infertility (Condorelli et al., 2011). ROS cause infertility by two main mechanisms. First, ROS damage the sperm membrane which in turn reduces the sperm motility and ability to fuse with the oocyte. Second, ROS directly damage sperm DNA, compromising the paternal genomic contribution to the embryo (Tremellen et al., 2008). A positive correlation between urinary TAC and different seminogram parameters including concentration, motility, morphology and vitality, as well as a negative correlation with round cells has been shown (Ortiz et al., 2011). Hence, antioxidant endogenous levels strengthen or ameliorate sperm parameters and diminish the number of round cells, which are responsible, at least in part, for the oxidant environment in seminal fluid due to ROS generation. Also endogenous melatonin exerts a role in semen quality improvement. Additionally, evidence supports that melatonin supplementation has a potential use to obtain more successful assisted reproductive technique outcomes (Ortiz et al., 2011.).

Although, orally-administered antioxidants improve sperm DNA damage and protamine packaging, and reduce seminal ROS generation and apoptosis, other researchers have not observed significant changes in routine sperm parameters (concentration, motility and morphology) (Tunc et al., 2009).

Infection in the genital tract usually results in leukocyte increase and a subsequent elevation of seminal ROS levels. If the number of leukocytes exceeds normality ($1x10^6$ leukocytes/mL) spermatozoa integrity may be compromised. However, at lower concentrations, leukocytes occasionally may cause oxidative stress (Kothary et al., 2010). Varicocele has adverse effects on spermatogenesis and sperm quality, but the responsible mechanisms remain little known. High levels of ROS, as well as low TAC levels, have been detected in semen from infertile varicocele patients and a decrease in ROS levels has been shown after varicocelectomia (Agarwal et al., 2004). ROS presence plays an important role causing asthenozoospermia. Given that some reactive species can induce peroxidation on membrane lipids, they affect negatively to axonemal structures compromising severely the sperm motility and the asthenozoospermia occurs. Interestingly, most men suffering from spinal cord injury suffer also from infertility (Lisenmeyer & Perkash, 1991). Both a polluted environment or lifestyle habits are quite often the causal origin of presence of ROS in sperm. Not only industrial air pollutants, such as those included in beauty products, heavy metals, pesticides, sulfur dioxide or food preservatives (Kothary et al., 2010), but also compounds of cigarette smoke have been reported to be harmful for health. More specifically, cigarette smoke produces ROS and decreases TAC and semen parameters (Saleh et al., 2002). In line with this, it is noteworthy that smokers' semen contains more ROS than non-smokers' semen. Thereby, fertility might be compromised by smoking-derived effects. Moreover, ethanol consumption may also have adverse effects for male fertility. Ethanol metabolism induces ROS generation damaging cellular molecules, including DNA, proteins and lipids (Vine, 1996). Given that antioxidant defenses play an essential role in apoptosis regulation, even when the death signal is not oxidative stress, supplementation which antioxidants, such as *N*-acetyl-L-cystein, both *in vitro* and *in vivo,* may diminish DNA-damage of spermatozoa, suggesting a new therapeutic strategy for oligospermic patients (Erkkilä et al., 1998).

Generally there are some anomalies in DNA of ejaculated spermatozoa. However the consequences that fertilization with anomalous DNA could cause in the development of the embryo are still not very well known. Intracytoplasmic sperm injection appears to be a growing risk to transfer damaged DNA (Sakkas et al., 1999b). In this regard, further studies are necessary to identify and select sperm with undamaged DNA or remove sperm with damaged DNA from samples, in order to improve the efficiency of pregnancy with *in vitro* fertilization methods. Although there is a negative correlation between quality of sperm parameters and DNA damage, breaks in DNA have been also found in normal parameters of seminograms. Two hypotheses define the most likely explanation for DNA damage in spermatozoa, a failed packaging of chromatin and induction of apoptosis (for review see Sakkas et al., 1999b). The main origin of DNA damage can be found in the anomalous packaging of chromatin. Protamines are proteins in charge of the DNA packaging, replacing histones in the haploid spermatogenesis. Furthermore they are believed to be essential for sperm condensation and DNA stabilization. Protamines are usually deficiently deposited in DNA during the packaging of spermatogenesis, remaining some vulnerable nicks along the chromatin. These nicks indicate incomplete maturation during spermatogenesis. Thus, DNA is susceptible to suffer damage by ROS or nucleases, which is in agreement with findings that showed a correlation between DNA damage and a deficient packaging due to underprotamination (Sailer et al., 1995). The tumor suppressor protein p53 is expressed when DNA is damaged. p53 promotes the transcription of some genes involved in apoptosis, including those that code for death receptors and pro-apoptotic Bcl-2 (Müller et al., 1998). Although p53 is not found in normal spermatogenesis, it has been found in spermatogonia under X-ray treatment, since germ cells from p53 knockout mice are not prone to trigger apoptosis of germ cells when DNA is irradiated. Evidence suggests that p53 is particularly involved at removing lethally damaged spermatogonia (Beumer et al., 1998).

4. Role of Ca^{2+} in sperm physiology

Cytosolic Ca^{2+} signals can control several physiological processes in excitable and non-excitable cells. These signals are produced by opening channels permeable to Ca^{2+} either in the plasma membrane or in the membrane of intracellular organelles containing high Ca^{2+} concentrations. Ca^{2+}-permeable channels can catalyze the flow of millions of Ca^{2+} ions through non-conducting lipid bilayers and, therefore, a small number of channels can cause significant changes in a tiny cell, such as the sperm, within milliseconds. In fact, changes in the intracellular concentration of Ca^{2+} due to the activation of such channels have been associated with different aspects of mammalian sperm function, including sperm motility, capacitation and the acrosome reaction.

4.1 Sperm capacitation

Capacitation of sperm is a prerequisite for successful fertilization. It comprises a series of complex and finely tuned changes that normally occur during transit in the female genital tract so that spermatozoa can reach and fuse with the oocyte. Changes associated with this process comprise, among others, an increase in respiration and subsequent changes in the sperm motility pattern, removal of cholesterol from the plasma membrane, increases in $[Ca^{2+}]_i$ in the sperm head and flagellum, and activation of second-messenger cascades (de Lamirande et al., 1997; Purohit et al., 1999; Darszon et al., 2001). Importantly, the most significant change in sperm after capacitation is its ability to undergo the acrosome reaction (AR).

Ion environment and ion fluxes through the sperm plasma membrane are highly important in capacitation. Particularly, intracellular Ca^{2+} has been shown to be increased during capacitation. This may be the result of (i) reduced Ca^{2+} efflux due to inhibition of the Ca^{2+} ATPase pump, (ii) increased leakage of Ca^{2+} across the membrane owing to instability caused by removal of cholesterol, and/or (iii) increased Ca^{2+} influx due to the activation of unidentified channels (Jagannathan et al., 2002). Nevertheless, regulation of voltage-gated Ca^{2+} (Ca_V) channels during sperm capacitation may also occur, although such a regulation has not been directly established (Espinosa et al., 2000; Darszon et al., 2001).

4.2 The acrosome reaction

The sperm acrosome reaction (AR) is a fundamental reproductive strategy which is a pre-requisite for successful fertilization. It involves exocytosis of the acrosomal vehicles contained in the head of the sperm. During this process, lytic enzymes and materials required for sperm binding are released into the extracellular space leading to the fusion of the gametes. Ca^{2+} influx is an absolute requirement for the physiological AR in sperm from all species examined to date (Vansudevan et al., 2010). In mammals, fertilization begins with the direct interaction of sperm and egg, a process mediated primarily by gamete surface proteins. Once the sperm has penetrated the cumulus cells and reaches the zona pellucida (ZP), it undergoes exocytosis, thus releasing the acrosomal content.

Sperm-ZP adhesion activity has been confirmed by gene knockout of one sperm surface enzyme that putatively binds ZP3 (a glycoprotein constituent of the ZP), i.e. beta-1,4-galactosyltransferase I (GalT I) (Rodeheffer & Shur, 2004). ZP3-induced exocytosis of the acrosomal contents proceeds through two sperm signaling pathways. In the first, ZP3 binding to GalT I and other potential receptors results in activation of a heterotrimeric guanosine-5'-trisphosphate (GTP)-binding protein and phospholipase C (PLC), thus elevating the concentration of intracellular Ca^{2+}. In the second pathway, ZP3 binding to the same receptor(s) stimulates a transient influx of Ca^{2+} through T-type Ca_V channels. The intracellular Ca^{2+} signal elicited by ZP3 is prolonged and the sperm AR occurs some minutes after the beginning of this signal. This initial intracellular Ca^{2+} entry, in a later phase of the signaling, induces a second, sustained Ca^{2+} influx through transient receptor potential cation (TRPC) family Ca^{2+} channels, thereby resulting in a sustained increase in intracellular Ca^{2+} that triggers exocytosis (Darszon et al., 2001; Primakoff and Myles, 2002).

4.3 Sperm motility

Although the external triggering mechanisms that initiate sperm motility are largely unknown, evidence supports a modification of the Ca^{2+} balance by several separate mechanisms. Elevation of intracellular Ca^{2+} can occur by entry of Ca^{2+} ions into cells through the plasma membrane or release of Ca^{2+} from internal stores. At this respect, it has been demonstrated that Ca_V channels are expressed in the sperm tail and may participate in the regulation of flagellar motility. Thus, these channels are present in the sperm flagella and compounds known to inhibit them induce a small decrease in human sperm motility, thereby indicating they might participate in regulating this function (Trevino et al., 2004). Additionally, confocal immunofluorescence experiments have shown that, at least, four distinct types of capacitative Ca^{2+} channels (TRPC1, 3, 4 and 6) are expressed and differentially localized in the human sperm. By analyzing the effects of distinct TRPC channel antagonists using a computer-assisted assay, evidence suggests that these proteins may play an important role in controlling human sperm flagellar movement (Castellano et al., 2003).

Likewise, at some time before fertilization, mammalian sperm undergoes a change in movement pattern, named hyperactivation, which is critical to the success of fertilization because it enhances the ability of sperm to penetrate the egg's ZP (Ho & Suarez, 2001a,b). Experimental evidence suggests that hyperactivated motility may be regulated by an inositol 1,4,5-trisphosphate receptor (IP_3R)-gated intracellular Ca^{2+} store in the neck region of mammalian sperm (Ho and Suarez, 2001b). Moreover, the unique sperm-specific cation channel, CatSper, is expressed by meiotic and post-meiotic spermatogenic cells but not by other cells, and is present in the sperm flagellum, thus suggesting a role in the regulation of sperm motility. In line with this, targeted disruption of mouse CatSper gene results in male sterility, mainly due to the inability of sperm to maintain normal patterns of motility and to penetrate the egg's ZP (Ren et al., 2001). Actually, disruption of CatSper2 seems to underlie highly reduced sperm motility in man, as ascertained in asthenoteratozoospermic patients (Avidan et al., 2003), which constitutes the first description of an autosomal gene associated with non-syndromic male infertility in humans.

4.4 Sperm apoptosis and its interaction with Ca^{2+} signaling

Apoptosis signaling in human sperm has been a controversially debated issue for a long time, because sperm are mainly transcriptionally inactive cells (Grunewald et al., 2005) and the knowledge gained from studies of somatic cells cannot be transferred without experimental evidence. Although initial studies denied the presence of apoptosis in ejaculated human sperm at all (Weil et al., 1998), and further studies suggested an abortive apoptosis as a remnant of incomplete spermatogenesis (Sakkas et al., 1999a), recent publications have suggested that human spermatozoa have the ability to undergo apoptosis or apoptosis-like conditions in response to a variety of stimuli (Grunewald et al., 2001; Paasch et al., 2003, Taylor et al., 2004; Eley et al., 2005; Barroso et al., 2006; Martin et al., 2007; Bejarano et al., 2008; Espino et al., 2011). Apoptosis signaling in human sperm is preferentially based on the mitochondria-associated pathway, the main features being activation of the initiator caspase, caspase-9, disruption of the transmembrane mitochondrial potential, activation of the major effector caspase, caspase-3, and consecutive cellular degradation (Paasch et al., 2004; Bejarano et al., 2008).

Although calcium is a key regulator of cell survival, the sustained and prolonged elevation of $[Ca^{2+}]_i$ plays a role in cell death (Demaurex & Distelhorst, 2003). The pro-apoptotic effects of calcium are mediated by a diverse range of calcium-sensitive factors that are compartmentalized in various intracellular organelles, including endoplasmic reticulum and mitochondria (Hajnoczky et al., 2003). Excessive calcium load to the mitochondria may induce apoptosis by stimulating the release of apoptosis-promoting factors from the mitochondrial intermembrane space to the cytosol and by impairing mitochondrial function (Wang, 2001). In this context, it has been demonstrated that H_2O_2 and progesterone are able to induce a mitochondria-dependent apoptosis program in ejaculated human spermatozoa, which requires increases in intracellular Ca^{2+} concentration and Ca^{2+} entry into mitochondria. In fact, both the $[Ca^{2+}]_i$ chelator, dimethyl BAPTA, and the specific blocker of calcium uptake into mitochondria, Ru360, were able to inhibit sperm apoptosis induced by both H_2O_2 and progesterone, as ascertained by experiments on caspase-3 activity and phosphatidylserine externalization (Bejarano et al., 2008).

Bcl-2 family members are reported to have an important role during testicular development (Yan et al., 2000). The members of the Bcl-2 family, composed of both death agonists and antagonists, differ in their structural features, and their expression pattern depends on the tissue of expression (Reed, 1997). A homologue of Bcl-2, Bcl-x, exists in two isoforms generated by alternative splicing. The large form, Bcl-xL, protects cells against death, whereas the short form, Bcl-xS, promotes cell death by inhibiting Bcl-2 or Bcl-xL function. In this context, it has been suggested that ionic alterations in the cell could signal a change in alternative splicing of Bcl-x leading to up-regulation of a given isoform. Thus, by using a well-known testicular toxin, 2,5-hexanedione (2,5-HD) (Akingbemi & Hardy, 2001), it has been proven that exposure to 2,5-HD causes an intracellular Ca^{2+} increase in spermatogenic cells, thus producing a shift toward a relative increase of Bcl-xS encoding isoform over the Bcl-xL isoform. Since the level of Bcl-2 and Bax remained unchanged after 2,5-HD exposure, the effect of 2,5-HD seems to be mediated by reversal of the ratio between apoptosis-inducing and -preventing isoforms of Bcl-x, leading to mitochondrial changes resulting in apoptotic death (Mishra et al., 2006). On the other hand, the Fas/FasL system has been strongly implicated in spermatogenic cell death during development (Hikim et al., 2003), adulthood (Koji et al., 2001), and after toxin exposure (Richburg et al., 2000). Actually, it has been showed that physiological apoptosis of spermatocytes during the first wave of spermatogenesis is associated with Fas up-regulation. Interestingly, up-regulation of Fas and subsequent activation of caspases were correlated with an increase in intracellular Ca^{2+} concentration (Lizama et al., 2007), thereby reaffirming the notion that apoptosis is linked to alterations in Ca^{2+} homeostasis.

5. Melatonin, a new advantage in fertility

Melatonin (N-acetyl-5-methoxytryptamine), the main secretory product of the pineal gland, acts as an antioxidant and a "scavenger" of free radicals, possesses anti-proliferative, oncostatic and anti-aging activity, and immunomodulatory and neuroprotective effects. Other organs and tissues can also produce melatonin, where it can be found in high concentrations. At the level of subcellular organelles, melatonin levels may vary. Some authors have reported levels of melatonin in the nucleus and mitochondria higher than those found in plasma (León et al., 2004). The number of articles reporting the role of melatonin in apoptosis has dramatically increased in the last decade. The fields of interest are grouped into two categories: i) the role of melatonin in preventing apoptosis in normal cells and ii) the role of melatonin increasing apoptosis in cancer cells. This pro-apoptotic role in tumor cells contrasts sharply with the anti-apoptotic actions in normal cells, implying a potential use of melatonin in the death of tumor cells, thus preserving cellular function of normal cells (Sainz et al., 2003; Bejarano et al., 2011).

It is known that human seminal plasma contains melatonin, which can exert important effects on sperm motility and sperm function, favoring and increasing fertility rates. In fact, it has been shown that melatonin is able to increase sperm hyperactivation acting through its receptor MT1 (Fujinoki, 2008). Melatonin also exerts beneficial effects in oocyte physiology and improves the fertilization rate. This means that melatonin has potential beneficial effects on fertility, for both male and female. It is worth noting that the supplementation with melatonin may be especially important in couples where one or both may be infertile. However, few clinical trials have been carried out in infertile patients treated with melatonin at medium/long-term periods.

Melatonin is known to regulate seasonal and circadian rhythms in mammals (Reiter et al., 2009), but emerging evidence also suggests that melatonin possesses protective effects against free radicals and apoptosis. This also seems to be the case for its metabolites (Hardeland et al., 2009). Results clearly indicate that the urinary metabolite of melatonin, 6-sulfatoxymelatonin is highly positively correlated with sperm quality, determined as sperm concentration, morphology, and sperm motility (Ortiz et al., 2010), while negatively correlated with round cells present in the ejaculate. The action of the indoleamine after the induction of apoptosis in human sperm using H_2O_2 and progesterone has been analyzed, reaching the conclusion that the use of melatonin inhibits the production of ROS and reverses various characteristics of apoptosis such as caspase activation or phosphatidylserine externalization (Espino et al., 2010). Antioxidant and detoxifying properties of melatonin have stimulated studies showing a reduction in molecular damage. In relation to this, the protective role of melatonin against oxidative damage and apoptosis in ejaculated human spermatozoa, as a result of its free radical scavenger action, has been recently reported (Espino et al., 2010).

This anti-apoptotic effect of melatonin is directly related to its known antioxidant capacity. Anti-apoptotic effects of melatonin are dose dependent, and depend on the activation of membrane receptor MT1. Moreover, the protective actions of melatonin on apoptosis induced by oxidative stress with H_2O_2 or $[Ca^{2+}]_i$ overload evoked by progesterone appears to be dependent on protein kinases ERK, which are related to cell survival (Espino et al., 2011). In addition, a recent study showed that melatonin and TAC nocturnal levels are positively correlated with several seminal parameters, including sperm concentration, motility and morphology, and negatively correlated with number of round cells present in seminal samples (Ortiz el al., 2011). An improvement in the *in vitro* sperm motility when spermatozoa are incubated for short periods of time with pharmacological concentrations of melatonin has been shown (Ortiz et al., 2011). The influence that the neurotransmitter serotonin (melatonin precursor) may have on seminal parameters, has been also determined through its urinary metabolite, 5-hydroxyindoleacetic acid in men with working rotating shifts, confirming that a mismatch in levels of serotonin may negatively affect the reproductive capacity of patients (Ortiz et al., 2010). Taken together, these results may contribute to a better understanding of the physiology and genesis of the pathological processes that affect human sperm, for example in asthenozoospermia or oligozoospermia, facilitating the establishment of guidelines and/or therapies for conditions related to human sperm, and by extension for the male reproductive physiology.

6. Conclusion

Although the relevance of understanding the mechanisms that control germ cell death is evident, male infertility treatment requires further investigation. Apoptosis is a well-characterized mechanism for removing redundant cells. The characterization of several apoptotic events as critical signals in damaged cells symbolizes a key advance in the knowledge of molecular aspects of male infertility. Detection of ROS overproduction is a faithful indicator of impaired spermatozoa. Seminal parameters including motility, morphology, velocity, concentration, and presence of rounds cells are closely related to oxidative status of germ cells. In fact, ROS damage DNA directly and indirectly triggering apoptosis, which subsequently leads to degradation of cellular substrates. Since imbalanced presence of ROS is common in many infertility-related disorders, antioxidant treatments are becoming relevant in protecting male germ cells from intracellular damage, increasing fertilization success rates. Additionally, sperm showing normal parameters experience an increase in ROS levels after manipulation, which decreases its quality. As discussed herein, antioxidants protect from damage caused when sperm is manipulated. On the other hand, Fas is present in plasma membrane of undesirable cells. Its expression may therefore help to localize immature spermatocytes or damaged germ cells. However, current fertilization techniques do not test this condition in spermatozoa. Cytometry sorting could help to rule out spermatozoa that show a positive profile for both Fas and ROS generation. In vitro fertilization techniques should take into account these hazardous signals to discard damaged spermatozoa that in normal conditions would have been eliminated. Knowledge on the effect of fertilization carried out with undesirable spermatozoa in embryo development still remains vague and controversial. Studies focused not only on seminogram parameters but also on the relationship between physiological status or apoptotic events and sperm quality are needed. Melatonin is an innocuous and antioxidant molecule that improves semen quality. Its supplementation may be potentially used to obtain successful results when assisted reproductive techniques are used. Further studies are required to clarify molecular mechanisms responsible for the beneficial effects of melatonin and to test whether the supplementation with the indoleamine is feasible to increase success rates in assisted reproductive technology.

7. Acknowledgement

This study was supported by Angelini Farmaceutica S.A. and Ministerio de Ciencia e Innovación-Fondo Europeo de Desarrollo Regional (BFU2010-15049). I. Bejarano is a beneficiary of a grant from Angelini Farmaceutica SA. S.D. Paredes was a beneficiary of a grant from Consejería de Economía, Comercio e Innovación-Fondo Social Europeo (Junta de Extremadura REI09009). J. Espino is a beneficiary of a grant from Ministerio de Ciencia e Innovación (AP2009-0753). The authors would like to express their thanks to Servicio de Técnicas Aplicadas a las Biociencias (STAB) of University of Extremadura for their excellent technical assistance.

8. References

Agarwal, A.; Ikemoto, I. & Loughlin, K.R. (1994) Relationship of sperm parameters with levels of reactive oxygen species in semen specimens. *The Journal of urology*. Vol.152, No.1, pp.107-110, ISSN 0022-5347.

Agarwal, A.; Nallella, K.P.; Allamaneni, SS. & Said, T.M. (2004). Role of antioxidants in treatment of male infertility: an overview of the literature. *Reproductive Biomedicine*. Vol.8, No.6, pp.616-627, ISSN 1472-6483.

Agarwal, A.; Prabakaran, S. & Allamaneni, S. (2006). What an andrologist/urologist should know about free radicals and why. *Urology*. Vol.67, No.1, pp.2–8, ISSN 0090-4295.

Aitken, R.J. & Curry, B.J. (2011). Redox regulation of human sperm function: from the physiological control of sperm capacitation to the etiology of infertility and DNA damage in the germ line. *Antioxidants & redox signaling*. Vol.14, No.3, pp.367-381, ISSN 1523-0864.

Aitken, R.J. & Koppers, A. (2011). Apoptosis and DNA damage in human spermatozoa. *Asian journal of andrology*. Vol.13, No.1, pp.36-42, ISSN 1008-682X.

Akingbemi, B.T. & Hardy, M.P. (2001). Oestrogenic and antiandrogenic chemicals in the environment: effects on male reproductive health. *Annals of medicine* Vol.33, No.6, pp.391-403, ISSN 0785-3890.

Alam, S.S.; Hafiz, N.A. & Abd El-Rahim, A.H. (2011) Protective role of taurine against genotoxic damage in mice treated with methotrexate and tamoxfine. *Environmental toxicology and pharmacology*. Vol.31, No.1, pp.143-152, ISSN 1382-6689.

Allison, J.; Georgiou, H.M.; Strasser, A. &Vaux, D.L. (1997). Transgenic expression of CD95 ligand on islet beta cells induces a granulocytic infiltration but does not confer immune privilege upon islet allografts. *Proceedings National Academy of Sciences of United States of America*. Vol.94, No.8, pp.3943-3947, ISSN 0027-8424.

Avidan, N.; Tamary, H.; Dgany, O.; Cattan, D.; Pariente, A.; Thulliez, M.; Borot, N.; Moati, L.; Barthelme, A.; Shalmon, L.; Krasnov, T.; Ben-Asher, E.; Olender, T.; Khen, M.; Yaniv, I.; Zaizov, R.; Shalev, H.; Delaunay, J.; Fellous, M.; Lancet, D. & Beckmann, J.S. (2003). CATSPER2, a human autosomal nonsyndromic male infertility gene. *European Journal Human Genetics*. Vol.11, No.7, pp. 497-502, ISSN 1018-4813.

Baker, T.G. (1963). A quantitative and cytological study of germ cells in human ovaries. *Proceedings of the royal society of london. Series b, biological sciences*. Vol.158, pp.417-433, ISSN 0080-4649.

Barroso, G.; Taylor, S.; Morshedi, M.; Manzur, F.; Gavino, F. & Oehninger, S. (2006). Mitochondrial membrane potential integrity and plasma membrane translocation of phosphatidylserine as early apoptotic markers: a comparison of two different sperm subpopulations. *Fertility and Sterility*. Vol.85, No.1, pp.149-154, ISSN 0015-0282.

Barroso, G.; Taylor, S.; Morshedi, M.; Manzur, F.; Gaviño, F. & Oehninger, S. (2006). Mitochondrial membrane potential integrity and plasma membrane translocation of phosphatidylserine as early apoptotic markers: a comparison of two different sperm subpopulations. *Fertility and sterility*. Vol.85, No.1, pp.149-154, ISSN 0015-0282.

Bejarano, I.; Espino, J.; Marchena, A.M.; Barriga, C.; Paredes, S.D.; Rodríguez, A.B. & Pariente, J.A. (2011). Melatonin enhances hydrogen peroxide-induced apoptosis in human promyelocytic leukaemia HL-60 cells. *Molecular and cellular biochemistry*. Vol.353, No.1-2, pp.167-176, ISSN 0300-8177.

Bejarano, I.; Lozano, G.M.; Ortiz, A.; Garcia, J.F.; Paredes, S.D.; Rodriguez, A.B.; Pariente, J.A.(2008). Caspase 3 activation in human spermatozoa in response to hydrogen peroxide and progesterone. *Fertility and Sterility*. Vol.90, pp.1340-1347, ISSN 0015-0282.

Bellgrau, D.; Gold, D.; Selawry, H.; Moore, J.; Franzusoff, A. & Duke, R.C. (1995). A role for CD95 ligand in preventing graft rejection. *Nature*. Vol.19, No.377, pp.630-632, ISSN 0028-0836.

Beumer, T.L.; Roepers-Gajadien, H.L.; Gademan, I.S.; Van Buul, P.P.; Gil-Gomez, G.; Rutgers, D.H. & De Rooij, D.G. (1998). The role of the tumor suppressor p53 in spermatogenesis. *Cell death and differentiation*. Vol.5, No.8, pp.669-677, ISSN 1350-9047.

Blake, D.R.; Allen, R.E. & Lunec, J. (1987). Free radicals in biological systems--a review orientated to inflammatory processes. *British medical bulletin*. ISSN 0007-1420.

Boumela, I.; Guillemin, Y.; Guérin, J.F. & Aouacheria, A. (2009). The Bcl-2 family pathway in gametes and preimplantation embryos. *Gynécologie, obstétrique & fertilité*. Vol.37, No.9, pp.720-732, ISSN 1297-9589.

Brookes, P.S.; Yoon, Y.; Robotham, J.L.; Anders, M.W. & Sheu, S.S. (2004). Calcium, ATP, and ROS: a mitochondrial love-hate triangle. *American journal of physiology. Cell physiology*. Vol.287, No.4, pp.C817–C833, ISSN 0363-6143.

Castellano, L.E.; Trevino, C.L.; Rodríguez, D.; Serrano, C.J.; Pacheco, J.; Tsutsumi, V.; Felix, R. & Darszon, A. (2003).Transient receptor potential (TRPC) channels in human sperm: expression, cellular localization and involvement in the regulation of flagellar motility. *FEBS Letter.* Vol.541, No.1-3, pp.69-74, ISSN 0014-5793.

Celik-Ozenci, C.; Sahin, Z.; Ustunel, I.; Akkoyunlu, G.; Erdogru, T.; Korgun, E.T.; Baykara, M. & Demir, R. (2006). The Fas system may have a role in male reproduction. *Fertility and Sterility.* Vol.85, No.1, pp.1168-78, ISSN 0015-0282.

Chandrasekaran, Y. & Richburg, J.H. (2005). The p53 protein influences the sensitivity of testicular germ cells to mono-(2-ethylhexyl) phthalate-induced apoptosis by increasing the membrane levels of Fas and DR5 and decreasing the intracellular amount of c-FLIP. *Biology of Reproduction.* Vol.72, No.1, pp.206-213, ISSN 0006-3363.

Condorelli, R.A.; La Vignera, S.; Di Bari, F.; Unfer, V. & Calogero, A.E. (2011). Effects of myoinositol on sperm mitochondrial function in-vitro. *European review for medical and pharmacological sciences.* Vol.15, No.2, pp.129-134, ISSN 1128-3602.

Darszon, A.; Beltrán, C.; Felix, R.; Nishigaki, T. & Treviño, C.L. (2001). Ion transport in sperm signaling. *Developmental of Biology.* Vol.240, No.1, pp.1-14, ISSN 0012-1606.

Davis, J.S. & Rueda, B.R. (2002). The corpus luteum: an ovarian structure with maternal instincts and suicidal tendencies. *Frontiers in bioscience : a journal and virtual library.* Vol.7, pp.d1949-d1978, ISSN 1093-9946.

De Lamirande, E.; Leclerc, P. & Gagnon, C. (1997). Capacitation as a regulatory event that primes spermatozoa for the acrosome reaction and fertilization. *Molecular Human. Reproduction.* Vol.3, No.3, pp.175-194, ISSN 1360-9947.

De Vries, K.J.; Wiedmer, T.; Sims, P.J. & Gazella, B.M. (2003). Caspase-independent expouse of aminophospholipids and tyrosine phosphorylation in bicarbonate responsive human sperm cells. *Biology of Reproduction.* Vol.68, No.6, pp. 2122-2134, ISSN 0006-3363 .

Demaurex, N. & Distelhorst, C. (2003). Apoptosis-the calcium connection. *Science.* Vol.300, No.5616, pp.65-67, ISSN 0036-8075.

Donnelly, E.T.; O'Connell, M.; McClure, N. & Lewis, S.E. (2000). Differences in nuclear DNA fragmentation and mitochondrial integrity of semen and prepared human spermatozoa. *Human reproduction.* Vol.15, No.7, pp.1552-1561, ISSN 0268-1161.

Eley, A., Hosseinzadeh, S.; Hakimi, H.; Geary, I. & Pacey, A.A. (2005). Apoptosis of ejaculated human sperm is induced by co-incubation with Clamydia trachomatis lipopolysaccharide. *Human Reproduction.* Vol.20, No.9, pp.2601-2607, ISSN 0268-1161.

Erkkilä, K.; Hirvonen, V.; Wuokko, E.; Parvinen, M. & Dunkel, L. (1998). N-acetyl-L-cysteine inhibits apoptosis in human male germ cells in vitro. *The Journal of clinical endocrinology and metabolism.* Vol.83, No.7, pp.2523-2531, ISSN 0021-972X.

Espino, J.; Bejarano, I.; Ortiz, A.; Lozano, G.M.; García, J.F.; Pariente, J.A. & Rodríguez, A.B. (2010). Melatonin as a potential tool against oxidative damage and apoptosis in ejaculated human spermatozoa. *Fertility and Sterility.* Vol.94, No.9, pp.1915-1917, ISSN 0015-0282.

Espino, J.; Ortiz, A.; Bejarano, I.; Lozano, G.M.; Monllor, F.; García, J.F.; Rodríguez, A.B. & Pariente, J.A. (2011). Melatonin protects human spermatozoa from apoptosis via melatonin receptor- and extracelular-regulated kinase-mediated pathways. *Fertility and Sterility*. Vol.95, No.7, pp.2290-2296, ISSN 0015-0282.

Espinosa, F.; López-González, I.; Muñoz-Garay, C.; Felix, R.; De la Vega-Beltrán, J.L.; Kopf, G.S.; Visconti, P.E. & Darszon, A. (2000). Dual regulation of the T-type Ca^{2+} current by serum albumin and betaestradiol in mammalian spermatogenic cells. *FEBS Letter*. Vol.475, No.3, pp.251-256, ISSN 0014-5793.

Espinoza, J.A.; Paasch, U. & Villegas, J.V. (2009). Mitochondrial membrane potential disruption pattern in human sperm. *Human reproduction*. Vol.24, No.9, pp.2079-2085, ISSN 0268-1161.

Francavilla, S.; D'Abrizio, P.; Cordeschi, G.; Pelliccione, F.; Necozione, S.; Ulises, S.; Properzi, G. & Francavilla, F. (2002). Fas expresión correlatos with human germ cell degeneration in meiotic and post-meiotic arrest of spermatogenesis. *Molecular Human Reproduction*. Vol.8, No.3, pp.213-220, ISSN 1360-9947.

Fujinoki, M. (2008). Melatonin-enhanced hyperactivation of hamster sperm. *Reproduction*. Vol.136, No.5, pp.533-541, ISSN 1470-1626.

Gallon, F.; Marchetti, C.; Jouy, N. & Marchetti, P. (2006). The functionality of mitochondria differentiates human spermatozoa with high and low fertilizing capability. *Fertility and sterility*. Vol.86, No.5, pp.1526-1530, ISSN 0015-0282.

Green, D.R. & Reed, J.C. (1998). Mitochondria and apoptosis. *Science*. Vol.281, No.5381, pp.1309-1312, ISSN 0036-8075.

Griveau, J.F.; Dumont, E.; Renard, P.; Callegari, J.P. & Le Lannou, D. (1995). Reactive oxygen species, lipid peroxidation and enzymatic defence systems in human spermatozoa. *Reproduction and Fertility*. Vol.103, No.1, pp.17-26, ISSN 0022-4251.

Grunewald, S.; Baumann, T.; Paasch, U. & Glander, H.J. (2006). Capacitation and acrosome reaction in nonapoptotic human spermatozoa. *Annals of the New York Academy of Sciences*. Vol.1090, pp.138-146, ISSN 0077-8923.

Grunewald, S.; Kriegel, C.; Baumann, T.; Glander, H.J. & Paasch, U. (2009a). Interactions between apoptotic signal transduction and capacitation in human spermatozoa. *Human reproduction*. Vol.24, No.9, pp.2071-2078, ISSN 0268-1161.

Grunewald, S.; Paasch, U. & Glander, H.J. (2001). Enrichment of non-apoptotic human spermatozoa after cryopreservation by immunomagnetic cell sorting. *Cell and Tissue Banking*. Vol.2, No. 3, pp.127-133, ISSN 1389-9333.

Grunewald, S.; Paasch, U.; Glander, H.J. & Anderegg, U. (2005). Mature human spermatozoa do not transcribe novel RNA. *Andrologia*. Vol.37, No.2-3, pp.69-71, ISSN 0303-4569.

Grunewald, S.; Sharma, R.; Paasch, U.; Glander, H.J. & Agarwal, A. (2009b). Impact of caspase activation in human spermatozoa. *Microscopy Research and Technology*. Vol.2, No.11, pp.878-888, ISSN 1059-910X.

Hajnoczky, G.; Davies, E. & Madesh, M. (2003). Calcium signaling and apoptosis. *Biochemical and biophysical research communications*. Vol.304, No.3, pp.445-454, ISSN 0006-291X.

Hardeland, R.; Tan, D.X. & Reiter, R.J. (2009). Kynuramines, metabolites of melatonin and other indoles: the resurrection of an almost forgotten class of biogenic amines. Journal *of pineal research.* Vol.47, No.2, pp.109-126, ISSN 0742-3098.

Ho, H.C. & Suarez, S.S. (2001a). Hyperactivation of mammalian spermatozoa: function and regulation. *Reproduction.* Vol.122, No.4, pp.519-526, ISSN 1470-1626.

Ho, H.C. & Suarez, S.S. (2001b). An inositol 1,4,5-trisphosphate receptor-gated intracellular Ca2+ store is involved in regulating sperm hyperactivated motility. *Bilogy of Reproduction.* Vol.65, No.5, pp.1606-1615, ISSN 0006-3363.

Hsueh, A.J.; Billing, H. & Tsafriri, A. (1994). Ovarian follicle atresia: a hormonally controlled apoptotic process. *Endocrine Reviews.* Vol.15, No.6, pp.707-724, ISSN 0163-769X.

Jagannathan, S.; Publicover, SJ.; Barratt, CL. (2000). Voltage-operated calcium channels in male germ cells. *Reproduction.* Vol.123, pp.203-215, ISSN1470-1626.

Jana, K.; Jana, N.; De, D.K. & Guha, S.K. (2010). Ethanol induces mouse spermatogenic cell apoptosis in vivo through over-expression of Fas/Fas-L, p53, and caspase-3 along with cytochrome c translocation and glutathione depletion. *Molecular Reproduction & Development.* Vol.77, No.9, pp.820-833, ISSN 1040-452X.

Jia, X.D.; Zhou, D.X. & Song, T.B. (2008). The reproductive system impairment of adult male rats induced by cocaine. *Journal of forensic medicine.* Vol.24, No.6, pp.411-413, ISSN 1004-5619.

Kerr, J.F.; Wyllie, A.H. & Currie, A.R. (1972). Apoptosis: a basic biological phenomenon with wide-ranging implications in tissue kinetics. *British Journal of Cancer.* Vol.26, No.4, pp.239-257, ISSN 0007-0920.

Khorsandi, L.S.; Hashemitabar, M.; Orazizadeh, M. & Albughobeish, N. (2008). Dexamethasone effects on fas ligand expression in mouse testicular germ cells. *Pakistan Journal of Biological Science.* Vol.15, No.11-18, pp.2231-2236, ISSN 1028-8880.

Koji, T. (2001). Male germ cell death in mouse testes: possible involvement of Fas and Fas ligand. *Medical electron microscopy : official journal of the Clinical Electron Microscopy Society of Japan.* Vol.34, No.4, pp.213-22, ISSN 0918-4287.

Koji, T.; Hishikawa, Y.; Ando, H.; Nakanishi, Y. & Kobayashi, N. (2001). Expression of Fas and Fas ligand in normal and ischemia-reperfusion testes: involvement of the Fas system in the induction of germ cell apoptosis in the damaged mouse testis. *Biology of Reproduction.* Vol.64, No.3, pp.946-954, ISSN 0006-3363.

Kothari, S.; Thompson, A.; Agarwal, A. & Du Plessis, S.S. (2010). Free radicals: their beneficial and detrimental effects on sperm function. *Indian Journal of Experimental Biology.* Vol.48. No.5, pp.425-35, ISSN 0019-5189.

Kumar, R.; Jagan Mohanarao, G.; Arvind. & Atreja, S.K. (2011). Freeze-thaw induced genotoxicity in buffalo (Bubalus bubalis) spermatozoa in relation to total antioxidant status. *Molecular biology reports.* Vol.38, No.3, pp.1499-1506, ISSN 0301-4851.

Kurosaka, K.; Takahashi, M.; Watanabe, N. & Kobayashi, Y. (2003). Silent cleaup of very early apoptotic cells by macrophages. *The Journal of Immunology.* Vol.171, No.9, pp.4672-4679, ISSN 0022-1767.

Leon, J.; Acuña-Castroviejo, D.; Sainz, R.M.; Mayo, J.C.; Tan, D.X. & Reiter, R.J. (2004). Melatonin and mitochondrial function. *Life sciences*. Vol.75, No.7, pp.765-790, ISSN 0024-3205.

Li, H.; Zhu, H.; Xu, CJ. & Yuan, J. (1998). Cleavage of BID by caspase 8 mediates the mitochondrial damage in the Fas pathway of apoptosis. *Cell*. Vol. 94, No.4, pp.491-501, ISSN 0092-8674.

Li, P.; Nijhawan, D.; Budihardjo, I.; Srinivasula, S.M.; Ahmad, M.; Alnemri, E.S. & Wang, X. (1997). Cytochrome c and dATP-dependent formation of Apaf-1/caspase-9 complex initiates an apoptotic protease cascade. *Cell*. Vol.91, No, 4, pp.479-489, ISSN 0092-8674.

Li, Z.; Lin, Q.; Liu, R.; Xiao, W. & Liu, W. (2010). Protective effects of ascorbate and catalase on human spermatozoa during cryopreservation. *Journal of andrology*. Vol.31, No.5, pp.437-444, ISSN 0196-3635.

Lin, W.W.; Lamb, D.J.; Wheeler, T.M.; Abrams, J.; Lipshultz, L.I. & Kim, E.D. (1997). Apoptotic frequency is increased in spermatogenic maturation arrest and hypospermatogenic states. *Journal of Urology*. Vol.158, No.5, pp.1791-1793, ISSN 0022-5347.

Linsenmeyer, T.A. & Perkash, I. (1991). Infertility in men with spinal cord injury. *Archives of physical medicine and rehabilitation*. Vol.72, No.10, pp.747-754, ISSN 0003-9993.

Lizama, C.; Alfaro, I.; Reyes, J.G. & Moreno, R.D. (2007). Up-regulation of CD95 (Apo-1/Fas) is associated with spermatocute apoptosis during the first round spermatogenesis in the rat. *Apoptosis* . Vol.12, No.3, pp.499-512, ISSN 1360-8185.

Lozano, G.M.; Bejarano, I.; Espino, J.; Gonzalez, D.; Ortiz, A.; Garcia, J.F.; Rodríguez, A.B. & Pariente, J.A. (2009). Relationship berween caspase activity and apoptotic markers in human sperm in response to hydrogen peroxide and progesterone. *Journal of Reproduction and Development* . Vol.55, No.6, pp.615-621, ISSN 0916-8818.

Makker, K.; Agarwal, A. & Sharma, R. (2009). Oxidative stress & male infertility. *The Indian journal of medical research*. Vol.129, No.4, pp.357-67, ISSN 0971-5916.

Marchetti, C.; Jouy, N.; Leroy-Martin, B.; Defossez, A.; Formstecher, P. & Marchetti, P. (2004). Comparison of four fluorochromes for the detection of the inner mitochondrial membrane potential in human spermatozoa and their correlation with sperm motility. *Human reproduction*. Vol.19, No.10, pp.2267-2276, ISSN 0268-1161.

Martin, G.; Cagnon, N.; Sabido, O.; Sion, B.; Grizard, G.; Durand, P. & Levy, R. (2007). Kinetics of occurrence of some features of apoptosis during the cryopreservation process of bovine spermatozoa. *Human Reproduction*. Vol.22, No.2, pp.380-388, ISSN 0268-1161.

Martin, G.; Sabido, O.; Durand, P. & Levy, R. (2005). Phosphatidylserine externalization in human sperm induced by calcium ionophore A23187: relationship with apoptosis, membrane scrambling and the acrosome reaction. *Human Reproduction*. Vol.20, No.12, pp.3459-3468, ISSN 0268-1161.

Martínez, RR.; Luna, M. & Chavarría, ME. (1987) Concentrations of calmodulin in sperm in relation to their motility in fertile euspermic and infertile asthenozoospermic men. *International journal of andrology*. Vol.10, No.3, pp.507-515, ISSN 0105-6263.

Meseguer, M.; Garrido, N.; Martínez-Conejero, JA.; Simón, C.; Pellicer, A. & Remohí, J. (2004). Relationship between standard semen parameters, calcium, cholesterol contents and mitochondrial activity in ejaculated spermatozoa from fertile and infertile males. *Journal of assisted reproduction and genetics.* Vol.21, No.12, pp. 445-451, ISSN 1058-0468.

Mishra, DP.; Pal, R. & Shaha, C. (2006). Changes in Cytosolic Ca^{2+} Levels Regulate Bcl-xS and Bcl-xL Expression in Spermatogenic Cells during Apoptotic Death. *The Journal of biological chemistry.* Vol.281, No.4, pp.2133-2143, ISSN 0021-9258.

Morita, Y. & Tilly, J.L. (1999). Oocyte apoptosis: like sand through an hourglass. *Developmental biology.* Vol.213, No.1, pp. 1-17, ISSN 0012-1606.

Mueller, T.; Voigt, W.; Simon, H.; Fruehauf, A.; Bulankin, A.; Grothey, A. & Schmoll, H.J. (2003). Failure of activation of caspase-9 induces a higher threshold for apoptosis and cisplatin resistance in testicular cancer. *American Association for Cancer Research.* Vol.63, No.2, pp.513-521, ISSN 0008-5472.

Müller, M.; Wilder, S.; Bannasch, D.; Israeli, D.; Lehlbach, K.; Li-Weber, M.; Friedman, S.L.; Galle, P.R.; Stremmel, W.; Oren, M. & Krammer, P.H. (1998). p53 activates the CD95 (APO-1/Fas) gene in response to DNA damage by anticancer drugs. *The Journal of experimental medicine.* Vol.188, No.11, pp.2033-2045, ISSN 0022-1007.

Murdoch, W.J. (2000). Proteolytic and cellular death mechanisms in ovulatory ovarian rupture. *Biological signals and receptors.* Vol.9, No.2, pp.102-114, ISSN 1422-4933.

Nicholson, D.W. (1999)Caspase structure, proteolytic substrates, and function during apoptotic cell death. *Cell death and differentiation.* Vol.6, No.11, pp.1028-1042, ISSN 1350-9047.

Oehninger, S.; Blackmore, P.; Mahony, M. & Hodgen, G. (1995). Effects of hydrogen peroxide on human spermatozoa. *Journal of assisted reproduction and genetics.* Vol.12, No.1, pp.41-47, ISSN 1058-0468.

Oehninger, S.; Morshedi, M.; Weng. S.L.; Taylor, S.; Duran, H. & Beebe, S. (2003). Presence and significance of somatic cell apoptosis markers in human ejaculated spermatozoa. *Reproductive biomedicine online.* Vol.7, No.4, pp.469-476, ISSN 1472-6483.

Oldereid, N.N.; Angelis, P.D.; Wiger, R. & Clausen, O.P. (2001). Expression of Bcl-2 family proteins and spontaneous apoptosis in normal human testis. *Molecular human reproduction.* Vol.7, No.5, pp.403-408, ISSN 1360-9947.

Omezzine, A.; Chater, S.; Mauduit, C.; Florin, A.; Tabone, E.; Chuzel, F.; Bars, R. & Benahmed, M. (2003) Long-term apoptotic cell death process with increased expression and activation of caspase-3 and -6 in adult rat germ cells exposed in utero to flutamide. *Endocrinology.* Vol.144, No.2, pp.648-661, ISSN 0013-7227.

Ozaki, Y.; Blomgren, K., Ogasawara, M.S.; Aoki, K.; Furuno, T.; Nakanishi, M.; Sasaki, M. & Suzumori, K. (2001). Role of calpain in human sperm activated by progesterone for fertilization. *Biological chemistry.* Vol.382, No.5, pp.831-838, ISSN 1431-6730.

Paasch, U.; Grunewald, S.; Dathe, S. & Glander, H.J. (2004). Mitochondria of human spermatozoa are preferentially susceptible to apoptosis. *Annals of the New York Academy of Sciences.* Vol.1030, pp.403-409, ISSN 0077-8923.

Paasch, U.; Grunewald, S.; Fitzl, G. & Glander, H.J. (2003). Deterioration of plasma membrane is associated with activation of caspases in human spermatozoa. *Journal of andrology.* Vol.24, No.2, pp.246-252, ISSN 0196-3635.

Paudel, K.P.; Kumar, S.; Meur, S.K. & Kumaresan, A. (2010). Ascorbic acid, catalase and chlorpromazine reduce cryopreservation-induced damages to crossbred bull spermatozoa. *Reproduction in domestic animals*. Vol.45, No.2, pp.256-262, ISSN 0936-6768.

Perticarari, S.; Ricci, G.; Boscolo, R.; De Santis, M.; Pagnini, G.; Martinelli, M. & Presani, G. (2008). Fas receptor is not present on ejaculated human sperm. *Human Reproduction*. Vol.23, No.6, pp.1271-1279, ISSN 0268-1161.

Plante, M.; de Lamirande, E. & Gagnon, C. (1994). Reactive oxygen species released by activated neutrophils, but not by deficient spermatozoa, are sufficient to affect normal sperm motility. *Fertility and sterility*. Vol.62, No.2, pp.387-393, ISSN 0015-0282.

Primakoff, P. & Myles, D.G. (2002). Penetration, adhesion, and fusion in mammalian sperm–egg interaction. *Science*. Vol. 296, No.5576, pp.2183-2185, ISSN 0036-8075.

Purohit, S.B.; Laloraya, M. & Kumar, G.P. (1999). Role of ions and ion channels in capacitation and acrosome reaction of spermatozoa. *Asian journal of andrology*. Vol.1, No.3, pp.95-107, ISSN 1008-682X.

Reed, J.C. (1997). Double identity for proteins of the Bcl-2 family. *Nature*. Vol.387, No.6635, pp.773-776, ISSN 0028-0836.

Reiter, R.J.; Tan, D.X.; Manchester, L.C.; Paredes, S.D; Mayo, J.C. & Sainz, R.M. (2009). Melatonin and reproduction revisited. *Biology of reproduction*. Vol.81, No.3, pp.445-456, ISSN 0006-3363.

Ren, D.; Navarro, B.; Pérez, G.; Jackson, A.C.; Hsu, S.; Shi, Q.; Tilly, J.L. & Clapham, D.E. (2001). A sperm ion channel required for sperm motility and male fertility. *Nature*. Vol.413, No.6856, pp:603-609, ISSN 0028-0836.

Riccioli, A.; Dal Secco, V.; De Cesaris, P.; Starace, D.; Gandini, L.; Lenzi, A.; Dondero, F.; Padula, F.; Filippini, A. & Ziparo, E. (2005). Presence of membrane and soluble forms of Fas ligand and of matrilysin (MMP-7) activity in normal and abnormal human semen. *Human Reproduction*. Vol.20, No.10, pp.2814-2820, ISSN 0268-1161.

Riccioli, A.; Salvati, L.; D'Alessio, A.; Starace, D.; Giampietri, C.; De Cesaris, P.; Filippini, A. & Ziparo, E. (2003). The Fas system in the seminiferous epithelium and its possible extra-testicular role. *Andrologia*. Vol.35, No.1, pp.64-70, ISSN 0303-4569.

Richburg, J.H.; Nañez, A.; Williams, L.R.; Embree, M.E. & Boekelheide, K. (2000). Sensitivity of testicular germ cells to toxicant-induced apoptosis in gld mice that express a nonfunctional form of Fas ligand. *Endocrinology*. Vol.141, No.2, pp.787-793; ISSN 0013-7227.

Rodeheffer, C. & Shur, B.D. (2004b). Sperm from beta-1,4-galactosyltransferase I-null mice exhibit precocious capacitation. *Development*. Vol.131, No.3, pp.491-501, ISSN 0950-1991.

Rodriguez, C.; Mayo, J.C.; Sainz, R.M.; Antolín, I.; Herrera, F.; Martín, V. & Reiter, R.J. (2004). Regulation of antioxidant enzymes: a significant role for melatonin. *Journal of pineal research*. Vol.36, No.1, pp.1-9, ISSN 0742-3098.

Rodriguez, I.; Ody, C.; Araki, K.; Garcia, I. & Vassalli, P. (1997). An early and massive wave of germinal cell apoptosis is required for the development functional spermatogenesis. *The EMBO journal*. Vol.16, No.9, pp.2262-2270, ISSN 0261-4189.

Rucker, E.B. 3rd.; Dierisseau, P.; Wagner, K.U.; Garrett, L.; Wynshaw-Boris, A.; Flaws, J.A. & Hennighausen, L. (2000). Bcl-x and Bax regulate mouse primordial germ cell survival and apoptosis during embryogenesis. *Molecular endocrinology.* Vol.14, No.7, pp.1038-1052, ISSN 0888-8809.

Ruwanpura, S.M.; McLachlan, R.I. & Meachem, S.J. (2010). Hormonal regulation of male germ cell development. *The Journal of endocrinology.* Vol.205, No.2, pp.117-131, ISSN 0022-0795.

Said, T.M.; Agarwal, A.; Grunewald, S.; Rasch, M.; Baumann, T.; Kriegel, C.; Li, L.; Glander, H.J.; Thomas, A.J. Jr. & Paasch, U. (2005). Selection of non-apoptotic spermatozoa as a new tool for enhancing assisted reproduction outcomes: an in vivo model. *Biology of reproduction.* Vol.74, No.3, pp.530-537, ISSN 0006-3363.

Sailer, B:L.; Jost, L.K. & Evenson, D.P. (1995). Mammalian sperm DNA susceptibility to in situ denaturation associated with the presence of DNA strand breaks as measured by the terminal deoxynucleotidyl transferase assay. *Journal of andrology.* Vol.16, No.1, pp.80-87, ISSN 0196-3635.

Sainz, R.M.; Mayo, J.C.; Rodriguez, C.; Tan, D.X.; Lopez-Burillo, S. & Reiter, R.J. (2003). Melatonin and cell death: differential actions on apoptosis in normal and cancer cells. *Cellular and molecular life sciences.* Vol.60, No.7, pp.1407-1426, ISSN 1420-682X.

Sakkas, D.; Mariethoz, E. & St John, J.C. (1999a). Abnormal sperm parameters in humans are indicative of an abortive apoptotic mechanism linked to the Fas-mediated pathway. *Experimental cell research.* Vol.251, No.2, pp.350-355, ISSN 0014-4827.

Sakkas, D.; Mariethoz, E.; Manicardi, G.; Bizzaro, D.; Bianchi, P:G. & Bianchi, U. (1999b). Origin of DNA damage in ejaculated human spermatozoa. *Reviews of reproduction.* Vol.4, No.1, pp.31-37, ISSN 1359-6004.

Saleh, R.A.; Agarwal, A.; Sharma, R.K.; Nelson, D.R. & Thomas, A.J. Jr. (2001). Effect of cigarette smoking on levels of seminal oxidative stress in infertile men: a prospective study. *Fertility and Sterility.* Vol.78, No.3, pp.491-499, ISSN 0015-0282.

Shaha, C. (2007). Modulators of spermatogenic cell survival. *Society of Reproduction and Fertility supplement.* Vol.63, pp.173-186.

Shekarriz, M.; Thomas, A.J. Jr. & Agarwal, A. (1995). Incidence and level of seminal reactive oxygen species in normal men. *Urology.* Vol.45, No.1, pp.103–107, ISSN0090-4295.

Sikka, S.C.; Rajasekaran, M. & Hellstrom, W.J. (1995). Role of oxidative stress and antioxidants in male infertility. *Journal of andrology.* Vol.16, No.6, pp.464-468, ISSN 0196-3635.

Sinha-Hikim, A.P. & Swerdloff, R.S. (1999). Hormonal and genetic control of germ cell apoptosis in the testis. *Reviews of reproduction.* Vol.4, No.1, pp.38-47, ISSN 1359-6004.

Sinha-Hikim, A.P.; Lue, Y.; Diaz-Romero, M.; Yen, P.H.; Wang, C. & Swerdloff, R.S. (2003). Deciphering the pathways of germ cell apoptosis in the testis. *The Journal of steroid biochemistry and molecular biology.* Vol.85, No.2-5, pp.175-182, ISSN 0960-0760.

Soleimani, M.; Tavalaee, M.; Aboutorabi, R.; Adib, M.; Bahramian, H.; Janzamin, E.; Kiani, A. & Nasr-Esfahani, M.H. (2010) Evaluation of Fas positive sperm and complement mediated lysis in subfertile individuals. *Journal of assisted reproduction and genetics.* Vol.27, No.8, pp.477-482, ISSN 1058-0468.

Stennicke, H.T. & Salvesen, G.S. (1997). Biochemical characteristics of capase-3, -6, -7, and -8. *The Journal of biological chemistry.* Vol.272, No.41, pp.25719-25723, ISSN 0021-9258.

Suda, T.; Takahashi, T.; Golstein, P. & Nagata, S. (1993). Molecular cloning and expression of the Fas ligand, a novel member of the tumor necrosis factor family. *Cell.* Vol.75, No.6, pp.1169-1178, ISSN 0092-8674.

Taylor, S.L.; Weng, S.L.; Fox, P.; Duran, E.H.; Morshedi, M.S.; Oehninger, S. & Beebe, S.J. (2004). Somatic cell apoptosis markers and pathways in human ejaculated sperm: potential utility as indicators of sperm quality. *Molecular human reproduction.* Vol.10, No.11, pp.825-834, ISSN 1360-9947.

Thuwanut, P.; Chatdarong, K.; Johannisson, A.; Bergqvist, A.S.; Söderquist, L. & Axnér, E. (2010). Cryopreservation of epididymal cat spermatozoa: effects of in vitro antioxidative enzymes supplementation and lipid peroxidation induction. *Theriogenology.* Vol.73, No.8, pp.1076-1087, ISSN 0093-691X.

Tremellen, K. (2008). Oxidative stress and male infertility - a clinical perspective. *Human reproduction update.* Vol.14, No.3, pp.243–258, ISSN 1355-4786.

Trevino, C.L.; Félix, R.; Castellano, L.E.; Gutiérrez, C.; Rodriguez, D.; Pacheco, J.; López-González, I.; Gomora, J.C.; Tsutsumi, V.; Hernández-Cruz, A.; Fiordelisio, T.; Scaling, A.L. & Darszon, A. (2004). Expression and differential cell distribution of low-threshold Ca^{2+} channels in mammalian male germ cells and sperm. *FEBS letters.* Vol.563, No.1-3, pp.87-92, ISSN 0014-5793.

Tripathi, D.N. & Jena, G.B. (2008). Astaxanthin inhibits cytotoxic and genotoxic effects of cyclophosphamide in mice germ cells. *Toxicology.* Vol.248, No.2-3, pp.96-103, ISSN 0300-483X.

Troiano, L.; Granata, A.R.; Cossarizza, A.; Kalashnikova, G.; Bianchi, R.; Pini, G.; Tropea, F.; Carani, C. & Franceschi, C. (1998). Mitochondrial membrane potential and DNA stainability in human sperm cells: a flow cytometry analysis with implications for male infertility. *Experimental cell research.* Vol.241, No.2, pp.384-393, ISSN 0014-4827.

Tunc, O.; Thompson, J. & Tremellen, K. Improvement in sperm DNA quality using an oral antioxidant therapy. (2009). *Reproductive biomedicine online.* Vol.18, No.6, pp.761-768, ISSN 1472-6483.

Vasudevan, S.R.; Lewis, A.M.; Chan, J.W.; Machin, C.L.; Sinha, D.; Galione, A. & Churchill, G.C. (2010). The calcium-mobilizing messenger nicotinic acid adenine dinucleotide phosphate participates in sperm activation by mediating the acrosome reaction. J *The Journal of biological chemistry.* Vol.285, No.24, pp.18262-18269. ISSN 0021-9258.

Vine, M.F. (1996). Smoking and male reproduction: a review. *International journal of andrology.* Vol.19, No.6, pp.323-337, ISSN 0105-6263.

Wang, K.K.; Posmantur, R.; Nadimpalli, R.; Nath, R.; Mohan, P.; Nixon, R.A.; Talanian, R.V.; Keegan, M.; Herzog, L. & Allen, H. (1998). Caspase-mediated fragmentation of calpain inhibitor protein calpastatin during apoptosis. *Archives of biochemistry and biophysics.* Vol.356, No.2, pp.187-196, ISSN 0003-9861.

Wang, Q.; Zhao, X.F.; Ji, Y.L.; Wang, H.; Liu, P.; Zhang, C.; Zhang, Y. & Xu, D.X. (2010). Mitochondrial signaling pathway is also involved in bisphenol A induced germ cell apoptosis in testes. *Toxicology letters.* Vol.199, No.2, pp.129-135, ISSN 0378-4274.

Wang, X. (2001). The expanding role of mitochondria in apoptosis. *Genes & development.* Vol.15, No.22, pp.2922-2933, ISSN 0890-9369.

Weil, M.; Jacobson, M.D. & Raff, M.C. (1998). Are caspases involved in the death of cells with a transcriptionally inactive nucleus? Sperm and chicken erythrocytes. *Journal of cell science.* Vol.111, No.Pt18, pp. 2707-2715, ISSN 0021-9533.

Yan, W.; Suominen, J.; Samson, M.; Jegou, B. & Toppari, J. (2000). Involvement of Bcl-2 family proteins in germ cell apoptosis during testicular development in the rat and pro-survival effect of stem cell factor on germ cells in vitro. *Molecular and cellular endocrinology.* Vol.165, No.1-2, pp.115-129, ISSN 0303-7207.

Yazawa, T.; Fujimoto, K.; Yamamoto, T. & Abé, S.I. (2001). Caspase activity in newt spermatogonial apoptosis induced by prolactin and cycloheximide. *Molecular reproduction and development.* Vol.59, No.2, pp.209-214, ISSN 1040-452X.

Yazawa, T.; Yamamoto, T. & Abé, S. (2000). Prolactin induces apoptosis in the penultimate spermatogonial stage of the testes in Japanese red-bellied newt (Cynops pyrrhogaster). *Endocrinology.* Vol.141, No.6, pp.2027-2032, ISSN 0013-7227.

Yudin, A.I.; Goldberg, E.; Robertson, K.R. & Overstreet, J.W. (2000). Calpain and calpastatin are located berween the plasma membrane and outer acrosomal membrane of cynomolgus macaque spermatozoa. *Journal of andrology.* Vol.21, No.5, pp.721-729, ISSN 0196-3635.

4

The Role of PDE5 Inhibitors in the Treatment of Testicular Dysfunction

Fotios Dimitriadis* et al.
Laboratory of Molecular Urology and Genetics of Human Reproduction, Department of Urology, Ioannina University School of Medicine, Ioannina
[1]*Greece*

1. Introduction

The cyclic nucleotide phosphodiesterases (PDEs) play the predominant role in the degradation of the cyclic adenosine monophosphate (cAMP) and cyclic guanosine monophosphate (cGMP). The PDEs function in conjunction with adenylate cyclase (AC) and guanylate cyclase (GC) to regulate the amplitude and duration of intracellular signaling mechanisms (mediated via cAMP and cGMP, respectively). Detailed sequence analyses suggest that there are at least 11 different families of mammalian PDEs. Most of the PDEs families include more than one gene product (Bender & Beavo, 2006). In addition, many of these genes can be alternatively spliced in a tissue specific manner. The overall result is the production of different mRNAs and proteins with altered regulatory properties or subcellular localization. This multiplicity of PDE proteins allows organ- and cell type-specific expression and even a specific intracellular localization of PDEs in the vicinity of various protein effectors inducing fine-tuning of compartmentalized regulation for cAMP and cGMP (Zaccolo & Pozzan, 2002; Bender & Beavo, 2006). For example, cGMP-hydrolyzing PDE5 is highly expressed in smooth muscle cells of the corpus cavernosum penis and vascular smooth muscle cells of the lung allowing the employment of PDE5 inhibitors for the pharmaceutical management of erectile dysfunction (Lue, 2000) and pulmonary hypertension (Ghofrani et al., 2002; Ghofrani et al., 2002; Ghofrani et al., 2003; Schermuly et al., 2004; Galie et al., 2005), respectively.

Phosphodiesterases, which hydrolyze cGMP or cAMP, play a major role in cell signaling by affecting the duration of cyclic nucleotide action (Bender & Beavo, 2006). Phosphodiesterases including PDE1A, PDE1B, PDE5, PDE6, PDE9 and PDE10 preferentially hydrolyze cGMP (Bender & Beavo, 2006). In contrast, PDE1C, PDE2 and PDE11 are dual

* Dimitrios Baltogiannis[1], Sotirios Koukos[1], Dimitrios Giannakis[1], Panagiota Tsounapi[2], Georgios Seminis[1], Motoaki Saito[3], Atsushi Takenaka[2] and Nikolaos Sofikitis[1]
[1]*Laboratory of Molecular Urology and Genetics of Human Reproduction, Department of Urology, Ioannina University School of Medicine, Ioannina, Greece*
[2]*Department of Urology, Tottori University School of Medicine, Yonago, Japan*
[3]*Division of Molecular Pharmacology, Department of Pathophysiological and Therapeutic Science, Tottori University School of Medicine, Yonago, Japan*

substrate-specific PDEs. In addition, PDE2, PDE5, PDE6 and PDE10 are cGMP-regulated by allosteric binding sites. On the other hand PDE3 represents a cGMP-inhibited PDE (Bender & Beavo, 2006). Exact analyses of tissue- and cell type-specific distribution of PDE gene families in the testis and epididymis are still missing. Published data on PDE expression in testis until now is primarily restricted to cAMP-hydrolyzing PDEs, such as PDE1C, PDE4A, PDE4C, PDE7B and PDE8A and their localization to male germ cells and spermatozoa (Bender & Beavo, 2006). With respect to cGMP pathways, transcripts of the cGMP-hydrolyzing PDE10 have been found in the human testis (Fujishige et al., 1999) and cGMP-hydrolyzing PDE5 has been recently localized to peritubular myoid cells of the rat (Scipioni et al., 2005).

2. Main heading expressions of PDEs in the male reproductive system

Till now, extra-vascular contractile cells of the male reproductive organs have been disregarded. In the testis and epididymis, smooth muscle cells and/or myofibroblasts, are known to surround the epithelium of the seminiferous tubules, the efferent ducts, and the epididymal duct (Setchell et al., 1994). These contractile cells are involved in the transport of immotile spermatozoa from the testis to the cauda epididymis, which ensures sperm maturation, (i.e. spermatozoa acquire their fertilization ability during this epididymal passage) (Setchell et al., 1994). In addition to its role in spermatozoal transport, the peritubular lamina propria of the human testis also affects spermatogenesis. In many cases of idiopathic male infertility the lamina propria is thickened with a reduction of contractile elements and an increase of extracellular components, resembling fibrotic changes in other organs (Davidoff et al., 1990). Moreover, the occurrence of segments of seminiferous tubules displaying pathological dilatations and a thin-walled lamina propria leads in impaired spermatogenesis. Most recently, the physiological significance of peritubular cells for spermatogenesis has been shown in tissue-selective knock-out mice with the androgen receptor gene deleted in peritubular myoid cells resulting in decreased total male germ cell number and oligozoospermia (Zhang et al., 2006).

Detailed analyses of tissue- and cell type-specific distribution of PDE gene families in the testis and epididymis are still lacking. The literature reveals data on PDE expression in testis restricted predominantly to cAMP-hydrolyzing PDEs such as PDE1C, PDE4A, PDE4C, PDE7B, and PDE8A (Table 1). Additionally it has been shown that PDE3 contributes to the regulation of epididymal contractility (Mewe et al., 2006). At least four genes encoding different isoforms of PDEs are differentially expressed in somatic and germ cells of the testis (Swinnen et al., 1989).

Several studies aiming to the localization of PDE in rat seminiferous tubules indicated that PDE1 and PDE2 are predominantly expressed in germ cells, whereas PDE3 and PDE4 are mainly restricted to Sertoli cells (Geremia et al., 1982; Morena et al., 1995). Three rat PDE3 mRNAs with divergent 5′ untranslated regions are present in Sertoli cells (Sette et al., 1994). The PDE of Sertoli cells may be a testis-specific enzyme because its cDNA only hybridizes to a 3.2-kb mRNA in Sertoli cells and in testicular RNA (Geremia et al., 1982; Swinnen et al., 1989).

Transcripts of the PDE10A has been demonstrated to be present in the human testis (Fujishige et al., 1999). cGMP-hydrolyzing-PDE5 has been localized in peritubular myoid cells of the rat (Scipioni et al., 2005). In another study by Coskran et al., (2006) PDE10A-immunoreactivity was detected in seminiferous tubules and epididymal spermatozoa of dog and cynomolgus macaque and in the testis of mouse, with no detectable immunoreactivity in testes or epididymes of rat or human (Coskran et al., 2006). Dog testis presented moderate specific PDE10A-immunoreactivity in round and elongated spermatids and to a lesser degree in the more mature spermatocytes (Coskran et al., 2006). In the cynomolgus macaque, testicular and epididymal spermatozoa exhibited the same pattern of PDE10A-immunoreactivity seen in the dog (Coskran et al., 2006). PDE10A-immunoreactivity in the mouse testis was similar to that observed in the cynomolgus macaque but was absent in mouse epididymal spermatozoa (Coskran et al., 2006). In the epididymes of dog and cynomolgus macaque, spermatozoal midsections, their tails, and distal cytoplasmic droplets were positive for PDE10A-immunoreactivity (Coskran et al., 2006). In the head of the epididymis spermatozoa contained PDE10A in their tails and distal droplets, whereas more mature spermatozoa in the tail of the epididymis expressed PDE10A only in the distal droplets (Coskran et al., 2006). Moreover, in other studies, PDE10A mRNA has been reported in the testis and in spermatozoa of humans and rats (Soderling et al., 1998; Fujishige et al., 1999; Fujishige et al., 1999; Baxendale & Fraser, 2005). The role of PDE10A in the spermatogenesis process is not fully elucidated. However, intact reproductive function in PDE10A knockout mice suggests that PDE10A is not essential for sperm fertilizing capacity (Siuciak et al., 2006).

The potential functions of PDE11 in the regulation of spermatogenesis process and sperm function has been an issue of major clinical importance since PDE11 serves as a substrate for the commonly used substance tadalafil (Francis, 2005). In fact the ejaculated spermatozoa from a knockout mouse model for PDE11 (PDE11-/-) displayed diminished sperm concentration, reduced rate of forward progression, and decreased percentage of a live spermatozoa (Wayman et al., 2005). Moreover, spermatozoa from the male reproductive tract from the same knockout animal model displayed enhanced premature/spontaneous capacitance (Wayman et al., 2005). The above data suggest a role for PDE11 in spermatogenesis and fertilization potential.

3. New horizons for PDE5 inhibitors

Male infertility represents not only a private but also a social problem. Although assisted reproductive technology (ART) represents a popular mode of therapeutic management of couple's infertility due to male factor, a significant subpopulation of infertile men remains childless after employment of intrauterine insemination, in vitro fertilization (IVF) or intracytoplasmic sperm injection (ICSI) techniques. An additional problem is that there are no widely accepted pharmaceutical agents effective for the treatment of the infertile male. Therefore the limitations of the success rate (i.e. live birth rate) of ART and the lack of effective pharmaceutical agents for the treatment of the infertile male represent the two main difficulties to solve the problem of male infertility.

Thus it appears that development of novel pharmaceutical agents with a positive impact on the alleviation of male infertility is of paramount importance. Recently studies have been published tending to justify a role for PDE5 inhibitors as an adjunct tool for male infertility therapeutic management. This review study aims to discuss and comment on the findings of all of the previous studies concerning the effect of PDE5 inhibitors on the male reproductive potential.

4. PDEs and hydrolysis of c-GMP in Leydig cells, Sertoli cells and peritubular cells

4.1 Hydrolysis of c-GMP in tunica albuginea, lamina propria, peritubular cells, and myofibroblasts

In male, the tunica albuginea has been shown to contain abundantly contractile elements (smooth muscle cells and myofibroblasts) as revealed by electron microscopy and immunohistochemical approaches (Middendorff et al., 2002). This tissue is characterized by extraordinarily high concentrations of cGMP-binding proteins including PKG I (Middendorff et al., 2002). In in vitro studies, atrial natriuretic peptide (ANP) and the nitric oxide (NO) donor sodium nitroprusside (SNP) have increased cGMP production in isolated strips of the tunica albuginea, and the underlying mechanism has been demonstrated (Middendorff et al., 2002). In fact, two cGMP-generating enzymes namely GC-A (the receptor for ANP) and soluble guanylate cyclase (sGC), could be identified in the tunica (Middendorff et al., 2002). Both the above enzymes have been found to be functionally active because ANP and SNP strongly enhance the production of cGMP in isolated pieces of the tunica (Middendorff et al., 2002). Contractile cells as well as Leydig cells located in the inner zone of the tunica have been identified as sites of NO synthase expression (Middendorff et al., 2002). Physiological studies have demonstrated spontaneous tunica contractions exclusively in regions close to the rete testis. These contractions could be attenuated by cGMP, SNP and ANP. Noradrenaline-induced contractions, detectable in all parts of the testicular capsule, could be abolished completely by SNP (Middendorff et al., 2002). These data, demonstrating complex contraction and relaxation activities, are indicative of a major physiological role of guanylate cyclase/cGMP pathway in the regulation of tunica albuginea function related to testicular sperm transport (Middendorff et al., 2002). In addition to its role in the tunica albuginea, ANP was found to affect spermatogenesis during postnatal development (Muller et al., 2004). In fact, a male germ specific cGK-anchoring protein, designed as GKAP42 (Yuasa et al., 2000) is expressed in a stage-dependent manner in spermatocytes and round spermatids. The latter protein interacts specifically with PKG Iα regulating germ cell development (Yuasa et al., 2000).

Moreover, recent studies demonstrated that GC-A can act as a regulator of cell size (Kishimoto et al., 2001) and proliferation (Lelievre et al., 2001). Thus growth regulation appears to represent an important aspect of the natriuretic peptide system (Silberbach & Roberts, 2001; Cameron & Ellmers, 2003). Considering that human spermatozoa can respond in a cGMP-dependent manner to ANP (Anderson et al., 1995) and that this peptide is capable of inducing acrosome reactions in spermatozoa (Rotem et al., 1998), there may be a probability for a role of GC-A in the regulation of the spermatozoal function (Muller et al., 2004).

The membrane-bound GC (GC-B) was found in Leydig cells as well as in the peritubular lamina propria (Middendorff et al., 2000) and in the tunica albuginea (Middendorff et al., 2002). The ligand of GC-B, C-type natriuretic peptide (CNP), is exclusively produced by Leydig cells (Middendorff et al., 1996) suggesting paracrine effects in contractile cells.

Middendorff et al., (2000) provided further data about the activation of sGC by carbon monoxide (CO) in the seminiferous tubules of the human testis (Middendorff et al., 2000). The CO-producing enzyme heme oxygenase-1 (HO-1) has been shown to be expressed in the adluminal compartments of Sertoli cells. Activation of sGC by HO-1-produced CO has resulted in increased cGMP levels (Middendorff et al., 2000). Since sGC has been found to be present in peritubular myofibroblasts, production of CO by HO-1 in the adluminal parts of Sertoli cells may trigger cGMP accumulation in peritubular lamina propria cells suggesting separation of the site of production and action of CO thereby mediating relaxation of myofibroblasts (Middendorff et al., 1997).

Scipioni et al., (2005) have reported that there is expression of PDE5 in Leydig cells and peritubular cells both in prepuberal and in adult rat testis. This gives additional strength to the idea that in mammalian testis cGMP-mediated processes influence not only the vessel dilatation but also the testosterone synthesis by Leydig cells and the transfer of spermatozoa, through the relaxation of peritubular lamina propria cells (Scipioni et al., 2005). In peritubular myoid cells, in particular, besides regulating contractility, cGMP modulation by PDE5 might affect the secretion of a number of substances, including extracellular matrix components (fibronectin, type I and IV collagens, proteoglycans) and growth factors (PModS, TGF beta, IGF-I, activin-A). The latter substances are known to affect the Sertoli cell function and to play a role in retinol processing (Maekawa et al., 1996). Retinol processing is essential for maintenance of the germinal epithelium and the process of spermatogenesis (Eskild & Hansson, 1994). Finally, the demonstration of PDE5 expression in both mature and differentiating rat peritubular cells (Scipioni et al., 2005) allows to suggest that in mammals this enzyme might play key roles in the acquisition and maintenance of the myoid cell contractile phenotype and more generally in the testis maturation.

4.2 Hydrolysis of cGMP and cAMP in Leydig cells

A few studies have suggested that administration of PDE5 inhibitors and in particular sildenafil and vardenafil in infertile men has either positive effects or lack of effects on the standard parameters of semen analysis (Dimitriadis et al., 2010). Leydig cells express PDE5 (Scipioni et al., 2005). Dimitriadis et al., (2010) investigated the effects of PDE5 inhibitors on Leydig cellular secretory function and on the standard parameters of semen analysis. The authors evaluated peripheral serum levels of Insl3 in patients with oligoasthenospermia prior to and after PDE5 administration. They reported that either sildenafil or vardenafil enhanced Leydig cell secretory function since serum Insl3 profiles were significantly larger after PDE5 inhibitor administration compared with Insl3 levels prior to administration of PDE5 inhibitors. Moreover the investigators have suggested that an increase in Leydig cell secretory function may contribute to the improvement in sperm parameters observed after administration of PDE5 inhibitors. An enhanced Leydig cell secretory function may result in a more optimal biochemical microenvironment within the seminiferous tubuli of oligoasthenospermic men stimulating spermatogenesis. In addition, an enhanced Leydig cell secretory function increasing probably intraepididymal testosterone concentrations may improve the epididymal sperm maturation process in oligoasthenospermic men increasing sperm motility (Dimitriadis et al., 2010). Additionally, it has been demonstrated that cAMP is the major intracellular messenger for LH action on steroidogenesis and that most, if not all, of the signaling action of cAMP is due to cAMP-dependent protein kinase (PKA)-mediated effects on proteins regulating the steroid biosynthetic pathway (Saez, 1994; Stocco et al., 2005). Substantial evidence for the regulatory function of PDEs in Leydig cells has been reported. A small stimulatory effect of non-selective PDE inhibitors on testosterone release by primary Leydig cells has been reported (Catt & Dufau, 1973; Mendelson et al., 1975). These observations have indicated that one or more PDEs additional to PDE5 might be active in Leydig cells to modulate the intensity, duration, and perhaps the desensitization of the LH-stimulated hormonal response (Vasta et al., 2006). Moreover, Vasta et al., (2006) have reported that PDE8A is expressed in mouse Leydig cells and have provided evidence that it is one of the PDEs that participates in the regulation of steroid production (Vasta et al., 2006). Although some biochemical, pharmacological, and genetic characteristics of PDE8A have been elucidated, its biological functions still remain largely unknown (Fisher et al., 1998; Soderling et al., 1998). Northern analysis has shown that PDE8A mRNA is highly expressed in testis (Soderling et al., 1998). The expression of PDE8A protein has been also reported for human CD4 T cells (Glavas et al., 2001) and mouse spermatozoa (Baxendale & Fraser, 2005). Vasta et al., (2006) have suggested that this enzyme plays an important role in setting the sensitivity to LH for testosterone production (Vasta et al., 2006).

4.3 Hydrolysis of cGMP in Sertoli cells

PDE5 inhibitors may also have a beneficial effect on Sertoli cell secretory function. Dimitriadis et al., (2011) evaluated the effect of vardenafil on Sertoli cell secretory function in obstructed azoospermic men and in non-obstructed azoospermic men who had had previously negative results in one or more trials of assisted reproduction technology (using frozen/thawed spermatozoa aspirated from the tail of the epididymis). The investigators showed that within the group of the obstructed azoospermic men, androgen-binding protein activity profiles (i.e., a marker of Sertoli cell secretory function) in the testicular cytosols, head epididymal-fluid samples, body epididymal-fluid samples and tail epididymal-fluid samples were significantly larger after vardenafil treatment than prior to vardenafil treatment. Likewise, within the group of the non-obstructed azoospermic men, androgen-binding protein activity profiles in testicular cytosols, epididymal head- fluid samples, epididymal body- fluid samples, and epididymal tail- fluid samples were significantly larger after vardenafil treatment than prior to vardenafil administration. Hence it appears that vardenafil administration enhances Sertoli cell secretory function both in obstructed azoospermic men and non-obstructed azoospermic men. Considering that PDE5 has not been demonstrated in Sertoli cells of several evaluated species, the increase of Sertoli cell secretory function after PDE5 inhibitors may be attributed to a positive action of inhibitors on Leydig cell secretory function or peritubular cells that subsequently enhance Sertoli cell secretory function.

Scipioni et al., (2005) could not detect any PDE5 expression in Sertoli cells in their experiments (Scipioni et al., 2005) suggesting that different PDEs are likely to contribute to the cGMP metabolism. Indeed, in Sertoli cells cGMP hydrolysis has been shown to occur in a calcium-calmodulin stimulated manner (Conti et al., 1982; Rossi et al., 1985; Conti et al., 1995) which identifies this hydrolytic activity as a result of a PDE1 family member. Enzymes of this family, though active towards both cAMP and cGMP, display a substantially higher affinity to the latter nucleotide (Zhao et al., 1997). PDE3 and PDE4 have been localized to Sertoli cells (Geremia et al., 1982; Morena et al., 1995).

5. Hydrolysis of cGMP and effects of PDE5 inhibitors on male accessory genital glands

5.1 Epididymis

Disturbances of the contractile activity in the epididymis have not yet been described (Ricker, 1998; Mewe et al., 2006). Concerning the contractility of the vas deferens, male infertility has already been described in a mouse model with disturbances in the contractile activity of the vas deferens (Mulryan et al., 2000).

The regulatory mechanisms responsible for the contraction and relaxation processes and thus for the transport of immotile spermatozoa through the epididymis are poorly understood. It has been shown that the messenger molecule cGMP, known to elicit smooth muscle relaxation, plays a crucial role in the regulation of contractility of the epididymal duct (Mewe et al., 2006). As it can be extrapolated from contractility studies and analyses of GC-B-knockouts (Tamura et al., 2004), differentiated cGMP-dependent relaxation processes appear to be fundamental to enable the transport and maturation of spermatozoa in the epididymis. As we have previously mentioned the second messenger cGMP can be generated in the male reproductive tract by different pathways involving either soluble (cytosolic) or particulate (plasma membrane-localized) GC activities (Lucas et al., 2000).

Mewe et al., (2006) using muscular tension recording and patch-clamp techniques analyzed the mechanisms underlying spontaneous phasic contractions (SCs) of the bovine epididymal duct (Glover & Nicander, 1971). SCs were demonstrated in the caput, the corpus and the proximal cauda region and found to be predominantly myogenic in origin. Removal of the luminal fluid induced a burst-like contraction pattern, and removal of the epithelium resulted in a complete loss of SC. Influx of extracellular Ca^{2+} through 'L-type' Ca^{2+} channels, but not Ca^{2+} release from intracellular stores was shown to be crucial for maintaining SCs (Mewe et al., 2006).

The functional role of cGMP-signaling in modulating SC in the bovine epididymal caput and corpus region has been examined by muscular tension recording, and immunological and autoradiographic techniques (Mewe et al., 2006). The cGMP-analogue 8-Br-cGMP, the NO donor SNP and the natriuretic peptides ANP and CNP have displayed distally increasing SC-relaxant effects (Mewe et al., 2006). Consistently a distally increasing epididymal expression of endothelial nitric oxide synthase (eNOS), GC-A, and PKG I has been found. Immunoreactivity for eNOS, sGC and PKG I is localized to the epididymal muscular cells (Mewe et al., 2006). The SC-relevant action of NO, ANP, and CNP is cGMP-dependent, and the action of 8-Br-cGMP, in turn, is modified by epithelial and luminal factors. The nitric oxide synthase (NOS) inhibitor L-NAME causes an increase in SC frequency. The SC-regulatory effect of 8-Br-cGMP was clearly reduced by the PKG inhibitor Rp-8-Br-cGMPS as well as by iberiotoxin, thapsigargin and indomethacin, pointing to PKG as main SC-relevant target of cGMP, and suggesting that large-conductance calcium-activated $K^{(+)}$ channels, the sarcoplasmic-endoplasmic reticulum Ca^{+}-ATPase, and cyclooxygenase-1 are possible targets of PKG (Mewe et al., 2006). These data support an essential role of cGMP signaling in the control of epididymal peristalsis allowing sperm transport and maturation (Mewe et al., 2006). Moreover, in the same study it has been suggested that phosphodiesterases also play a role in the epididymal peristalsis (Mewe et al., 2006) since as contraction-relevant target of cGMP in smooth muscle, the cGMP-inhibited cAMP-degrading PDE3 has been proposed (Lucas et al., 2000). Mewe et al., (2006) have found an SC-modulatory effect of the specific inhibitor of this cGMP-dependent PDE, milrinone, in the corpus of epididymis (Mewe et al., 2006).

On the other hand, Dimitriadis et al., (2011) evaluated the effects of the PDE5 inhibitor vardenafil administration (10 mg daily for at least 45 days) on male epididymal secretory function. Vardenafil has not influenced the secretory function of epididymis (Dimitriadis et al., 2011). Additionally, Dimitriadis et al., (2011) investigated the effects of sildenafil (50mg) on epididymal secretory function (Dimitriadis et al., 2011). A group of oligozoospermic infertile men provided three semen samples prior to sildenafil administration and three semen samples after sildenafil administration (50mg). The investigators evaluated the semen levels of α-glucosidase as a marker of the epididymal secretory function prior to and after sildenafil treatment and found absence of significant difference (Dimitriadis et al., 2011).

5.2 Vas deferens

Anatomical and physiological findings suggest a role for the nitric oxide/cGMP (NO/cGMP) phosphodiesterase signaling pathway in the modulation of ejaculation. Several studies have suggested that sildenafil could act beneficially in the alleviation of premature ejaculation (Abdel-Hamid, 2004). Chen et al., (2003) have shown that in patients with premature ejaculation, sildenafil plus paroxetine have a significantly higher therapeutic success rate (98%) than paroxetine alone (42%) (Chen et al., 2003). The inhibitory effect of sildenafil on PDE5, the destructive enzyme of cGMP, increases the level of cGMP in the vas deferens muscular fibers achieving the relaxation of the smooth muscle cells in vas deferens. This prolongs the time necessary for the achievement of ejaculation.

Studies with human erythrocytes have shown that the organic anionic pump which transports cGMP to extracellular area is dependent on a) ATP, b) its hydrolysis, and on c) the stimulation of ATPase activity by the cGMP itself (Sundkvist et al., 2002). PDE inhibitors block this transport. Sildenafil inhibiting PDE5 increases cGMP in the vas deferens muscular fibers and additionally blocks the activity of this organic anion pump. The overall result is an increase in the intracellular cGMP by a) prevention of the destruction of cGMP and b) inhibition of cGMP extracellular export (Sundkvist et al., 2002).

It has been suggested that sildenafil activates the opening of prejunctional potassium channels to reduce adrenergic neurotransmission by using NO-independent mechanisms (Medina et al., 2000). If this is true, this sildenafil induced reduction in adrenergic neurotransmission in smooth muscular fibers may alter the adrenergic tone in vas deferens muscular fiber and may reduce its pattern of contraction. Studies have demonstrated the expression of PDE5 in vas deferens (Bilge et al., 2005).

5.3 Seminal vesicles

Dimitriadis et al., (2008) reported the effects of sildenafil on seminal vesicular function. Three semen samples were collected from a group of 13 oligozoospermic infertile men prior to and after sildenafil treatment (50 mg). The authors evaluated seminal fructose as a marker of the seminal vesicular function and they found no significant difference (Dimitriadis et al., 2008) in seminal fructose profiles between samples collected prior to sildenafil and after sildenafil therapy.

In addition the effects of another PDE5 inhibitor namely vardenafil on seminal vesicular function has been evaluated (Dimitriadis et al., 2008). Eighteen infertile men participating in an assisted reproduction program were treated daily with vardenafil (10 mg every day) for at least 45 days. All these men had previously undergone at least one in vitro fertilization trial without success. Prior to and after the vardenafil-treatment six semen samples from each man were collected. The investigators showed that administration of vardenafil resulted in no significant difference in the secretory function of seminal vesicles (as measured by the fructose concentration in the seminal plasma) (Dimitriadis et al., 2008). This finding is consistent with the observation that there are no reports in the literature supporting the presence of PDE5 in seminal vesicles.

5.4 Prostate

Citrate, the major anion of human seminal fluid is important for maintaining the osmotic equilibrium of the seminal plasma and is secreted by the prostate (Ponchietti et al., 1984). A zinc compound (probably a salt) is a potent antibacterial factor which is excreted from the human prostate providing for the high content of zinc in the sperm nucleus and contributes to the stability of the quaternary structure of the sperm nucleus chromatin (Fair et al., 1973). Spermine, a substance in seminal fluid, secreted by the prostate, is correlated with the sperm motility. Semen cholesterol content is synthesized in human prostate and is important for stabilizing the sperm membrane against temperature and environmental shock (Meares, 1991). All the above substances having beneficial effects on sperm quality are secreted by the prostate and their secretions are up-regulated by either sildenafil (Dimitriadis et al., 2008) or vardenafil (Dimitriadis et al., 2008).

Nitric oxide synthase has been localized biochemically and immunohistochemically in both the transitional and peripheral zones of the human prostate (Burnett et al., 1995). Specifically NOS has been found in the nerve fibres and ganglia located in the prostatic smooth musculature indicating that NO is important for the prostatic smooth muscular function (Takeda et al., 1995). This is supported by the action of NO donors which have been shown to mediate relaxation of human prostatic smooth muscle in vitro (Takeda et al., 1995).

PDE4 and PDE5 have been demonstrated immunohistochemically in the prostatic transitional zone (Uckert et al., 2001). In vitro sildenafil and rolipram, a PDE4 inhibitor, have been shown to reverse tension in prostatic smooth muscle strips from the transitional zone (Uckert et al., 2001). This information could lead to further investigations aiming to recruit PDE4 inhibitors and PDE5 inhibitors to the pharmacologic management of benign prostatic hyperplasia (Uckert et al., 2001). Furthermore PDE5 inhibitors may have some beneficial effects in patients with chronic prostatitis. Grimsley et al., (2007) postulated that PDE5 inhibitors relax prostatic smooth muscular fibers altering the retrograde urinary flow in prostatic ducts allowing greater washout of the ducts and reducing accumulation of irritative urinary contents. The final result may be a reduction of the prostatic inflammation.

Moreover, previous reports have shown that human PDE11 and particularly its splice variant PDE11A4 is abundantly expressed in the prostate, suggesting that the PDE11A gene undergoes tissue-specific alternative splicing that generates structurally distinct gene products (Yuasa et al., 2001; Loughney et al., 2005).

6. The influence of PDE5 inhibitors on standard parameters of semen analysis

6.1 The development of in vivo studies

The influence of PDE inhibitors on the sperm parameters has been investigated by several authors. The positive effect of the PDE inhibition on sperm motility may suggest an association between the intracellular levels of cAMP or cGMP and the sperm ability to move (Sikka & Hellstrom, 1991; Fisch et al., 1998). However the majority of studies evaluating the effects of PDE inhibitors on spermatozoa have employed non-selective PDE inhibitors. Only few of the above studies have employed a selective PDE5 inhibitor such as sildenafil, vardenafil, or tadalafil.

Many chemical molecules have been studied to evaluate their effects on human sperm functions. Methylxanthines (Tesarik et al., 1992; Tournaye et al., 1995) belong to the first generation of PDE inhibitors and represent a chemical group of drugs derived from xanthine (a purine derivative) including among others: theophylline, caffeine, and pentoxifylline. Their beneficial effects on sperm motility has been recognized since 1970 (Haesungcharern & Chulavatnatol, 1973; Schill, 1975; De Turner et al., 1978; Schill et al., 1979). Jaiswal and Majumder (1996) in an in vitro study investigated the role of theophylline demonstrating that this PDE inhibitor markedly increased (10-fold or greater) the motility of goat spermatozoa derived from proximal corpus, mid-corpus, distal-corpus, and proximal-cauda epididymes. In another in vitro study caffeine has been also shown to increase sperm motility and metabolism when it has been added into the semen (Levin et al., 1981; Rees et al., 1990). However this compound promotes the spontaneous sperm acrosomal reactions. This effect of caffeine on sperm acrosomal cup counteracts the benefits from its role as a motility stimulant (Tesarik et al., 1992). Pentoxifylline (PTX), is the most widely non-selective PDE inhibitor that has been used in assisted reproductive technology programs (Wang et al., 1983; Marrama et al., 1985; Shen et al., 1991; Tesarik et al., 1992; Fuse et al., 1993; Pang et al., 1993; Tournaye et al., 1994). Although its beneficial effect on the outcome of IVF trials in normozoospermic subjects and oligo-asthenozoospermic patients is well documented (Yovich et al., 1988; Yovich et al., 1990; Tasdemir et al., 1993; Yunes et al., 2005) the efficacy of its oral administration to increase sperm fertilizing ability is controversial (Tournaye et al., 1994). PTX has been considered to stimulate flagellar motility by increasing sperm intracellular cAMP (Stefanovich, 1973; Garbers & Kopf, 1980; Tash & Means, 1983; Ward & Clissold, 1987) as well as by reducing sperm intracellular superoxide anion and reactive oxygen species known to damage DNA (Lopes et al., 1998; Twigg et al., 1998). In particular PTX in both in vivo and in vitro studies, appears to increase significantly beat cross frequency, curvilinear velocity, and the percentage of hyperactivated spermatozoa (Rees et al., 1990; Shen et al., 1991; Tesarik et al., 1992; Lewis et al., 1993; Moohan et al., 1993; Pang et al., 1993; Tournaye et al., 1994; Centola et al., 1995; Paul et al., 1996; Nassar et al., 1999).

It should be mentioned that PDE4 inhibitors, as well, increase sperm motility. As it has been demonstrated in an in vitro study (Fisch et al., 1998), PDE4 inhibitors do not have an obvious effect on the sperm acrosome reaction. On the other hand PDE1 inhibitors seem to selectively stimulate the acrosome reaction (Fisch et al., 1998).

In a double-blinded, four-period, two-way, crossover study encompassing 17 sexually healthy male volunteers, Purvis et al., (2002) examined the effect of sildenafil on sperm motility and morphology parameters. The authors compared an 100-mg dose of sildenafil with placebo. Both sildenafil and placebo were administered as single oral doses for two periods separated by a washout period of at least 5–7 days. The authors reported a lack of influence of sildenafil on sperm motility. The authors observed no significant differences between the sildenafil group and the placebo group for the percentage of motile spermatozoa, the percentage of static spermatozoa, the percentage of rapidly moving spermatozoa, and the percentage of progressively moving spermatozoa. Mean values of sperm count, morphology, and viability, as well as seminal plasma volume and viscosity were not significantly different between the placebo group and the control group.

The above study by Purvis et al., (2002) has confirmed earlier findings published by Aversa et al., (2000). The authors have conducted a prospective double-blind, placebo-controlled, cross-over, two-period-investigation study, embracing 20 male subjects, which were treated with sildenafil or placebo. After a washout period of seven days all subjects were crossed over to receive the alternative treatment. The authors found no statistically significant differences in the mean values of sperm number, sperm motility, and percentage of morphologically abnormal spermatozoa between the two groups. In that study the investigators emphasized the potential usage of sildenafil in assisted reproductive programs when a temporary erectile dysfunction may occur due to the stress and the psychological pressure for semen production. The last suggestion had been expressed earlier by Tur-Kaspa et al., (1999) who reported their experience on the usage of sildenafil in men with proven erectile dysfunction during assisted reproductive technologies cycles. It appears that the stress and psychological pressure for semen collection becomes larger if more than one semen samples are necessary during the day of oocyte pick-up.

In contrast to the above study by Aversa et al., (2000) a positive effect of sildenafil on some sperm motility parameters was proven in another study. In a prospective double-blind, placebo-controlled, crossover, two-period-administration, clinical investigation, du Plessis et al., (2004) determined the effect of in vivo sildenafil citrate administration on semen parameters and sperm function. Twenty healthy male subjects randomly were asked to ingest a single dose of 50-mg of sildenafil or placebo. The authors reported no significant differences in the percentage of spermatozoa with progressive motility and in the sperm track velocity, sperm amplitude of lateral head displacement, sperm beat cross frequency, sperm straightness, and sperm linearity between the sildenafil treated group and the placebo group. However borderline statistically significant differences were observed in sperm smoothed path velocity and sperm straight-line velocity. In addition there was a statistically significant increase in the percentage of rapidly moving spermatozoa after sildenafil administration.

In an open-label pilot study, Jannini et al., (2004) investigated the effect of 50-mg orally administered sildenafil in a group of sexually healthy men who participated in an intrauterine artificial insemination program or planned sexual intercourses to perform a post-coital test. The authors found no effect of sildenafil administration on sperm motility, on the sperm concentration, or on the total number of spermatozoa ejaculated. Similarly no effect of sildenafil administration was demonstrated on the percentage of non-linear progressive motile spermatozoa. However, a significant increase was seen in the linear progressive motility after sildenafil administration. The authors have additionally suggested that the administration of sildenafil prior to semen collection in ART programs reduces the stress that is experienced by the male in the ejaculation room. Similar conclusions have been raised by the same group of authors in an earlier study (Lenzi et al., 2003). In that earlier study the authors noted that sildenafil is effective in increasing compliance of male patients facing infertile couple management procedures, and also in improving cervical mucus sperm penetration assay (Lenzi et al., 2003).

Evaluation of the effects of sildenafil on semen quality has been the aim of a study conducted by Dimitriadis et al., (2008). The authors found that the mean values of total sperm count, percentage of motile spermatozoa and seminal plasma citrate levels were significantly larger in semen samples collected after sildenafil administration compared with semen samples collected prior to usage of sildenafil (Dimitriadis et al., 2008). The authors have suggested that the increase in prostatic secretory function after administration of sildenafil provides an explanation for the enhanced sperm motility. This is consistent with other reports that have demonstrated that secretory dysfunction of the male accessory genital glands due to prostatic infections impairs male fertility potential (Sofikitis & Miyagawa, 1991). The seminal fluid may contain factors that are not absolutely essential to fertilization (Portnoy, 1946). However, optimal concentrations of prostatic secretory markers may provide an environment ideal for sperm motility and transport (Sofikitis & Miyagawa, 1993). The increase in the prostate secretory function, sperm motility, and total sperm count in the study by Dimitriadis and co-workers (Dimitriadis et al., 2008) may be attributable to the higher sexual satisfaction observed in samples collected after sildenafil treatment. The importance of the positive effects of sexual satisfaction and orgasm on the semen quality and sperm fertilizing capacity have been emphasized in another study comparing masturbation with videotaped sexual images and masturbation without videotaped sexual images. Masturbation with videotaped sexual images resulted in recovery of spermatozoa of greater fertilizing potential (Yamamoto et al., 2000). In addition in a similar report Sofikitis and Miyagawa (1993) demonstrated improved spermatozoal motility in the semen samples collected via sexual intercourse versus masturbation in infertile men. Sofikitis and Miyagawa (1993) have suggested that the higher the sexual stimulation is, the larger the prostatic secretory function is and the larger the vas deferens loading during ejaculation is. The latter suggestion is supported by a study showing that restraint of bulls or false mounts prior to semen collection increases the number of motile spermatozoa by as much as 50% (Salisbury & Vandermark, 1961). Furthermore in bulls, it has been suggested that oxytocin and prostaglandin F2a may be at least partly responsible for the improvement of the ejaculate after sexual stimulation (Hafs et al., 1962; Sharma & Hays, 1973).

Few other studies support the findings of the above investigation by Dimitriadis et al., (2008). Ali et al., (2007) administered 100-mg sildenafil citrate in diabetic neuropathic patients. The authors found that sperm motility and semen volume were increased in men treated with sildenafil. On the other hand sperm morphology remained unaffected. In addition the authors have proposed that sildenafil administration is associated with an improvement in the entire smooth musculature architecture of the male reproductive and urinary tract which has been altered due to neuropathy. Sildenafil administration resulted in reduction in the excessive accumulation of interstitial collagen and calcification in the smooth muscles which leaded to bladder atonia in the diabetic men. On the other hand the authors have noticed that long time sildenafil treatment is associated with a significant decrease in total sperm output and sperm concentration.

Pomara et al., (2007) performed a prospective, double-blind, randomized, crossover study describing the acute effect of both sildenafil (50 mg) and tadalafil (20 mg) in young infertile men. Eighteen young infertile men were asked to ingest a single dose of either sildenafil or tadalafil in a blind, randomized order. Semen samples were collected one or two hours after the administration of each PDE-5 inhibitor. The authors reported a significant increase in sperm progressive motility in semen samples collected after sildenafil administration compared with semen samples collected prior to sildenafil administration. The authors have suggested that the stimulatory effect of sildenafil on sperm motility may be due to a direct action of sildenafil on sperm mitochondria and calcium channels. Another report (Nomura & Vacquier, 2006) has demonstrated that PDE5A is localized mainly on sea urchin sperm flagella regulating intracellular cGMP levels. Thus a direct effect of sildenafil on sperm flagella cannot be ruled out (Nomura & Vacquier, 2006). Interestingly, the study by Pomara et al., (2007) revealed a significant decrease in the sperm motility after a single dose of tadalafil (Pomara et al., 2007). These latter findings are inconsistent with an earlier study conducted by Hellstrom and colleagues (2003) who investigated the effects of tadalafil on semen characteristics and serum concentrations of reproductive hormones in healthy men and men with mild erectile dysfunction. Hellstrom et al., (2003) performed two randomized, double-blind, placebo controlled, parallel group studies (one study for a 10-mg dose tadalafil and one study for a 20-mg dose tadalafil) enrolling 204 subjects in the 10 mg tadalafil-study and 217 subjects in the 20-mg tadalafil-study. The investigators assessed the effect of daily tadalafil or placebo administration for six months on semen samples and serum levels of reproductive hormones (testosterone, luteinizing hormone, and follicle-stimulating hormone). The investigators demonstrated that in each study the proportion of participants with a 50% or greater decrease in sperm concentration was relatively small and similar for the placebo group and the 10 mg-tadalafil group or the 20 mg-tadalafil group. Similarly there were no significant alterations in sperm morphology or sperm motility after treatment with 10 mg or 20 mg tadalafil. In addition, the authors demonstrated that there were no significant alterations in the serum levels of reproductive hormones after tadalafil administration concluding that administration of tadalafil at doses of 10 mg and 20 mg for six months did not adversely affect testicular spermatogenesis process or serum levels of reproductive hormones. However other investigators have emphasized their dilemma concerning the administration of tadalafil on a daily basis, as they believe that up today the available data confirming the safety of tadalafil administered on a daily basis are not yet adequate (Pomara et al., 2007). Taking in consideration the above dilemma Hellstrom et al., (2008) expanded their investigation efforts in a double-blind, placebo-controlled, noninferiority study, assessing the effects of tadalafil (20mg) on spermatogenesis over three spermatogenesis cycles in men elder than 45-year-old. The investigators demonstrated no deleterious effects of 9-month daily tadalafil (20mg) administration on spermatogenesis.

Bauer et al., (2002) performed a randomized, placebo control, double-blind, crossover study to determine the effects of a single dose of vardenafil (20 mg) on sperm parameters. Sixteen healthy males participated in this study. The scientists found no statistically significant effects of vardenafil on sperm motility, sperm concentration, sperm viability, and sperm morphology.

In another study, Dimitriadis et al., (2008) evaluated the effects of vardenafil administration (10 mg) on semen quality. The investigators noted that semen samples from infertile men treated with 10 mg of vardenafil presented a significantly larger total number of spermatozoa, quantitative sperm motility, qualitative sperm motility, and percentage of morphologically normal spermatozoa compared with semen samples collected prior to vardenafil administration from the same individuals. The authors suggested that vardenafil stimulated the prostatic secretory function due to an enhanced sexual stimulation increasing the quantitative and qualitative motility of spermatozoa and decreasing sperm abnormalities.

Jarvi et al., (2008) performed a randomized, double-blind, placebo controlled, parallel group, multicenter study investigating the effect of vardenafil and sildenafil on sperm characteristics. A total of 200 men with or without erectile dysfunction, able to produce semen samples without therapy for erectile dysfunction, 25 to 64 years old, were randomized to daily treatment with vardenafil, sildenafil or placebo for 6 months. Vardenafil or sildenafil had no effect vs. placebo on the percentage of patients with 50% or greater decrease in sperm concentration (Jarvi et al., 2008). Additionally, vardenafil or sildenafil did not affect any sperm parameters or peripheral serum gonadotropin profiles (Jarvi et al., 2008).

6.2 The development of in vitro studies

After the introduction of sildenafil in the market, several studies have evaluated the in vitro effects of this compound on sperm parameters. Burger et al., (2000) in an ex vivo study investigated the effect of sildenafil on the motility and viability of human spermatozoa. The above spermatozoal parameters were evaluated in sperm samples of both healthy donors (n=6) and clinically infertile men (n=6). Separate sperm aliquots were incubated for 0 h, 1 h and 3 h in the absence or presence of sildenafil (125 ng/mL, 250 ng/mL, and 750 ng/mL), PTX (as a positive control), or Ham's medium (as a reagent control). The authors have reported no statistically significant effect of sildenafil on sperm viability, sperm motility, and sperm forward progression after incubation of spermatozoa with various doses of sildenafil.

Similarly, in another study, the group of Andrade et al., (2000) attempted to evaluate a direct effect of sildenafil or phentolamine on sperm motility. Using samples of either unwashed or washed spermatozoa, the investigators added directly to the sperm samples sildenafil at a concentration of 20 mg/mL or phentolamine in various doses and incubated the samples for 30 minutes. The authors demonstrated a dose-related inhibition of sperm motility in sperm samples treated with phentolamine, whereas sildenafil (at a concentration of 200 μg/mL) did not adversely affect sperm motility either in unwashed or washed sperm. In contrast the highest dose of sildenafil (2000 μg/mL) reduced the sperm motility approximately at a level of 50% of the original value. However, it should be emphasized that at this concentration sildenafil caused a marked acidification of the medium which may be the reason for the reduced sperm motility (Su & Vacquier, 2006).

In an experimental study Su and Vacquier (2006) cloned and characterized a sea urchin spermatozoal PDE (suPDE5) which is an ortholog of human PDE5. The authors have found that phospho-suPDE5 localizes mainly on sperm flagella and that the PDE5 phosphorylation increases when spermatozoa contact the jelly layer that surrounds the eggs. Since the in vitro dephosphorylation of suPDE5 decreases its activity, the authors have suggested that PDE5 inhibitors such as sildenafil may inhibit the activity of suPDE5 and increase sperm motility.

A concentration-dependent stimulatory effect of sildenafil on sperm motility was also demonstrated by Mostafa (2007) when 85 semen specimens from asthenozoospermic patients were exposed to different concentrations of sildenafil (4.0 mg/mL, 2.0 mg/mL, 1.0 mg/mL, 0.5 mg/mL, and 0.1 mg/mL). However, the evaluation of sperm motility in that study was performed 3 hours only after the spermatozoal exposure to sildenafil.

Lefièvre et al., (2000) have investigated whether PDE5 is present in human spermatozoa and whether sildenafil affects sperm function. The authors have demonstrated that this PDE5 inhibitor stimulates human sperm motility with an increase in intracellular cAMP suggesting an inhibitory action on a PDE that is different to PDE5.

Cuadra et al., (2000) evaluated the effect of sildenafil on sperm motility. Spermatozoa were exposed to sildenafil at either 0 nmol/L, 0.4 nmol/L, 4.0 nmol/L, or 40 nmol/L. The investigators observed increased sperm motility parameters in the presence of 0.4 nmol/L sildenafil compared with the control sample four hours after the exposure to sildenafil. However, the motility parameters decreased 48 hours after the exposure to sildenafil. Spermatozoa exposed to higher concentration of sildenafil (40 nmol/L) showed decreased sperm motility parameters. cGMP regulates calcium entry into microdomains along the sperm flagellum affecting sperm motility. Since PDE5 hydrolyzes cGMP, the authors have suggested that inhibition of PDE5 by sildenafil citrate enhances the effects of cGMP on sperm motility. The data provided by the authors (Cuadra et al., 2000) suggest that there is a stimulatory effect on sperm motility when PDE5 is moderately inhibited; however, extensive inhibition of PDE5 appears to lead to decreased sperm motility.

Another group of researchers (Glenn et al., 2007) attempted to determine the influence of sildenafil on sperm motility. Semen samples from 57 unselected men with asthenozoospermic profiles were prepared and then exposed to 0.67 µmol/L of sildenafil which is equivalent to the plasma concentration of sildenafil, one hour after oral ingestion of 100 mg of sildenafil (Glenn et al., 2007). The authors found that both the number and the velocity of progressively motile spermatozoa were significantly increased. The investigators have suggested that the elevated levels of cGMP, attributable to the inhibitory effect of sildenafil, may affect calcium transport into spermatozoa which potentially affects the sperm motion.

The effects of tadalafil on human sperm motility in vitro have been investigated. Mostafa (2007) assessed the effects of tadalafil on human sperm motility in 70 asthenozoospermic semen specimens. The semen samples were exposed to three different concentrations of tadalafil (4.0, 1.0, 0.5 mg/mL) and it was found that sperm samples treated with 4 mg/mL tadalafil solution demonstrated a significant decrease in sperm motility compared with the control samples. On the other hand, sperm samples treated with 1.0 or 0.5 mg/mL tadalafil solution demonstrated a significant increase in sperm progressive forward motility. The authors have suggested that the concentration of tadalafil is an important factor in such studies.

Alternatively, the effect of tadalafil on sperm motility may be related additionally to the inhibitory effect of this compound on PDE11. In fact, PDE11 is highly expressed in the testis, prostate, and developing sperm cells even if its physiological role is not known (Table 1). Wayman et al., (2005) in an effort to investigate the role of PDE11 in spermatozoa physiology, retrieved spermatozoa from PDE11 knockout mice (PDE11-/-). The authors found a reduced sperm concentration, decreased forward motility, and lower percentage of alive spermatozoa in the latter animals which suggest a role for PDE11 in spermatogenesis and fertilization potential.

Taken together the results of the above ex vivo studies, we may postulate a dose dependent effect of sildenafil and tadalafil on sperm motility. In fact this effect seems to be enhanced at low doses of PDE5 inhibitors but it may be reduced at high concentrations. Definitely further investigations are required to evaluate the mechanisms mediating the effects of PDE5 selective inhibitors on sperm motility.

7. The effect of PDE5 inhibitors on sperm capacitation and acrosome reaction process

Lefièvre et al., (2000) investigated the potential effect of PDE5 inhibitor sildenafil on spermatozoal ability to undergo capacitation process. The authors showed that sildenafil at 30 µmol/L, 100 µmol/L, and 200 µmol/L triggered the capacitation process of washed spermatozoa. Capacitated spermatozoa underwent an acrosome reaction when challenged with lysophosphatidylcholine (LPC) alone or LPC plus IBMX (a non selective PDE inhibitor), but not with sildenafil alone. The authors have suggested that PDE inhibitors by themselves cannot initiate the acrosome reaction nor can they potentiate the acrosome reaction of capacitated spermatozoa.

Cuadra et al., (2000) investigated the effect of sildenafil on sperm acrosomal reaction. Spermatozoa were exposed to different doses of sildenafil (from 0 nmol/L to 40 nmol/L). The authors reported that sildenafil affected the sperm acrosomal reaction with an increase in the percentage of acrosomally reacted spermatozoa of almost 50% compared to the control samples. It is known that cGMP directly opens cyclic nucleotide-gated channels for calcium entry into the spermatozoa initiating the acrosome reaction (Biel et al., 1998). Since PDE5 hydrolyzes cGMP, inhibition of PDE5 by sildenafil citrate enhances the effects of cGMP on sperm acrosome reaction.

Glenn et al., (2007) evaluated the influence of sildenafil on sperm acrosomal reaction. The study included fifty-seven unselected men with asthenozoospermic profiles who provided semen samples which were further processed for sperm isolation. Then spermatozoa were exposed to 0.67 µmol/L of sildenafil. The investigators (Glenn et al., 2007) noticed that sildenafil caused a significant increase in the proportion of acrosome-reacted spermatozoa. In a case report, sildenafil was administered for semen collection for ART purposes. The investigators failed to fertilize oocytes despite the intracytoplasmic injection of the sperm (Tur-Kaspa et al., 1999). Although this fertilization failure was attributed to the advanced age of oocytes due to the delay in obtaining the semen sample, a deleterious effect of sildenafil on spermatozoal function can not be excluded.

8. The effects of PDE5 inhibitors on sperm functional assays

Several studies have evaluated the in vitro effects of PDE5 inhibitors on sperm functional assays. Burger et al., (2000) performed an in vitro study investigating and comparing the effects of sildenafil on the membrane integrity, and functional sperm capacity between healthy donors and clinically infertile men. The authors noted a marked decrease of sperm membrane integrity in spermatozoa of infertile patients treated with sildenafil (Burger et al., 2000). This observation may be taken into consideration when treatment with sildenafil is planed in subfertile couples with a male factor infertility (Burger et al., 2000). However, sperm penetration assay data has suggested that there is neither a beneficial nor a detrimental effect of sildenafil on its outcome (Burger et al., 2000).

9. Conclusions

The expression of PDEs has been documented in several regions of the male reproductive tract. Increasing evidence based on several studies tend to suggest that PDE5 inhibitors may have a therapeutic effect in some disorders of semen parameters. Moreover, PDE5 inhibitors may promote sperm capacitation process. In addition PDE5 inhibitors may affect sperm transfer through the male reproductive tract by affecting the contractility of the tunica albuginea and the epididymis. However, the current evidence needs further confirmation by additional studies that are necessary to suggest unequivocally a therapeutic role of PDE5 inhibitors in the management of defects in testicular or epididymal function.

<table>
<tr><th colspan="2">Type of cell/ Tissue</th><th>PDE</th><th>Species</th><th>Relative References</th></tr>
<tr><td colspan="2" rowspan="3">Testis</td><td>PDE5
PDE8A
PDE8B
PDE1A
PDE11A
PDE11A2
PDE11A3</td><td>Human</td><td>Foresta et al., (2008)
Baxendale et al., (2005)
Dousa et al., (1999)
Michibata et al., (2001)
Fawcett et al., (2000)
Kotera et al., (1999)
Yuasa et al., (2001)
D'Andrea et al., (2005)
Horvath et al., (2006)</td></tr>
<tr><td>PDE1A
PDE1B
PDE1C
PDE3B
PDE4A
PDE4B
PDE4C
PDE4D
PDE5A
PDE6γ′
PDE7A
PDE8A
PDE10A</td><td>Mouse</td><td>Baxendale et al., (2005)</td></tr>
<tr><td>PDE1C</td><td>Rat</td><td>Dousa (1999)</td></tr>
<tr><td colspan="5"></td></tr>
<tr><td rowspan="4">Germ cells</td><td rowspan="2"></td><td>PDE11A</td><td>Human</td><td>D'Andrea et al., (2005)</td></tr>
<tr><td>PDE1
PDE2</td><td>Rat</td><td>Swinnen et al., (1989)</td></tr>
<tr><td rowspan="2">Spermatogonia</td><td>PDE11</td><td>Human</td><td>Baxendale et al., (2001)</td></tr>
<tr><td>PDE11</td><td>Mouse</td><td>Baxendale et al., (2001)</td></tr>
</table>

Germ cells	**Spermatocytes**		PDE11	Human	Baxendale et al., (2001)
	Developing spermatocytes		PDE3B	Rat	Degerman et al.,(1997)
	Pachytene spermatocytes		PDE4D PDE4A PDE1C	Rat	Salanova et al., (1999) Yan et al., (2001)
	Spermatids		PDE11	Human	Baxendale et al., (2001)
			PDE11	Mouse	Baxendale et al., (2001)
			PDE4A	Rat	Farooqui et al., (2001)
		Round	PDE4A PDE4D	Rat	Salanova et al., (1999) Farooqui et al., (2001)
		Round~ Elongating	PDE1A PDE1C	Mouse	Yan et al., (2001)
		Elongating	PDE4D	Rat	Salanova et al., (1999)
	Spermatozoa		PDE1 PDE1A PDE3A PDE4 PDE5	Human	Fisch et al., (1998) Aversa et al., (2000) Lefievre et al., (2002)
			PDE6 PDE3B	Mouse	Baxendale et al., (2005)
		Acrosomal region/ head	PDE4D	Mouse	Baxendale et al., (2005)
		Flagellum	PDE1A PDE4D PDE10A	Mouse	Baxendale et al., (2005)
Sertoli cells			PDE3 PDE4	Rat	Swinnen et al., (1989)
			PDE4B	Rat	Farooqui et al., (2001)
			PDE4D	Rat	Levallet et al., (2007)
Peritubular myoid cells			PDE5	Rat	Scipioni et al., (2005)

Leydig cells		PDE11A	Human	D'Andrea et al., (2005)
		PDE4B	Rat	Farooqui et al., (2001)
		PDE5	Rat	Scipioni et al., (2005)
		PDE8A PDE11	Mouse	Vasta et al., (2006) Baxendale et al., (2001)
Vascular myocytes		PDE11	Human	Baxendale et al., (2001)
		PDE5	Rat	Scipioni et al., (2005)
		PDE11	Mouse	Baxendale et al., (2001)
Epididymis		PDE3	Bull	Mewe et al., (2006)
Vas Deferens		PDE5	Human Rabbit	Mancina et al., (2005)
Prostate		PDE4 PDE5A PDE11A4 PDE11A1	Human	Kotera et al., (1999) Yuasa et al., (2001) Fawcett et al., (2000) Uckert et al., (2001)
	Epithelial cells	PDE11A	Human	Loughney et al., (2005) D'Andrea et al., (2005)
	Endothelial cells	PDE11A	Human	D'Andrea et al., (2005)
	Smooth muscle cells	PDE11A	Human	D'Andrea et al., (2005)
Penis		PDE2 PDE3 PDE4 PDE5	Human	Milhoua et al., (2007)
	Corpus cavernosum	PDE1A PDE1B PDE1C PDE2A	Human	D'Andrea et al., (2005) Kuthe et al., (2001) Foresta et al., (2008)

Penis	**Corpus cavernosum**	PDE3A PDE4A PDE4B PDE4C PDE4D PDE5A PDE6 PDE7A PDE8A PDE9A PDE11A	Human	
	Endothelial cells	PDE11A	Human	D'Andrea et al., (2005) Kuthe et al., (2001) Foresta et al., (2008)
	Tunica Albuginea	PDE4 PDE5	Rat	Valente et al., (2003)

Table 1. Expression of phosphodiesterases PDEs in the male reproductive tract.

10. Abbreviations

AC = adenylate cyclase
ANP = atrial natriuretic peptide
ART = assisted reproductive technology
cAMP = cyclic adenosine monophosphate
cGMP = cyclic guanosine monophosphate
CNP = C-type natriuretic peptide
CO = carbon monoxide
eNOS = endothelial nitric oxide synthase
GC = guanylate cyclase
GC-B = membrane-bound GC
HO-1= heme oxygenase-1
ICSI = intracytoplasmic sperm injection
IVF = in vitro fertilization
LPC = lysophosphatidylcholine
NO = nitric oxide
NOS = nitric oxide synthase
PDEs = phosphodiesterases
PKA = protein kinase
PTX = pentoxifylline
SCs = spontaneous phasic contractions
sGC = soluble guanylate cyclase
SNP = sodium nitroprusside
suPDE5= sea urchin spermatozoal PDE

11. References

Abdel-Hamid, I.A. (2004). Phosphodiesterase 5 inhibitors in rapid ejaculation: potential use and possible mechanisms of action. *Drugs*, Vol. 64, No. 1, pp. 13-26, ISSN 0012-6667 (Print)

Ali, S.T. & Rakkah, N.I. (2007). Neurophysiological role of sildenafil citrate (Viagra) on seminal parameters in diabetic males with and without neuropathy. *Pak J Pharm Sci*, Vol. 20, No. 1, pp. 36-42

Anderson, R.A., Jr., Feathergill, K.A., et al. (1995). Atrial natriuretic peptide: a chemoattractant of human spermatozoa by a guanylate cyclase-dependent pathway. *Mol Reprod Dev*, Vol. 40, No. 3, pp. 371-378, ISSN 1040-452X (Print)

Andrade, J.R., Traboulsi, A., et al. (2000). In vitro effects of sildenafil and phentolamine, drugs used for erectile dysfunction, on human sperm motility. *Am J Obstet Gynecol*, Vol. 182, No. 5, pp. 1093-1095

Aversa, A., Mazzilli, F., et al. (2000). Effects of sildenafil (Viagra) administration on seminal parameters and post-ejaculatory refractory time in normal males. *Hum Reprod*, Vol. 15, No. 1, pp. 131-134

Bauer, R.J. & Rohde, G. (2002). A single oral dose of vardenafil had no acute effect on sperm motility in healthy males. 27th Annual Meeting of the American Society of Andrology. April 24-27, 2002. Seattle, Washington, USA. *J Androl*, Vol. Suppl, pp. 26, ISSN 0196-3635 (Print)

Baxendale, R., Burslem, F., et al. (2001). Phosphodiesterase type 11 (PDE11) cellular localisation: progress towards defining a physiological role in testis and/or reproduction. *J Urol*, Vol. 165 (suppl 5), pp. 340

Baxendale, R.W. & Fraser, L.R. (2005). Mammalian sperm phosphodiesterases and their involvement in receptor-mediated cell signaling important for capacitation. *Mol Reprod Dev*, Vol. 71, No. 4, pp. 495-508, ISSN 1040-452X (Print)

Bender, A.T. & Beavo, J.A. (2006). Cyclic nucleotide phosphodiesterases: molecular regulation to clinical use. *Pharmacol Rev*, Vol. 58, No. 3, pp. 488-520, ISSN 0031-6997 (Print)

Biel, M., Sautter, A., et al. (1998). Cyclic nucleotide-gated channels--mediators of NO:cGMP-regulated processes. *Naunyn Schmiedebergs Arch Pharmacol*, Vol. 358, No. 1, pp. 140-144, ISSN 0028-1298 (Print)

Bilge, S.S., Kesim, Y., et al. (2005). Possible role of sildenafil in inhibiting rat vas deferens contractions by influencing the purinergic system. *Int J Urol*, Vol. 12, No. 9, pp. 829-834, ISSN 0919-8172 (Print)

Burger, M., Sikka, S.C., et al. (2000). The effect of sildenafil on human sperm motion and function from normal and infertile men. *Int J Impot Res*, Vol. 12, No. 4, pp. 229-234

Burnett, A.L., Maguire, M.P., et al. (1995). Characterization and localization of nitric oxide synthase in the human prostate. *Urology*, Vol. 45, No. 3, pp. 435-439, ISSN 0090-4295 (Print)

Cameron, V.A. & Ellmers, L.J. (2003). Minireview: natriuretic peptides during development of the fetal heart and circulation. *Endocrinology*, Vol. 144, No. 6, pp. 2191-2194, ISSN 0013-7227 (Print)

Catt, K.J. & Dufau, M.L. (1973). Spare gonadotrophin receptors in rat testis. *Nat New Biol*, Vol. 244, No. 137, pp. 219-221, ISSN 0090-0028 (Print)

Centola, G.M., Cartie, R.J., et al. (1995). Differential responses of human sperm to varying concentrations of pentoxifylline with demonstration of toxicity. *J Androl*, Vol. 16, No. 2, pp. 136-142, ISSN 0196-3635 (Print)

Chen, J., Mabjeesh, N.J., et al. (2003). Efficacy of sildenafil as adjuvant therapy to selective serotonin reuptake inhibitor in alleviating premature ejaculation. *Urology*, Vol. 61, No. 1, pp. 197-200, ISSN 1527-9995 (Electronic)

Conti, M., Iona, S., et al. (1995). Characterization of a hormone-inducible, high affinity adenosine 3'-5'-cyclic monophosphate phosphodiesterase from the rat Sertoli cell. *Biochemistry*, Vol. 34, No. 25, pp. 7979-7987, ISSN 0006-2960 (Print)

Conti, M., Toscano, M.V., et al. (1982). Regulation of follicle-stimulating hormone and dibutyryl adenosine 3',5'-monophosphate of a phosphodiesterase isoenzyme of the Sertoli cell. *Endocrinology*, Vol. 110, No. 4, pp. 1189-1196, ISSN 0013-7227 (Print)

Coskran, T.M., Morton, D., et al. (2006). Immunohistochemical localization of phosphodiesterase 10A in multiple mammalian species. *J Histochem Cytochem*, Vol. 54, No. 11, pp. 1205-1213, ISSN 0022-1554 (Print)

Cuadra, D.L., Chan, P.J., et al. (2000). Type 5 phosphodiesterase regulation of human sperm motility. *Am J Obstet Gynecol*, Vol. 182, No. 5, pp. 1013-1015

D'Andrea, M.R., Qiu, Y., et al. (2005). Expression of PDE11A in normal and malignant human tissues. *J Histochem Cytochem*, Vol. 53, No. 7, pp. 895-903

Davidoff, M.S., Breucker, H., et al. (1990). Cellular architecture of the lamina propria of human seminiferous tubules. *Cell Tissue Res*, Vol. 262, No. 2, pp. 253-261, ISSN 0302-766X (Print)

De Turner, E., Aparicio, N.J., et al. (1978). Effect of two phosphodiesterase inhibitors, cyclic adenosine 3':5'-monophosphate, and a beta-blocking agent on human sperm motility. *Fertil Steril*, Vol. 29, No. 3, pp. 328-331, ISSN 0015-0282 (Print)

Degerman, E., Belfrage, P., et al. (1997). Structure, localization, and regulation of cGMP-inhibited phosphodiesterase (PDE3). *J Biol Chem*, Vol. 272, No. 11, pp. 6823-6826

Dimitriadis, F., Giannakis, D., et al. (2008). Effects of phosphodiesterase-5 inhibitors on sperm parameters and fertilizing capacity. *Asian J Androl*, Vol. 10, No. 1, pp. 115-133, ISSN 1008-682X (Print)

Dimitriadis, F., Tsambalas, S., et al. (2010). Effects of phosphodiesterase-5 inhibitors on Leydig cell secretory function in oligoasthenospermic infertile men: a randomized trial. *BJU Int*, Vol. 106, No. 8, pp. 1181-1185, ISSN 1464-410X (Electronic) 1464-4096 (Linking)

Dimitriadis, F., Tsampalas, S., et al. (2011). Effects of phosphodiesterase-5 inhibitor vardenafil on testicular androgen-binding protein secretion, the maintenance of foci of advanced spermatogenesis and the sperm fertilising capacity in azoospermic men. *Andrologia*, ISSN 1439-0271 (Electronic) 0303-4569 (Linking)

Dousa, T.P. (1999). Cyclic-3',5'-nucleotide phosphodiesterase isozymes in cell biology and pathophysiology of the kidney. *Kidney Int*, Vol. 55, No. 1, pp. 29-62

du Plessis, S.S., de Jongh, P.S., et al. (2004). Effect of acute in vivo sildenafil citrate and in vitro 8-bromo-cGMP treatments on semen parameters and sperm function. *Fertil Steril*, Vol. 81, No. 4, pp. 1026-1033

Eskild, W. & Hansson, V. (1994). Vitamin A functions in the reproductive organs, In: *Vitamin A in Health and Disease*, R. Blomhoff, (Ed.), 531-559, ISBN, Marcel Dekker, Inc., New York

Fair, W.R., Couch, J., et al. (1973). The purification and assay of the prostatic antibacterial factor (PAF). *Biochem Med*, Vol. 8, No. 2, pp. 329-339

Farooqui, S.M., Al-Bagdadi, F., et al. (2001). Surgically induced cryptorchidism-related degenerative changes in spermatogonia are associated with loss of cyclic adenosine monophosphate-dependent phosphodiesterases type 4 in abdominal testes of rats. *Biol Reprod*, Vol. 64, No. 6, pp. 1583-1589

Fawcett, L., Baxendale, R., et al. (2000). Molecular cloning and characterization of a distinct human phosphodiesterase gene family: PDE11A. *Proc Natl Acad Sci U S A*, Vol. 97, No. 7, pp. 3702-3707, ISSN 0027-8424 (Print) 0027-8424 (Linking)

Fisch, J.D., Behr, B., et al. (1998). Enhancement of motility and acrosome reaction in human spermatozoa: differential activation by type-specific phosphodiesterase inhibitors. *Hum Reprod*, Vol. 13, No. 5, pp. 1248-1254, ISSN 0268-1161 (Print)

Fisher, D.A., Smith, J.F., et al. (1998). Isolation and characterization of PDE8A, a novel human cAMP-specific phosphodiesterase. *Biochem Biophys Res Commun*, Vol. 246, No. 3, pp. 570-577, ISSN 0006-291X (Print)

Foresta, C., Caretta, N., et al. (2008). Expression of the PDE5 enzyme on human retinal tissue: new aspects of PDE5 inhibitors ocular side effects. *Eye*, Vol. 22, No. 1, pp. 144-149

Francis, S.H. (2005). Phosphodiesterase 11 (PDE11): is it a player in human testicular function? *Int J Impot Res*, Vol. 17, No. 5, pp. 467-468, ISSN 0955-9930 (Print)

Fujishige, K., Kotera, J., et al. (1999). Cloning and characterization of a novel human phosphodiesterase that hydrolyzes both cAMP and cGMP (PDE10A). *J Biol Chem*, Vol. 274, No. 26, pp. 18438-18445

Fujishige, K., Kotera, J., et al. (1999). Striatum- and testis-specific phosphodiesterase PDE10A isolation and characterization of a rat PDE10A. *Eur J Biochem*, Vol. 266, No. 3, pp. 1118-1127, ISSN 0014-2956 (Print)

Fuse, H., Sakamoto, M., et al. (1993). Effect of pentoxifylline on sperm motion. *Arch Androl*, Vol. 31, No. 1, pp. 9-15, ISSN 0148-5016 (Print)

Galie, N., Ghofrani, H.A., et al. (2005). Sildenafil citrate therapy for pulmonary arterial hypertension. *N Engl J Med*, Vol. 353, No. 20, pp. 2148-2157, ISSN 1533-4406 (Electronic)

Garbers, D.L. & Kopf, G.S. (1980). The regulation of spermatozoa by calcium cyclic nucleotides. *Adv Cyclic Nucleotide Res*, Vol. 13, pp. 251-306

Geremia, R., Rossi, P., et al. (1982). Cyclic nucleotide phosphodiesterase in developing rat testis. Identification of somatic and germ-cell forms. *Mol Cell Endocrinol*, Vol. 28, No. 1, pp. 37-53, ISSN 0303-7207 (Print)

Ghofrani, H.A., Olschewski, H., et al. (2002). [Sildenafil for treatment of severe pulmonary hypertension and commencing right-heart failure]. *Pneumologie*, Vol. 56, No. 11, pp. 665-672, ISSN 0934-8387 (Print)

Ghofrani, H.A., Schermuly, R.T., et al. (2003). Sildenafil for long-term treatment of nonoperable chronic thromboembolic pulmonary hypertension. *Am J Respir Crit Care Med*, Vol. 167, No. 8, pp. 1139-1141, ISSN 1073-449X (Print)

Ghofrani, H.A., Wiedemann, R., et al. (2002). Combination therapy with oral sildenafil and inhaled iloprost for severe pulmonary hypertension. *Ann Intern Med*, Vol. 136, No. 7, pp. 515-522, ISSN 1539-3704 (Electronic)

Glavas, N.A., Ostenson, C., et al. (2001). T cell activation up-regulates cyclic nucleotide phosphodiesterases 8A1 and 7A3. *Proc Natl Acad Sci U S A*, Vol. 98, No. 11, pp. 6319-6324, ISSN 0027-8424 (Print)

Glenn, D.R., McVicar, C.M., et al. (2007). Sildenafil citrate improves sperm motility but causes a premature acrosome reaction in vitro. *Fertil Steril*, Vol. 87, No. 5, pp. 1064-1070

Glover, T.D. & Nicander, L. (1971). Some aspects of structure and function in the mammalian epididymis. *J Reprod Fertil Suppl*, Vol. 13, pp. Suppl 13:39-50, ISSN 0449-3087 (Print)

Grimsley, S.J., Khan, M.H., et al. (2007). Mechanism of Phosphodiesterase 5 inhibitor relief of prostatitis symptoms. *Med Hypotheses*, Vol. 69, No. 1, pp. 25-26, ISSN 0306-9877 (Print)

Haesungcharern, A. & Chulavatnatol, M. (1973). Stimulation of human spermatozoal motility by caffeine. *Fertil Steril*, Vol. 24, No. 9, pp. 662-665, ISSN 0015-0282 (Print)

Hafs, H.D., Knisely, R.C., et al. (1962). Sperm output of dairy bulls with varying degrees of sexual preparation. *J Dairy Sci*, Vol. 35, pp. 359-362

Hellstrom, W.J., Gittelman, M., et al. (2008). An evaluation of semen characteristics in men 45 years of age or older after daily dosing with tadalafil 20mg: results of a multicenter, randomized, double-blind, placebo-controlled, 9-month study. *Eur Urol*, Vol. 53, No. 5, pp. 1058-1065, ISSN 0302-2838 (Print)

Hellstrom, W.J., Overstreet, J.W., et al. (2003). Tadalafil has no detrimental effect on human spermatogenesis or reproductive hormones. *J Urol*, Vol. 170, No. 3, pp. 887-891

Horvath, A., Boikos, S., et al. (2006). A genome-wide scan identifies mutations in the gene encoding phosphodiesterase 11A4 (PDE11A) in individuals with adrenocortical hyperplasia. *Nat Genet*, Vol. 38, No. 7, pp. 794-800

Jaiswal, B.S. & Majumder, G.C. (1996). Cyclic AMP phosphodiesterase: a regulator of forward motility initiation during epididymal sperm maturation. *Biochem Cell Biol*, Vol. 74, No. 5, pp. 669-674, ISSN 0829-8211 (Print)

Jannini, E.A., Lombardo, F., et al. (2004). Treatment of sexual dysfunctions secondary to male infertility with sildenafil citrate. *Fertil Steril*, Vol. 81, No. 3, pp. 705-707

Jarvi, K., Dula, E., et al. (2008). Daily vardenafil for 6 months has no detrimental effects on semen characteristics or reproductive hormones in men with normal baseline levels. *J Urol*, Vol. 179, No. 3, pp. 1060-1065, ISSN 1527-3792 (Electronic)

Kishimoto, I., Rossi, K., et al. (2001). A genetic model provides evidence that the receptor for atrial natriuretic peptide (guanylyl cyclase-A) inhibits cardiac ventricular myocyte hypertrophy. *Proc Natl Acad Sci U S A*, Vol. 98, No. 5, pp. 2703-2706, ISSN 0027-8424 (Print)

Kotera, J., Fujishige, K., et al. (1999). Genomic origin and transcriptional regulation of two variants of cGMP-binding cGMP-specific phosphodiesterases. *Eur J Biochem*, Vol. 262, No. 3, pp. 866-873

Kuthe, A., Wiedenroth, A., et al. (2001). Expression of different phosphodiesterase genes in human cavernous smooth muscle. *J Urol*, Vol. 165, No. 1, pp. 280-283, ISSN 0022-5347 (Print) 0022-5347 (Linking)

Lefievre, L., De Lamirande, E., et al. (2000). The cyclic GMP-specific phosphodiesterase inhibitor, sildenafil, stimulates human sperm motility and capacitation but not acrosome reaction. *J Androl*, Vol. 21, No. 6, pp. 929-937

Lefievre, L., de Lamirande, E., et al. (2002). Presence of cyclic nucleotide phosphodiesterases PDE1A, existing as a stable complex with calmodulin, and PDE3A in human spermatozoa. *Biol Reprod,* Vol. 67, No. 2, pp. 423-430

Lelievre, V., Pineau, N., et al. (2001). Proliferative actions of natriuretic peptides on neuroblastoma cells. Involvement of guanylyl cyclase and non-guanylyl cyclase pathways. *J Biol Chem,* Vol. 276, No. 47, pp. 43668-43676, ISSN 0021-9258 (Print)

Lenzi, A., Lombardo, F., et al. (2003). Stress, sexual dysfunctions, and male infertility. *J Endocrinol Invest,* Vol. 26, No. 3 Suppl, pp. 72-76

Levallet, G., Levallet, J., et al. (2007). Expression of the cAMP-phosphodiesterase PDE4D isoforms and age-related changes in follicle-stimulating hormone-stimulated PDE4 activities in immature rat sertoli cells. *Biol Reprod,* Vol. 76, No. 5, pp. 794-803

Levin, R.M., Greenberg, S.H., et al. (1981). Quantitative analysis of the effects of caffeine on sperm motility and cyclic adenosine 3',5'-monophosphate (AMP) phosphodiesterase. *Fertil Steril,* Vol. 36, No. 6, pp. 798-802, ISSN 0015-0282 (Print)

Lewis, S.E., Moohan, J.M., et al. (1993). Effects of pentoxifylline on human sperm motility in normospermic individuals using computer-assisted analysis. *Fertil Steril,* Vol. 59, No. 2, pp. 418-423

Lopes, S., Jurisicova, A., et al. (1998). Reactive oxygen species: potential cause for DNA fragmentation in human spermatozoa. *Hum Reprod,* Vol. 13, No. 4, pp. 896-900

Loughney, K., Taylor, J., et al. (2005). 3',5'-cyclic nucleotide phosphodiesterase 11A: localization in human tissues. *Int J Impot Res,* Vol. 17, No. 4, pp. 320-325, ISSN 0955-9930 (Print)

Lucas, K.A., Pitari, G.M., et al. (2000). Guanylyl cyclases and signaling by cyclic GMP. *Pharmacol Rev,* Vol. 52, No. 3, pp. 375-414, ISSN 0031-6997 (Print)

Lue, T.F. (2000). Erectile dysfunction. *N Engl J Med,* Vol. 342, No. 24, pp. 1802-1813, ISSN 0028-4793 (Print)

Maekawa, M., Kamimura, K., et al. (1996). Peritubular myoid cells in the testis: their structure and function. *Arch Histol Cytol,* Vol. 59, No. 1, pp. 1-13, ISSN 0914-9465 (Print)

Mancina, R., Filippi, S., et al. (2005). Expression and functional activity of phosphodiesterase type 5 in human and rabbit vas deferens. *Mol Hum Reprod,* Vol. 11, No. 2, pp. 107-115

Marrama, P., Baraghini, G.F., et al. (1985). Further studies on the effects of pentoxifylline on sperm count and sperm motility in patients with idiopathic oligo-asthenozoospermia. *Andrologia,* Vol. 17, No. 6, pp. 612-616, ISSN 0303-4569 (Print)

Meares, E.M., Jr. (1991). Prostatitis. *Med Clin North Am,* Vol. 75, No. 2, pp. 405-424

Medina, P., Segarra, G., et al. (2000). Inhibition of neuroeffector transmission in human vas deferens by sildenafil. *Br J Pharmacol,* Vol. 131, No. 5, pp. 871-874, ISSN 0007-1188 (Print)

Mendelson, C., Dufau, M., et al. (1975). Gonadotropin binding and stimulation of cyclic adenosine 3':5'-monophosphate and testosterone production in isolated Leydig cells. *J Biol Chem,* Vol. 250, No. 22, pp. 8818-8823, ISSN 0021-9258 (Print)

Mewe, M., Bauer, C.K., et al. (2006). Regulation of spontaneous contractile activity in the bovine epididymal duct by cyclic guanosine 5'-monophosphate-dependent pathways. *Endocrinology,* Vol. 147, No. 4, pp. 2051-2062, ISSN 0013-7227 (Print)

Mewe, M., Bauer, C.K., et al. (2006). Mechanisms regulating spontaneous contractions in the bovine epididymal duct. *Biol Reprod,* Vol. 75, No. 4, pp. 651-659, ISSN 0006-3363 (Print)

Michibata, H., Yanaka, N., et al. (2001). Human Ca2+/calmodulin-dependent phosphodiesterase PDE1A: novel splice variants, their specific expression, genomic organization, and chromosomal localization. *Biochim Biophys Acta,* Vol. 1517, No. 2, pp. 278-287

Middendorff, R., Davidoff, M.S., et al. (2000). Multiple roles of the messenger molecule cGMP in testicular function. *Andrologia,* Vol. 32, No. 1, pp. 55-59, ISSN 0303-4569 (Print)

Middendorff, R., Kumm, M., et al. (2000). Generation of cyclic guanosine monophosphate by heme oxygenases in the human testis--a regulatory role for carbon monoxide in Sertoli cells? *Biol Reprod,* Vol. 63, No. 2, pp. 651-657, ISSN 0006-3363 (Print)

Middendorff, R., Muller, D., et al. (2002). The tunica albuginea of the human testis is characterized by complex contraction and relaxation activities regulated by cyclic GMP. *J Clin Endocrinol Metab,* Vol. 87, No. 7, pp. 3486-3499, ISSN 0021-972X (Print)

Middendorff, R., Muller, D., et al. (1996). Natriuretic peptides in the human testis: evidence for a potential role of C-type natriuretic peptide in Leydig cells. *J Clin Endocrinol Metab,* Vol. 81, No. 12, pp. 4324-4328, ISSN 0021-972X (Print)

Middendorff, R., Muller, D., et al. (1997). Evidence for production and functional activity of nitric oxide in seminiferous tubules and blood vessels of the human testis. *J Clin Endocrinol Metab,* Vol. 82, No. 12, pp. 4154-4161, ISSN 0021-972X (Print)

Milhoua, P., Lowe, D., et al. (2007). Normal Anatomy and Physiology, In: *Male Sexual Function,* J.J. Mulcahy, (Ed.), 1-45, ISBN 978-1-58829-747-1 (Print) 978-1-59745-155-0 Humana Press Inc, Totowa, NJ

Moohan, J.M., Winston, R.M., et al. (1993). Variability of human sperm response to immediate and prolonged exposure to pentoxifylline. *Hum Reprod,* Vol. 8, No. 10, pp. 1696-1700

Morena, A.R., Boitani, C., et al. (1995). Stage and cell-specific expression of the adenosine 3',5' monophosphate-phosphodiesterase genes in the rat seminiferous epithelium. *Endocrinology,* Vol. 136, No. 2, pp. 687-695, ISSN 0013-7227 (Print)

Mostafa, T. (2007). In vitro sildenafil citrate use as a sperm motility stimulant. *Fertil Steril,* Vol. 88, No. 4, pp. 994-996

Mostafa, T. (2007). Tadalafil as an in vitro sperm motility stimulant. *Andrologia* Vol. 39, No. 1, pp. 12-15

Muller, D., Mukhopadhyay, A.K., et al. (2004). Spatiotemporal regulation of the two atrial natriuretic peptide receptors in testis. *Endocrinology,* Vol. 145, No. 3, pp. 1392-1401, ISSN 0013-7227 (Print)

Mulryan, K., Gitterman, D.P., et al. (2000). Reduced vas deferens contraction and male infertility in mice lacking P2X1 receptors. *Nature,* Vol. 403, No. 6765, pp. 86-89, ISSN 0028-0836 (Print)

Nassar, A., Mahony, M., et al. (1999). Modulation of sperm tail protein tyrosine phosphorylation by pentoxifylline and its correlation with hyperactivated motility. *Fertil Steril,* Vol. 71, No. 5, pp. 919-923

Nomura, M. & Vacquier, V.D. (2006). Proteins associated with soluble adenylyl cyclase in sea urchin sperm flagella. *Cell Motil Cytoskeleton,* Vol. 63, No. 9, pp. 582-590

Pang, S.C., Chan, P.J., et al. (1993). Effects of pentoxifylline on sperm motility and hyperactivation in normozoospermic and normokinetic semen. *Fertil Steril*, Vol. 60, No. 2, pp. 336-343, ISSN 0015-0282 (Print)

Paul, M., Sumpter, J.P., et al. (1996). Factors affecting pentoxifylline stimulation of sperm kinematics in suspensions. *Hum Reprod*, Vol. 11, No. 9, pp. 1929-1935

Pomara, G., Morelli, G., et al. (2007). Alterations in sperm motility after acute oral administration of sildenafil or tadalafil in young, infertile men. *Fertil Steril*, Vol. 88, No. 4, pp. 860-865

Ponchietti, R., Raugei, A., et al. (1984). Calcium, zinc, magnesium, concentration in seminal plasma of infertile men with prostatitis. *Acta Eur Fertil*, Vol. 15, No. 4, pp. 283-285

Portnoy, L. (1946). The diagnosis and prognosis of male infertility: a study of 44 cases with special reference to sperm morphology. *J Urol*, Vol. 48, pp. 735

Purvis, K., Muirhead, G.J., et al. (2002). The effects of sildenafil on human sperm function in healthy volunteers. *Br J Clin Pharmacol*, Vol. 53 Suppl 1, pp. 53S-60S

Rees, J.M., Ford, W.C., et al. (1990). Effect of caffeine and of pentoxifylline on the motility and metabolism of human spermatozoa. *J Reprod Fertil*, Vol. 90, No. 1, pp. 147-156, ISSN 0022-4251 (Print)

Ricker, D.D. (1998). The autonomic innervation of the epididymis: its effects on epididymal function and fertility. *J Androl*, Vol. 19, No. 1, pp. 1-4, ISSN 0196-3635 (Print)

Rossi, P., Pezzotti, R., et al. (1985). Cyclic nucleotide phosphodiesterases in somatic and germ cells of mouse seminiferous tubules. *J Reprod Fertil*, Vol. 74, No. 2, pp. 317-327, ISSN 0022-4251 (Print)

Rotem, R., Zamir, N., et al. (1998). Atrial natriuretic peptide induces acrosomal exocytosis of human spermatozoa. *Am J Physiol*, Vol. 274, No. 2 Pt 1, pp. E218-223, ISSN 0002-9513 (Print)

Saez, J.M. (1994). Leydig cells: endocrine, paracrine, and autocrine regulation. *Endocr Rev*, Vol. 15, No. 5, pp. 574-626, ISSN 0163-769X (Print)

Salanova, M., Chun, S.Y., et al. (1999). Type 4 cyclic adenosine monophosphate-specific phosphodiesterases are expressed in discrete subcellular compartments during rat spermiogenesis. *Endocrinology*, Vol. 140, No. 5, pp. 2297-2306

Salisbury, G.W. & Vandermark, N.L. (1961). Physiology of Reproduction and Artificial Insemination of Cattle, In: *A Series of books in animal science*, NoEditors., (Ed.), 395–396, ISBN, Freeman, San Francisco and London

Schermuly, R.T., Kreisselmeier, K.P., et al. (2004). Chronic sildenafil treatment inhibits monocrotaline-induced pulmonary hypertension in rats. *Am J Respir Crit Care Med*, Vol. 169, No. 1, pp. 39-45, ISSN 1073-449X (Print)

Schill, W.B. (1975). Caffeine- and kallikrein-induced stimulation of human sperm motility: a comparative study. *Andrologia*, Vol. 7, No. 3, pp. 229-236, ISSN 0303-4569 (Print)

Schill, W.B., Pritsch, W., et al. (1979). Effect of caffeine and kallikrein on cryo-preserved human spermatozoa. *Int J Fertil*, Vol. 24, No. 1, pp. 27-32, ISSN 0020-725X (Print)

Scipioni, A., Stefanini, S., et al. (2005). Immunohistochemical localisation of PDE5 in Leydig and myoid cells of prepuberal and adult rat testis. *Histochem Cell Biol*, Vol. 124, No. 5, pp. 401-407, ISSN 0948-6143 (Print)

Setchell, B.P., Maddocks, S., et al. (1994). Anatomy, vasculature, innervation, and fluids of the male reproductive tract, In: *The Physiology of Reproduction*, E. Knobil & J.D. Neill, (Ed.), 1063-1175, ISBN, Raven Press, New York

Sette, C., Iona, S., et al. (1994). The short-term activation of a rolipram-sensitive, cAMP-specific phosphodiesterase by thyroid-stimulating hormone in thyroid FRTL-5 cells is mediated by a cAMP-dependent phosphorylation. *J Biol Chem*, Vol. 269, No. 12, pp. 9245-9252, ISSN 0021-9258 (Print)

Sharma, O.P. & Hays, R.L. (1973). Release of an oxytocic substance following genital stimulation in bulls. *J Reprod Fertil*, Vol. 35, No. 2, pp. 359-362, ISSN 0022-4251 (Print)

Shen, M.R., Chiang, P.H., et al. (1991). Pentoxifylline stimulates human sperm motility both in vitro and after oral therapy. *Br J Clin Pharmacol*, Vol. 31, No. 6, pp. 711-714, ISSN 0306-5251 (Print)

Sikka, S.C. & Hellstrom, W.J. (1991). The application of pentoxifylline in the stimulation of sperm motion in men undergoing electroejaculation. *J Androl*, Vol. 12, No. 3, pp. 165-170, ISSN 0196-3635 (Print)

Silberbach, M. & Roberts, C.T., Jr. (2001). Natriuretic peptide signalling: molecular and cellular pathways to growth regulation. *Cell Signal*, Vol. 13, No. 4, pp. 221-231, ISSN 0898-6568 (Print)

Siuciak, J.A., McCarthy, S.A., et al. (2006). Genetic deletion of the striatum-enriched phosphodiesterase PDE10A: evidence for altered striatal function. *Neuropharmacology*, Vol. 51, No. 2, pp. 374-385, ISSN 0028-3908 (Print)

Soderling, S.H., Bayuga, S.J., et al. (1998). Cloning and characterization of a cAMP-specific cyclic nucleotide phosphodiesterase. *Proc Natl Acad Sci U S A*, Vol. 95, No. 15, pp. 8991-8996, ISSN 0027-8424 (Print)

Sofikitis, N. & Miyagawa, I. (1991). Secretory dysfunction of the male accessory genital glands due to prostatic infections and fertility; a selected review of the literature. *Jpn J Fertil Steril* Vol. 36, pp. 690-699

Sofikitis, N.V. & Miyagawa, I. (1993). Endocrinological, biophysical, and biochemical parameters of semen collected via masturbation versus sexual intercourse. *J Androl*, Vol. 14, No. 5, pp. 366-373

Stefanovich, V. (1973). Effect of 3,7-dimethyl-1-(5-oxo-hexyl)xanthine and 1-hexyl-3,7-dimethyl xanthine on cyclic AMP phosphodiesterase of the human umbilical cord vessels. *Res Commun Chem Pathol Pharmacol*, Vol. 5, No. 3, pp. 655-662

Stocco, D.M., Wang, X., et al. (2005). Multiple signaling pathways regulating steroidogenesis and steroidogenic acute regulatory protein expression: more complicated than we thought. *Mol Endocrinol*, Vol. 19, No. 11, pp. 2647-2659, ISSN 0888-8809 (Print)

Su, Y.H. & Vacquier, V.D. (2006). Cyclic GMP-specific phosphodiesterase-5 regulates motility of sea urchin spermatozoa. *Mol Biol Cell*, Vol. 17, No. 1, pp. 114-121

Sundkvist, E., Jaeger, R., et al. (2002). Pharmacological characterization of the ATP-dependent low K(m) guanosine 3',5'-cyclic monophosphate (cGMP) transporter in human erythrocytes. *Biochem Pharmacol*, Vol. 63, No. 5, pp. 945-949, ISSN 0006-2952 (Print)

Swinnen, J.V., Joseph, D.R., et al. (1989). Molecular cloning of rat homologues of the Drosophila melanogaster dunce cAMP phosphodiesterase: evidence for a family of genes. *Proc Natl Acad Sci U S A*, Vol. 86, No. 14, pp. 5325-5329, ISSN 0027-8424 (Print)

Takeda, M., Tang, R., et al. (1995). Effects of nitric oxide on human and canine prostates. *Urology*, Vol. 45, No. 3, pp. 440-446, ISSN 0090-4295 (Print)

Tamura, N., Doolittle, L.K., et al. (2004). Critical roles of the guanylyl cyclase B receptor in endochondral ossification and development of female reproductive organs. *Proc Natl Acad Sci U S A*, Vol. 101, No. 49, pp. 17300-17305

Tasdemir, M., Tasdemir, I., et al. (1993). Pentoxifylline-enhanced acrosome reaction correlates with fertilization in vitro. *Hum Reprod*, Vol. 8, No. 12, pp. 2102-2107

Tash, J.S. & Means, A.R. (1983). Cyclic adenosine 3',5' monophosphate, calcium and protein phosphorylation in flagellar motility. *Biol Reprod*, Vol. 28, No. 1, pp. 75-104

Tesarik, J., Mendoza, C., et al. (1992). Effect of phosphodiesterase inhibitors, caffeine and pentoxifylline, on spontaneous and stimulus-induced acrosome reactions in human sperm. *Fertil Steril* Vol. 58, No. 6, pp. 1185-1190

Tesarik, J., Thebault, A., et al. (1992). Effect of pentoxifylline on sperm movement characteristics in normozoospermic and asthenozoospermic specimens. *Hum Reprod*, Vol. 7, No. 9, pp. 1257-1263, ISSN 0268-1161 (Print)

Tournaye, H., Devroey, P., et al. (1995). Use of pentoxifylline in assisted reproductive technology. *Hum Reprod*, Vol. 10 Suppl 1, pp. 72-79, ISSN 0268-1161 (Print)

Tournaye, H., Van Steirteghem, A.C., et al. (1994). Pentoxifylline in idiopathic male-factor infertility: a review of its therapeutic efficacy after oral administration. *Hum Reprod*, Vol. 9, No. 6, pp. 996-1000, ISSN 0268-1161 (Print)

Tur-Kaspa, I., Segal, S., et al. (1999). Viagra for temporary erectile dysfunction during treatments with assisted reproductive technologies. *Hum Reprod*, Vol. 14, No. 7, pp. 1783-1784

Twigg, J., Fulton, N., et al. (1998). Analysis of the impact of intracellular reactive oxygen species generation on the structural and functional integrity of human spermatozoa: lipid peroxidation, DNA fragmentation and effectiveness of antioxidants. *Hum Reprod*, Vol. 13, No. 6, pp. 1429-1436

Uckert, S., Kuthe, A., et al. (2001). Characterization and functional relevance of cyclic nucleotide phosphodiesterase isoenzymes of the human prostate. *J Urol*, Vol. 166, No. 6, pp. 2484-2490, ISSN 0022-5347 (Print)

Valente, E.G., Vernet, D., et al. (2003). L-arginine and phosphodiesterase (PDE) inhibitors counteract fibrosis in the Peyronie's fibrotic plaque and related fibroblast cultures. *Nitric Oxide*, Vol. 9, No. 4, pp. 229-244

Vasta, V., Shimizu-Albergine, M., et al. (2006). Modulation of Leydig cell function by cyclic nucleotide phosphodiesterase 8A. *Proc Natl Acad Sci U S A*, Vol. 103, No. 52, pp. 19925-19930, ISSN 0027-8424 (Print)

Wang, C., Chan, C.W., et al. (1983). Comparison of the effectiveness of placebo, clomiphene citrate, mesterolone, pentoxifylline, and testosterone rebound therapy for the treatment of idiopathic oligospermia. *Fertil Steril*, Vol. 40, No. 3, pp. 358-365, ISSN 0015-0282 (Print)

Ward, A. & Clissold, S.P. (1987). Pentoxifylline. A review of its pharmacodynamic and pharmacokinetic properties, and its therapeutic efficacy. *Drugs*, Vol. 34, No. 1, pp. 50-97

Wayman, C., Phillips, S., et al. (2005). Phosphodiesterase 11 (PDE11) regulation of spermatozoa physiology. *Int J Impot Res*, Vol. 17, No. 3, pp. 216-223

Yamamoto, Y., Sofikitis, N., et al. (2000). Influence of sexual stimulation on sperm parameters in semen samples collected via masturbation from normozoospermic men or cryptozoospermic men participating in an assisted reproduction programme. *Andrologia*, Vol. 32, No. 3, pp. 131-138

Yan, C., Zhao, A.Z., et al. (2001). Stage and cell-specific expression of calmodulin-dependent phosphodiesterases in mouse testis. *Biol Reprod*, Vol. 64, No. 6, pp. 1746-1754

Yovich, J.M., Edirisinghe, W.R., et al. (1988). Preliminary results using pentoxifylline in a pronuclear stage tubal transfer (PROST) program for severe male factor infertility. *Fertil Steril*, Vol. 50, No. 1, pp. 179-181

Yovich, J.M., Edirisinghe, W.R., et al. (1990). Influence of pentoxifylline in severe male factor infertility. *Fertil Steril*, Vol. 53, No. 4, pp. 715-722

Yuasa, K., Kanoh, Y., et al. (2001). Genomic organization of the human phosphodiesterase PDE11A gene. Evolutionary relatedness with other PDEs containing GAF domains. *Eur J Biochem*, Vol. 268, No. 1, pp. 168-178

Yuasa, K., Omori, K., et al. (2000). Binding and phosphorylation of a novel male germ cell-specific cGMP-dependent protein kinase-anchoring protein by cGMP-dependent protein kinase Ialpha. *J Biol Chem*, Vol. 275, No. 7, pp. 4897-4905, ISSN 0021-9258 (Print)

Yunes, R., Fernandez, P., et al. (2005). Cyclic nucleotide phosphodiesterase inhibition increases tyrosine phosphorylation and hyper motility in normal and pathological human spermatozoa. *Biocell*, Vol. 29, No. 3, pp. 287-293

Zaccolo, M. & Pozzan, T. (2002). Discrete microdomains with high concentration of cAMP in stimulated rat neonatal cardiac myocytes. *Science*, Vol. 295, No. 5560, pp. 1711-1715, ISSN 1095-9203 (Electronic)

Zhang, C., Yeh, S., et al. (2006). Oligozoospermia with normal fertility in male mice lacking the androgen receptor in testis peritubular myoid cells. *Proc Natl Acad Sci U S A*, Vol. 103, No. 47, pp. 17718-17723, ISSN 0027-8424 (Print)

Zhao, A.Z., Yan, C., et al. (1997). Recent advances in the study of Ca2+/CaM-activated phosphodiesterases: expression and physiological functions. *Adv Second Messenger Phosphoprotein Res*, Vol. 31, pp. 237-251, ISSN 1040-7952 (Print)

5

Effectiveness of Assisted Reproduction Techniques as an Answer to Male Infertility

Sandrine Chamayou and Antonino Guglielmino
Unità di Medicina della Riproduzione – Via Barriera del Bosco
Sant'Agata Li Battiati (CT)
Italy

1. Introduction

The assisted reproductive technologies (ART) are of huge help in the resolution of couple infertility especially for male factor. For an evaluation of male fertility, the semen exam is the first analysis requested. All the procedures for an objective exam and parameters of normality have been worldwide established and described in a manual written by the World Health Organization (WHO).

In the application of ART to obtain the pregnancy of healthy children, there are different levels of invasiveness that take in account both male and female factors. For moderate alteration of semen values, the ART called *intra* uterine insemination (IUI) is easy to perform because fertilization occurs *in vivo*. In case of intermediate alteration of semen values, metaphase II oocytes are incubated in a solution of motile spermatozoa in a process called *in vitro* fertilization (IVF). One spermatozoon penetrates by itself the oocyte membranes and fertilizes it. The development of embryos generated in the laboratory is followed until embryos are *in utero* transferred or stored in liquid nitrogen. Intra-cytoplasmic sperm injection (ICSI) is a variation of IVF in which the fertilization process is assisted. The elective field of ICSI application is a severe male factor. ICSI can be performed with fresh or thawed, motile or immotile, ejaculated or surgically retrieved (microsurgical epididymal sperm aspiration-MESA, sperm aspiration from the epididymis-PESA or testicle-TESA) spermatozoa. Recently, a new technique called IMSI (morphologically selected sperm injection) was introduced in the clinically assisted reproduction. In this case, the spermatozoon to micro-inject in the ooplasm is accurately chosen according to its morphology and particularly to the number and volume of vacuoles in the head of the cell.

Numerous studies related *in vivo* and *in vitro* ART outcomes with male infertility and semen characteristics. The aim of this chapter is to present the effectiveness of ART as an answer to male infertility according to semen alterations (number, motility, morphology), the extraction of the spermatozoa (ejaculated/surgically extracted) and the process it underwent (cryopreservation). Furthermore, it has to be underlined that spermatozoa cryopreservation combined with ART represents a huge opportunity of fertility preservation for cancer patients. The genetic analysis of cells from biopsied embryos produced after ICSI (preimplantation genetic diagnosis-PGD) is an alternative mode of reproduction for couples with high risk in the transmission of male genetic disorder.

2. Semen characteristics

The semen analysis is the basic exam in the determination of male fertility or infertility as it has been early determined a positive correlation between normal semen parameters and male infertility potential (WHO, 1987, 1992).

The semen is a mixture of spermatozoa suspended in secretions from the testis and epididymis which are combined with seminal liquid. The seminal liquid is secreted in 90% by the prostate and the seminal vesicles, and a small proportion is secreted by bulb urethral glands. The final semen is a viscous fluid that comprises the ejaculate. The total number of spermatozoa reflects the sperm production by the testes and the patency of the post-testicular duct system. The volume of the sample, produced by the accessory glands reflect the secretary activity of the glands. Other important parameters of the sperm function are represented by the vitality, the motility, the morphology and composition of the semen. The semen analysis must be standardized and objective. To emphasize the standardization of analysis procedures and to establish reference values, the WHO wrote a manual where the procedure of semen collection, analysis and the parameters of normality are described. Nowadays the fifth edition is available where the criteria of male infertility has been revised (WHO, 2010).

2.1 Semen analysis

This paragraph resumes the procedures for a correct semen collection and laboratory analysis as described by the WHO manual (2010).

Commonly, the semen sample is obtain by masturbation. The semen sample should be collected after a minimum of 48 hours but no longer than seven days of sexual abstinence. The semen sample collection should be completed and two samples should be collected for initial evaluation within an interval of time that should not be less than 7 days or more than 3 weeks. In case of markedly differences between two assessments, additional samples should be analyzed.

The semen analysis is divided in macroscopic analysis and microscopic analysis.

The macroscopic parameters are the semen aspect, the viscosity, liquefaction, the volume and the pH.

The microscopic parameters are the sperm concentration calculated per millilitre (ml), the total number of spermatozoa per ejaculate, the percentage of motile spermatozoa, the sperm vitality, the agglutination of spermatozoa, the spermatozoa morphology and the presence of cellular elements other than spermatozoa. It is recommended to execute all microscopic examinations using a phase-contrast microscope.

The semen analysis must be carried out on a fixed 20 um depth preparation. Depths less than 20 um constrain the rational movement of spermatozoa. Since sperm motility is highly dependent on temperature, the assessment of the motility should be performed at 37°C.

The concentration of spermatozoa should be determined using the haemocytometer chamber as the 'Newbauer haemocytometer' on a diluted preparation of semen covered with a coverslip. The sperm count should be made of complete spermatozoa (heads with tails). Defective spermatozoa (pinheads and tailless heads) should also be counted but recorded separately. If no spermatozoa is detected by microscopy, the entire sample should be centrifuged at 3000*g* for 15 minutes. If no spermatozoa is found after the complete analysis of the centrifuged sample, the semen is qualified as 'azoospermic'. The total sperm number refers to the total number of spermatozoa in the entire ejaculate. This number is obtained by multiplying the sperm concentration by the semen volume.

The grade of progressive motility of the spermatozoa is correlated with the pregnancy rate (Jouannet *et al.* 1988; Larsen *et al.* 2000; Zinaman *et al.* 2000). The sperm motility valuation should be performed close to the liquefaction of the sample, between 30 minutes and one hour after sperm collection. At least five microscopic fields are assessed in a systematic way to classify 200 spermatozoa. The motility of each spermatozoon is graded as 'progressive', 'non-progressive', 'immotile', according to whether it shows:

- Progressive motility (PR): spermatozoa moving actively, either linearly or in a large circle, regardless of speed;
- Non progressive motility (NP): Swimming in small circles, the flagellar forces hardly displacing the head, or when only a flagellar beat can be observed;
- Immotility (IM): no movement.

The vitality is estimated by assessing the membrane vitality of the cells. It is routinely determined for the samples with less than 40% of progressively motile spermatozoa. The percentage of viable cells normally exceeds that of motile cells. The presence of a large proportion of vital but immotile spermatozoa may be indicative of structural defects in the flagellum (Cheme and Rawe, 2003); a high percentage of immotile and non-viable spermatozoa (necrozoospermia) may indicate epididymal pathology (Wilton *et al.* 1988; Correa-Perrez *et al.* 2004).

The term of 'Agglutination of spermatozoa' means that motile spermatozoa stick to each other head-to-head, tail-to tail or in a mixed way, e.g. head-to-tail. The presence of agglutination is suggestive, but not sufficient evidence for, an immunological cause of infertility.

The spermatozoa morphology is determined after cell staining. The most widely recommended staining recommended method used is the Papanicolaou stain. For a spermatozoa to be normal, the sperm head, neck, midpiece and tail must be normal. The head should be oval in shape. Allowing for the slight shrinkage induced by fixation and staining, the length of the head should be 4.0-5.0 um and the width 2.5-3.5 um. The length-to-width ratio should be 1.50 to 1.75. There should be a well-defined acrosomal region comprising 40-70% of the head area. The midpiece should be slender, less than 1 um in width, about one and a half times the length of the head, and attached axially to the head. The morphological sperm defects should be noted as head defects, neck and midpiece defects, tail defects and cytoplasmic droplets. Abnormal spermatozoa generally have a lower fertilizing potential. Morphologically defects are associated with chromosomal abnormalities.

In the microscopic analysis the non- nemaspermic cellular components are also valuated. There are referred as 'round cells' and compound of leukocytes, spermatogenic cells, epithelium cells, red cells, prostate cells. A normal ejaculate should not contain more than 5 x 10^6 round cells/ml.

The semen analysis can be computer-assisted (Computeur-assisted semen analysis-CASA) (Yeung *et al.* 1997). The advantage of a computer assisted system for sperm analysis is the ability to obtain precise quantitative data as wells as the potential for the standardization of semen analysis procedures. Nevertheless, the main disadvantages are the lack of standardization procedures and the significant expense of equipment requirement. CASA is a valuable tool for research but the manual semen analysis remains the reference (Amann *et al.* 2004). Other tests can be made on semen such as the detection of sperm antibodies, sperm vitality, hypo-osmotic swelling test, assays of the sperm acrosome, sperm penetration assay, hemizona assay, mannose binding assay and assays of sperm DNA integrity and fragmentation.

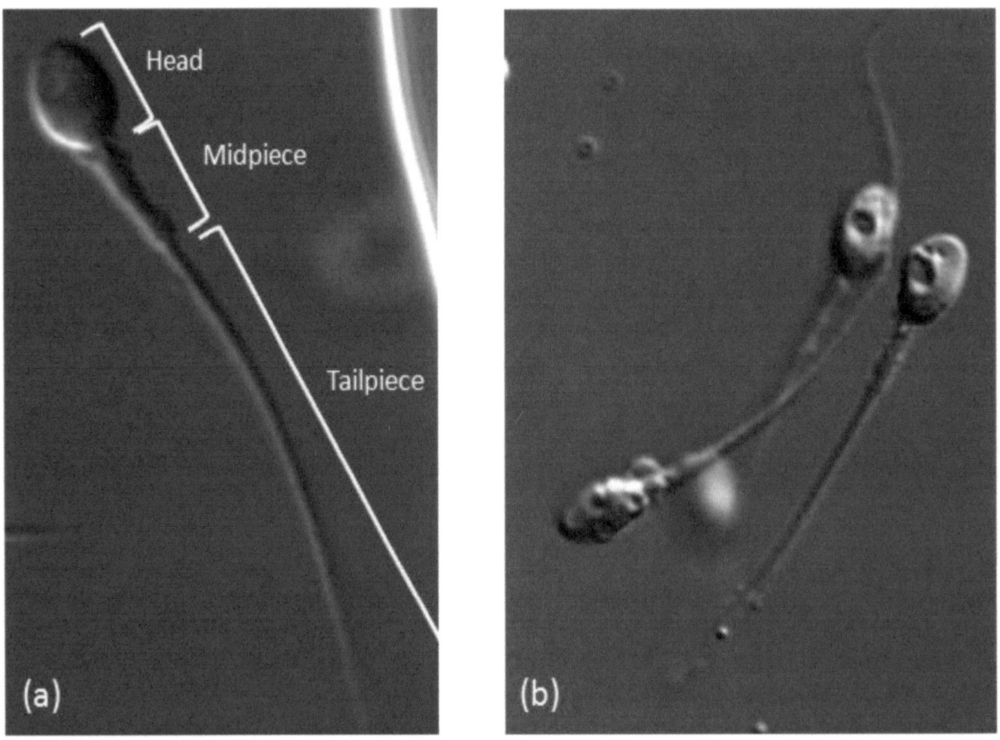

Fig. 1. Spermatozoon with normal morphology (a) and spermatozoa with vacuoles into the head (b).

2.1.1 Reference values of semen analysis and semen variables

Tables 1 and 2 summarise the lower references limits of semen characteristics as defined in the fifth edition of WHO manual, and the nomenclature of semen variables.

Parameter	Lower reference limit
Semen volume (ml)	1.5 (1.4-1.7)
Total sperm number (10^6 per ejaculate)	39 (33-46)
Sperm concentration (10^6 per ml)	15 (12-16)
Total motility (PR+NP, %)	40 (38-42)
Progressive motility (PR, %)	32 (31-34)
Vitality (live spermatozoa, %)	58 (55-63)
Sperm morphology (normal form, %)	4 (3.0-4.0)
pH	$\geq$ 7.2
Peroxidase-positive leucocytes (10^6 per ml)	< 1.0
MAR test (motile spermatozoa with bound particles, %)	< 50
Immunobead test (motile spermatozoa with bound beads, %)	< 50
Seminal zinc (umol/ejaculate)	$\geq$ 2.4
Seminal fruttose (umol/ejaculate)	$\geq$ 13
Seminal neutral glucosidase (mU/ejaculate)	$\geq$ 20

Table 1. Lower reference limits of semen characteristics (5th centiles, 95% confidence intervals)

Aspermia	No ejaculate
Asthenozoospermia	Less than the reference value for motility
Asthenoteratozoospermia	Less than the reference values for motility and morphology
Azoospermia	No spermatozoa in the ejaculate
Cryptozoospermia	No spermatozoa is observed in the fresh preparation but only after centrifuged pellet
Hemospermia (Hematospermia)	Presence of leukocytes in the ejaculate
Leukospermia (Leukocytospermia, pyospermia)	Presence of leukocytes in the ejaculate above the threshold value
Necrozoospermia	Low percentage of live and high percentage of immotile spermatozoa in the ejaculate
Normozoospermia	Normal ejaculate as defined by the reference values
Oligoastenoteratozoospermia	Signifies disturbance of all three variables (concentration or total number, motility, morphology)
Oligoteratozoospermia	Less than the reference values for concentration or total number and morphology
Oligozoospermia	Sperm concentration (or total number) less than the reference value
Teratozoospermia	Less than the reference value for morphology

Table 2. Nomenclature related to semen variations.

2.1.2 Sperm preparation techniques

In a view to apply diagnostic tests of functions or to use the spermatozoa for therapeutic recovery for intra-uterine insemination (IUI) or *in vitro* ART, the spermatozoa must be separated from the seminal liquid. While the seminal liquid support the cervical mucus penetration in natural intercourse, the elimination of part of its compounds is necessary to perform IUI or *in vitro* fertilization (IVF). In the separation of spermatozoa from the seminal liquid, the final preparation concentrates morphologically normal and motile spermatozoa, free from debris, non-germ cells and dead spermatozoa. The separation and concentration of those spermatozoa is done performing a sperm preparation. Three methods are mainly used. The choice of a method is leaded by the semen characteristics. These methods are the simple washing, the direct swim-up and the density gradients. In all the sperm preparations, balanced salt solutions supplemented with proteins and containing an appropriate buffer are used as culture medium.

The 'Sperm washing' is a simple sperm preparation, performed for good quality semen, often used for IUI. The principal is in the washing of the semen to remove the secretive part (WHO, 2010).

The direct swim-up select the spermatozoa on their ability to swim out of the seminal liquid to the culture medium. It is the preferred method for the extraction of motile spermatozoa especially when their percentage is low e.g. for IVF and intracytoplasmic sperm injection (ICSI) (WHO, 2010).

The discontinuous density gradient consists in the centrifugation of the semen on a column of colloidal silica coated with silane which separate the cells according to their density. Furthermore, the motile spermatozoa swim through the gradients and concentrate at the bottom of the tube. This method selects a high fraction of motile spermatozoa and is selective against the debris, the leukocytes, non-germ cells and degenerating germs cells. The discontinuous density gradient is mainly used for IVF and ICSI (WHO, 2010).

If the patient is infected by the human immunodeficiency virus (HIV), the viral RNA and proviral DNA can be found in the seminal liquid and in non-sperm cells. In a view to prevent female partner contamination, a combination of density-gradient centrifugation followed by swim-up can be performed (Gilling-Smith *et al.* 2006; Savasi *et al.* 2007). With this combination of procedures, the motile spermatozoa are separated from the seminal liquid and virus-affected non-sperm cells.

3. ART and results

In the IUI practice, the female patient is monitored to determine the moment of ovulation; the semen is collected and prepared to select the best spermatozoa to transfer *in utero*. The fertilization process is *in vivo*. In IVF and ICSI protocols, the fertilization process is followed and *in vitro* assisted. Embryos are produced in the laboratory and are subsequently transferred *in utero*.

3.1 IUI

IUI is one of the earliest technique of assisted conception to be applied. It derives from intra-cervical insemination in which the principle was to deposit a sample of semen (fresh or thawed) into the vagina using a catheter. With the development of new sperm preparation and the separation of the motile spermatozoa from the secretive part (Mortimer, 1994), the IUI could be attempted. Concentrated preparation of sperm were attempted directly into the Fallopian tubes, peritoneal cavity, or ovarian follicles of the women, before to reach the consensus that IUI was the most effective method, providing a maximum pregnancy rate with a minimum of complications (Sacks and Simon, 1991). Although IUI can be performed in the natural cycle, nowadays it is combined with ovarian stimulation to increase the pregnancy rate.

The clinical indications for IUI are couples with unexplained infertility, mild or moderate male-factor infertility. This technique can be applied in certain female factors infertility such as antisperm antibodies or hostile cervical environment. In case of male infertility, the presence of ten million of motile spermatozoa is a prerequisite but good results can be obtained with 5 and even one million of motile spermatozoa injected in uterus.

From a technical point of view, on the day of IUI, the patient is asked to produce sperm into a sterile cup. After liquefaction and semen analysis, the sample is treated as previously described to select a high concentration of good motility spermatozoa. The final suspension of selected spermatozoa is concentrated in a maximal final volume of 500 ul of culture medium. IUI can be performed on natural cycle or on female patient that underwent a mild ovarian stimulation. Around the moment of pharmacologically monitored ovulation, the spermatozoa are deposited into the uterus without neither local anesthetic nor antibiotic prophylaxis using polyethylene catheter attached to a plastic syringe. After IUI, the female patient can resume normal activity.

The success rates of IUI depends on the female patient age (De Sutter *et al.* 2005), the presence of comorbid conditions, ovulation method and the male factor (Burr *et al.* 1996). Abnormal spermatozoa morphology is associated with poor IUI outcomes on natural cycles and IUI with clomiphene or gonadotropin stimunation (Van Waart *et al.* 2001). Furthermore, abnormal sperm morphology has been associated with higher IUI complication rates such as miscarriage. Motility and concentration play also an important role in the pregnancy rate expectancy (Montanaro *et al.* 2001; Ombelet *et al.* 1997). Patients with percentage of a sperm motility superior to 30 percent have a four time increase cumulative pregnancy rate than patients with sperm motility less than 30 percent (Yalti *et al.* 2004).

In conclusion, IUI is the most commonly performed ART procedure, a low cost technique and straightforward to perform.

3.2 IVF

The first world birth after IVF was obtained but Steptoe and Edwards in 1978 (Steptoe and Edwards, 1978). In 2006, it was estimated that more than three million of babies had been born using this procedure (ESHRE, 2006). The indications for IVF treatment include long-standing infertility due to tubal disease, endometriosis, unexplained infertility, infertility involving male factor.

The principle of IVF is the following: the female partner is given stimulatory drugs (gonadotrophin) in the weeks leading up to the procedure and in a view to trigger the development of several follicules. The follicular fluid are collected in a tube and under sedation. The follicular fluid is carefully read in the IVF laboratory and the oocytes that have grown inside the follicules are isolated and incubated. On the same day, the mature oocytes are incubated with an aliquot of fresh (or frozen) motile partner 'spermatozoa. The test-tubes or dishes containing the oocytes in the solution of spermatozoa are incubated up to 18 hours at 37°C and 5% CO2. A reduced concentration of O2 (5-6%) can also be applied. Between 16 and 18 hours, the fertilization process is checked with the observation of two pronuclei. Tipically, between 60 and 70% of the oocytes are fertilized. In the following hours, a large majority of fertilized oocytes (now called 'zygotes') reach the embryo-stage with the first cell division. The embryo quality is evaluated on the base the number of cells according to the time of incubation, the absence of extra-cellular fragments, the capacity of the cells to compact at the morula stage and the blastocyst to expanse. The embryos can be maintained in *in vitro* culture until 5-6 days. Within this period, any embryo can be in utero transferred, discarded or frozen for a successive *in utero* transfer.

Oehninger *et al.* (1988) studied the correlation between normal sperm morphology and insemination concentration. By increasing the insemination concentration in samples of severe teratozoospermia, the fertilization rate can be improved.

The couples with male factor and undergoing conventional IVF have a lower fertilization and pregnancy rate expectancy. On the same trend, very low pregnancy rates are obtained with surgical retrieved sperm (Hirsh *et al.* 1994). As a consequence and if a sufficient number of progressive motility spermatozoa is not available, the assisted reproductive technology called 'Intra-cytoplasmic sperm injection' (ICSI) must be applied as alternative and in a view to assist the fertilization process. The clinical pregnancy rate of IVF across Europe is 26.1% per egg collection and 29.6% per embryo-transfer (Andersen *et al.* 2007), although the success rates decrease according to female age over 35 (HFEA, 2005).

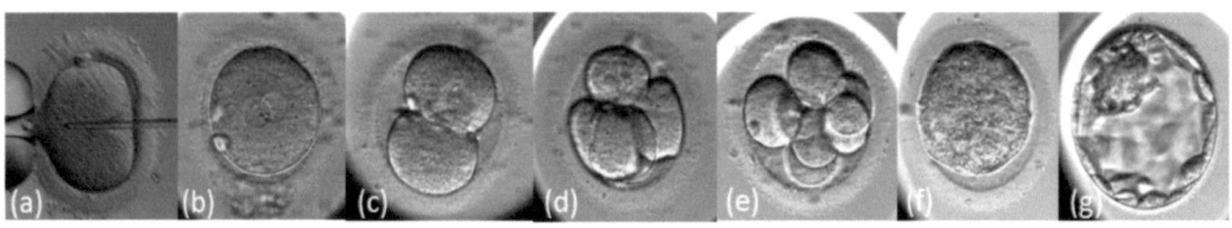

Fig. 2. Embryo development. (a)Time of micro-injection: 0 hour (h); (b) zygote at 17 ± 1 h; (c) 2 cells at 23 ± 1 h ; (d) 4 cells at 44 ± 1 h; (e) 8 cells at 68 ± 1h; (f) compacting morula at 92 ± 2h; (g) blastocyst at 116 ± 2h post ICSI or IVF.

3.3 ICSI

3.3.1 ICSI: History and indications

On the process of micro-manipulation history that lead to ICSI, the techniques that were previously applied were the partial zona dissection (PZD) to facilitate the sperm penetration (Cohen *et al.* 1989), the subzonal insemination (SUZI) where the motile spermatozoa were micro-injected under the peri-vitelline space and were in direct contact with the oolemma (Laws-King *et al.* 1987). Subsequently ICSI of which the principle is the direct micro-injection of a single preferably with good morphology spermatozoon into the ooplasma was invented. The first pregnancies and births was obtained in 1992 (Palermo *et al.* 1992). Since the beginning, ICSI appeared a superior technique due to higher resutls compared to SUZI in terms of oocyte fertilization rate, number of embryos produced and implantation rates (Palermo *et al.* 1993; Van Steirteghem AC *et al.* 1993a; Van Steirteghem *et al.* 1993b).

ICSI can be applied in extremely low sperm counts, impair of motility, poor morphology (oligo-astheno-teratozoospermia) or azoospermia due to impaired testicular function or obstructed excretory ducts. ICSI can also be applied with non progressive motility or immotile spermatozoa. ICSI is the ultimate and only option for successful treatment of male infertility due to obstruction of the excretory ducts and impair of testicular functions.

Table 3 shows the indications for ICSI.

Ejaculated spermatozoa
Oligozoospermia
Asthenozoospermia (caveat for 100% immotile spermatozoa)
Teratozoospermia (even globozoospermia and acrosomeless spermatozoa)
High titers of antisperm antibodies
Repeated fertilization failure after conventional IVF
Autoconserved frozen sperm from cancer patients in remission
Ejaculatory disorders (e.g. electroejaculation, retrograde ejaculation)
Epidydimal spermatozoa
Congenital bilateral absence of the vas deferens
Young syndrome
Failed vaso-epididymosotomy
Failed vasovasostomy
Obstruction of both ejaculatory ducts
Testicular spermatozoa
All indications for epididymal sperm
Failure of epididymal sperm recovery because of fibrosis
Azoospermia caused by testicular failure (maturation arrest, germ-cell aplasia)
Necrozoospermia

(Van Steirteghem, 2007)

Table 3. Indications for clinical application of ICSI.

The clinical pregnancy rates by use of ICSI are similar to those obtained with IVF, 26.5% of pregnancy rate according to egg collection and 28.7% according to embryo-transfer (Andersen *et al.* 2007). High fertilization and pregnancy rates can be obtained from motile spermatozoa (Nagy *et al.* 1995) while immotile and dead spermatozoa result in lower fertilization rate (Tournaye *et al.* 1996).

3.3.2 ICSI protocol

As for the IVF procedure, the patient is stimulated and the follicle fluids containing mature (Metafase II) oocytes are aspirated. The retrieved oocytes are incubated in 5%CO2 at 37°C. The difference between IVF and ICSI lays in fertilization method. In a view to perform micro-injection, the cumulus and corona cells surrounding the oocytes must be removed using a combination of enzymatic and mechanical procedures. The assessment of the zona pellucida and the presence or absence of a germinal vesicle and of the first polar body are verified at the microscopic observation. The presence and orientation of the meiotic spindle can be assessed when exposed to polarized light. 3.9% of the intact oocytes are at the metaphase I stage because they underwent germinal vesicle (GV) breakdown but they have not expelled the first polar; 10.3% of the intact oocytes are at the GV stage, and around 85.8% of the intact oocytes are in the metaphase II stage, reaching the haploid stage and therefore available for micro-injection (Bonduelle *et al.* 1999). Matured, denuded and rinsed oocytes are incubated until the time of micro-injection. ICSI can be performed with spermatozoa that have been ejaculated, extracted from epipydimus or testis. As it has been described previously, the sperm is prepared to select motile and good morphology spermatozoa.

The micro-injection of single spermatozoa inside the ooplasm is performed under an inverted microscope equipped with micro-manipulators, microinjectors and heating stage to maintain the temperature at 37°C. The magnification of 400X is recommended for the selection of moving spermatozoa. Micromanipulators give the possibility to move the two microinjectors in the 3 directions. The microinjectors can be filled with air or mineral oil and a micrometer controls the plunger. Generally, the holding is fixed to the microinjector on the left of the operator, and the injection pipette is fixed on the right. The oocyte can be fixed, positioned and released by the holding pipette, the spermatozoa is immobilized, injected and released using the injection pipette. It is recommended to position the microscope on a vibration-proof table.

For the micro-injection setting, the gametes (metaphase II oocytes to be micro-injected and spermatozoa to micro-inject) are deposed within micro-droplets of buffered medium and on the same plastic micro-injection dish. The micro-droplets are covered by mineral oil. The micro-drop containing the spermatozoa is a mixture of spermatozoa plus PVP. The PVP slows down the spermatozoa motility and facilitates the manipulation and the control of the fluids. For ejaculated spermatozoa, they should be deposited on a single micro-drop, while extracted spermatozoa from testis or epididymis can be deposited on several micro-droplets. Each denuded oocytes is placed on a single micro-drop-droplet (usually eight micro-droplets contain eight oocytes on the micro-injection dish). After the preparation of the dish with the gametes to use, the ICSI is performed. Step by step, ICSI can be described as follows:

- the spermatozoa to micro-inject is chosen on the basis of its good morphology and motility.
- The spermatozoa is immobilised using the injection pipette. Its immobilization is necessary to make the membrane permeable and to allow the release of sperm cytosolic factor which activates the oocyte (Palermo *et al.* 1993). For spermatozoa immobilization, the cell is positioned at 90° to the tip of the pipette, which is then lowered gently to compress the sperm flagellum. The shape of the tail should be maintained.
- The immobilized psermatozoon is entered and maintained inside the micro-injection pipette by the flagellum. In other terms, the head is close to the way out of the micropipette.
- The holding pipette is moved slowly to the oocyte.
- The oocyte is held by the suction applied to the holding pipette.
- The oocyte is slowly positioned: the polar body is at the 12 or 6 o'clock position. Nowadays, it is not the polar body that is taken in consideration as reference for oocyte

orientation but the meiotic spindle. During the oocyte denudation, the polar body can move within the peri-vitellin space. As a consequence, the position of the polar body could not correspond to the meiotic spindle position and the micro-injection can disturb the chromosomes alignment on the equatorial plane of the meiotic spindle and generate aneuploidies.

- The oocyte is maintained in this position and the micro-injection pipette carrying the immobilized spermatozoa is moved slowly to the oocyte.
- The spermatozoa is positioned at the end of the injection pipette.
- The micro-injection pipette penetrates the zona pellucida and the ooplasma at the 3 o'clock position.
- The ooplasma is aspirated gently inside the micro-injection pipette until the observation of the sudden oolemma break.
- The aspiration is immediately stopped.
- The ooplasma is released from the micro-injection pipette and this way out movement is completed when the spermatozoon is completely released into the ooplasma.
- The micro-injection pipette is slowly removed from the oocyte.
- The oocyte is released from the holding pipette.

When all of the oocytes of the dish have been microinjected, the dish is removed from the microscope and the oocytes are incubated in non-buffered medium in 5% of CO_2 at 37°C.

Differences in the oolemma breakage have been observed. The immediate break of the oolemma without any aspiration is associated with lower oocyte survival rates (Palermo *et al.* 1996).

As in the IVF protocol, the fertilization process is checked 16-18 hours after micro-injection and embryo culture is prolonged until the destiny of each embryo is decided (transferred, frozen or discarded). As in IVF, abnormal fertilization can be observed with the formation of one pronucleus (about 3% of the micro-injected oocytes), and the finding of three pronuclear (3PN-about 4% of micro-injected oocytes) after the micro-injection of one single spermatozoon can be the consequence of extrusion failure of the second polar body at the time of fertilization (Staessen *et al.* 1997). No embryo generated from 1PN and 3PN oocytes must be transferred. About 90% of the 2PN-oocytes cleave and become embryos.

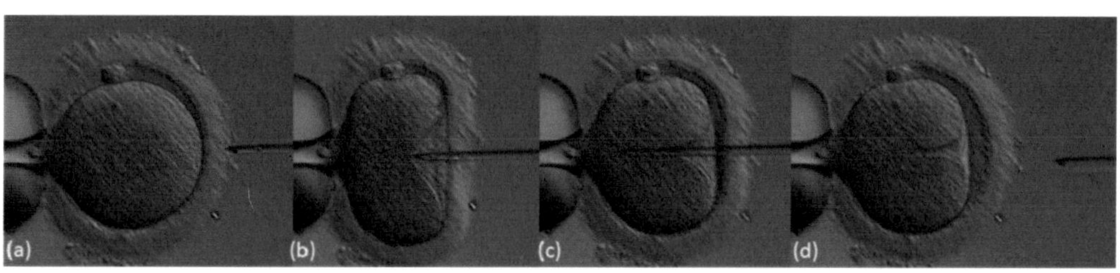

Fig. 3. Intracytoplasmic sperm injection procedure. The oocyte and the micro-injection pipette with the spermatozoon are positioned (a). The micro-injection pipette with the spermatozoon at its end goes through the zona pellucida, the peri-vitellin space (b) and penetrates the oolemma (c). The micro-injection pipette is removed after that the spermatozoon has been released into the ooplasma (d) (with the kind collaboration of C. Ragolia).

3.4 ICSI with surgical spermatozoa

In patients that appear to be azoospermic after semen analysis, the surgical sperm retrieval is the last option to collect spermatozoa. The different techniques are percutaneous epididymal sperm aspiration (PESA), testicular sperm aspiration (TESA), testicular sperm extraction (TESE), and microsurgical epididymal sperm aspiration (MESA). The choice of the technique depends on the type of patient and of the diagnosis.

In all surgical sperm retrieval, ICSI is the method of choice to obtain a pregnancy using fresh or frozen/thawed spermatozoa.

3.4.1 PESA

PESA is the least invasive surgical sperm retrieval technique. The patient is in conscious sedation and/or spermatic cord blockage with marcaine or lidocaine. The testis is immobilized and the aspiration is carried out with a 25-G butterfly needle. The fluid is aspirated and examined under microscope to check for motile spermatozoa. The recovered spermatozoa can be subsequently cryopreserved. The percentage of motile spermatozoa retrieval is 93% (Ramos *et al.* 2004).

3.4.2 TESA, TESE and micro-TESE

Testicular sperm retrieval can be performed either on open surgical biopsy or as a percutaneous procedure. The term 'Testicular sperm extraction' (TESE) qualifies the open biopsy, and the term 'testicular sperm aspiration' (TESA) qualifies the percutaneous retrieval (Schlegel *et al.* 1998). The open surgical biopsy provides a higher quantity of tissue for harvesting spermatozoa than as aspiration procedure does. Nevertheless, TESA is generally sufficient for spermatozoa retrieval in patients with obstructive infertility and normal spermatogenesis. TESA is performed under local anesthesia. The transcutaneous aspiration uses a needle of 19-21 gauge directly into the testicular parenchyma and using negative pressure. In case of severely crompromised spermatogenesis, TESE should be the preferred method for harvesting spermatozoa.

TESE is performed after spermatic cord anesthesia with marcaine and a transversal 1 cm incision through the scrotum and tunica vaginalis down to the tunica albuginea and tissue from the mid anterior surface of the testis.

Microscopic TESE is a conjunction between open biopsy and it is conceptually similar to multibiopsy TESE, with the following differences: a single long testis incision is made to expose a large area of the testicular parenchyma and to access germ cells tubules, and a microscope is used to select the seminiferous tubules to be excised (Schlegel 1999). Since the number of spermatozoa obtained from micro-TESE is low, this procedure is generally performed the same day as eggs retrieval during ICSI.

3.4.3 MESA

The microsurgical epididymal sperm aspiration (MESA) is an advance in the therapy of non-reconstructable obstructive azoospermia (Schroeder-Printzen *et al.* 2000). The epididymis is exposed to a 12 mm incision made in the scrotal skin, an operating microscope is used to identify and open the epidydimal tubule to carry out the epididymal sperm aspiration. In 90 percent of obstructive azoospermia cases, spermatozoa were retrieved from epididymis (Silber *et al.* 1990, Holden *et al.* 1997; Patrizio 2000). Nowadays this technique has been substitute by the less invasive PESA method.

3.5 ICSI Results from surgical retrieved sperm

The patients with obstructive azoospermia and non-obstructive azoospermia are successfully treated with ICSI using surgically retrieved spermatozoa from epididymis or testis. Numerous literature report ICSI with spermatozoa recovered from epididymis (Silber *et al.* 1994; Tournaye *et al.* 1994; Mansour *et al.* 1996) or testis (Schyosman *et al.* 1993; Silber *et al.* 1995). The fertilization and pregnancy rates from obstructive azoospermic patients are comparable to those obtained from patients with ejaculated sperm (Aboughar *et al.* 1997). In those patients, only the etiology can influence ICSI outcomes. The patients with acquired causes of obstructive azoospermia have higher fertilization (Nicopoullos *et al.* 2004a). The patients with non-obstructive azoospermia have a statistically significant decrease of fertilization and pregnancy rate when compared to osbstructive azoospermic patients (Nicopoullos *et al.* 2004b).

3.6 IVF and ICSI results

Beyond the male factor, the efficacy of all assisted reproductive technique is directly correlated with female age with a significant pregnancy expectancy over 40 years old (Oehninger *et al.* 1995; Devroey *et al.* 1996).

With ICSI, lower rated in terms of fertilization and pregnancy rates can be expected when no motile spermatozoa are available.

It is now an overall consensus that the health of the children born from ART is the most important outcome parameter that has to be considered (Wennerholm *et al.* 2004). Pregnancy complications, major malformations, possible reasons for adverse outcome as well as the increase of multiple ART pregnancies must be taken under consideration. According to Jackson *et al.* (2004) and when compared to spontaneous conceived singleton children, the IVF and ICSI pregnancies are associated with higher odds of each perinatal mortality, pre-term delivery, low birth weight, very low birth weight and small gestation age. In twin pregnancies, the perinatal mortality is lower in assisted conception compared to spontaneous twins conceptions (Helmerhost *et al.* 2004). There is an overall increase for major congenital malformations after IVF and ICSI compared to spontaneously conceived children (Hansen *et al.* 2005) but no significant differences when IVF and ICSI are compared among them (Rimm *et al.* 2004). The possible causes of malformations are the abnormal caryotypes of infertile patients and properly in abnormal spermatozoa (Bonduelle *et al.* 1999). A significative 2.1% of *de novo* anomalies are observed when sperm concentrations used for ICSI was below 20 million/ml (Bonduelle *et al.* 2002). It is possible that ART is associated with a higher risk of imprinting disorder, especially Angelman syndrome and Beckwith-Wiedemann syndrome. However, children born with ART are healthy and develop similar to children spontaneously conceived. General health, growth, and mental and psychomotor development of IVF children do not differ from spontaneously conceived children, even if lower birth weight and prematurity may contribute to some health problems observed (Ludwig *et al.* 2006).

3.7 IMSI

The first findings on ICSI showed no influence of spermatozoa morphology on ICSI outcomes in terms of fertilization, embryo transfer and pregnancy rate (Hammadeh *et al.* 1996; Svalander *et al.* 1996; Gomez *et al.* 2000). But successively, De Vos *et al.* (2003) underlined lower fertilization, pregnancy and implantation rates when the injected spermatozoa were morphologically abnormal. These data are supported by evaluating the aneuploidy rate in abnormal spermatozoa. The aneuploidy rates for chromosomes X, Y and 18 was 29% in morphologically abnormal spermatozoa compared to 1.8%-5.5% in morphologically normal spermatozoa from the same sample (Ryu *et al.* 2004).

In 2002, the method of motile sperm organelle morphology examination was developed (MSOME-Bartoov *et al.* 2002). The examination is performed using an inverted microscope equipped with high-power Nomarski optics enhanced by digital imaging to achieve a magnification up to 6600X. The ICSI performed with a morphologically selected spermatozoa is called 'intracytoplasmic morphologically selected spermatozoa' (IMSI). In 2009, Nadalini *et al.* reviewed the benefice of this technique on fertilization rate, embryo quality, implantation and pregnancy rates. Furthermore, the application of IMSI lead to a decrease of abortion rate and major congenital malformation (Berkovitz *et al.* 2007). As a consequence, the clinical application of IMSI technique highlights the early and late paternal effects on embryo development (Vanderzwalmen *et al.* 2008). Several studies showed that the correlation between morphologically abnormal head of the spermatozoa and incorrect DNA packaging (Berkowitz *et al.* 2005; Hazout *et al.* 2006), DNA-protamine organization (Larson *et al.* 2000), DNA fragmentation (Franco *et al.* 2008), numerical and structural chromosome abnormalities (Calogero, 2003; Carrell *et al.* 2004).

In conclusion, IMSI seems to improve *in vitro* results in selected group of patients with male factor infertility (Balaban *et al.* 2011).

4. Sperm cryopreservation

4.1 History and indications for sperm banking

The history of human sperm cryobiology starts in the late 1940s with the discovery that glycerol protected the spermatozoa from freezing injury (Polge *et al.* 1949). In 1953, the first pregnancies were reported with the use of artificial insemination in combination with frozen-thawed sperm (Sherman and Bunge, 1953). Finally it was discovered that liquid nitrogen (LN2) leads to a better storage of human sperm with no subsequent loss of the motility when thawed after a long period of banking (Sherman, 1963).

The semen cryopreservation has an important role in the male fertility preservation. Usually, the patients that undergo sperm banking are those that have a high risk in becoming infertile due to surgical or medical treatments such as chemo- or radiotherapy for cancer treatment but it is nowadays commonly used for areas of medicine that rely on the use of potentially cytotoxic drugs including treatments of progressive loss of muscular or neurological function, or for autoimmune conditions (Ranganathan *et al.* 2002). The oncological treatments can have detrimental effects on the gonad and preclude the survivors from having genetically related children. In these individuals, some degree of fertility can return post-treatment but it cannot be predicted. The incidence of azoospermia is high and only 20 to 50 percent of these men eventually recover spermatogenesis (Shin *et al.* 2005). For these reasons, sperm banking is highly recommended for all patients with malignant disease that wish to preserve their fertility potential (Schover *et al.* 2002).

Sperm banking can be applied before contraceptive measure (vasectomy), for precautionary measure of fertility because of high risk occupation or activity such as military forces, to prevent infertility due to surgeries for recurrent varicocele or hydrocele (Anger *et al.* 2003), or in a view to ensure a sample available the day of *in vitro* treatment. The patients that need special collection such as assisted ejaculated patients with spinal injury, spermatozoa from retrograde ejaculation in urine or surgical collection from the genital tract, found in sperm banking the possibility to cryopreserve spermatozoa for clinical and reproductive subsequent use.

For all the patients that are at risk in losing the fertility due to pre-cited reasons, sperm banking gives a significant psychological support in the hope of future paternity. As a consequence, all males requiring chemo- or radiotherapy, including adolescents should have offered the possibility to store spermatozoa (Kamischke *et al.* 2004).

Finally, sperm banking plays a crucial role in sperm donation programs.

4.2 Sperm banking protocols and results

The success of sperm cryopreservation depends on the maintenance of post-thaw structural and functional integrity. The compartments (i.e. acrosome, flagella, midpiece) of the spermatozoon must be protected in a view to undergo normal fertilization under either *in vivo* or *in vitro* conditions. Human spermatozoa are not very sensitive to damage caused by rapid initial cooling (cold shock) and they may be more resistant than other cells to cryopreservation damage because of their low water content (50%). Nevertheless, the post-thaw motility of human spermatozoa can be ranged between 20 and 50 percent (Sbracia *et al.* 1997). It is believed that the cause of this decrease could be multiple including diminished integrity of the membranes and cryodamage to the membranes of the intracellular compartments, which affects energy metabolism and synthesis.

Pregnancy rates after IUI with cryopreserved donor semen are often related to sperm quality after thawing, timing of insemination and recipient factors such as age, previous pregnancy with sperm donor and ovulatory and uterine tubal disorders (Le Lannou and Lansac, 1993). If the semen is stored in appropriate conditions, no obvious deterioration of sperm quality should occur depending on the time of storage. Feldschuh *et al.* (2005) and Clarke *et al.* (2006) obtained children born after 28 years of sperm storage in liquid nitrogen.

As a single spermatozoa is needed for each single oocyte to micro-inject, cryopreservation of any live spermatozoa is worthwhile. The assisted reproductive technique to apply for the research of pregnancy and using thawed semen depends on the quality of post-thaw semen parameters.

Sperm cryopreservation is a complex process with a special responsibility and potential liability on the laboratory staff. The resources such as vessels, banks, storage room, liquid nitrogen containment and removal, the staff safety and protection, the safety of sample storage in a view to ensure sterility, very stable conditions of temperature and to avoid the cross-contamination with infectious agents between samples in storage (e.g. transmission of

HIV, or hepatitis B or C via cryopreservation vessels) must be considered. The labeling and traceability of stored samples must be supported by written, validated and applied procedures in a view to insure the safety of its clinical use.

The common practice to obtain sperm to freeze is masturbation but surgical retrieved samples can also be frozen. Every freezing procedure is successive to a semen analysis that states the quality of the sample especially for spermatozoa concentration (and number) and motility. Nowadays, the human sperm storage can be performed in vapor phase or in direct contact with liquid nitrogen itself. The vapor phase may reduce the chances to cross-contamination between siero-discordant samples but at the same time, it can be subject to large temperature gradients inside the vessels. In a view to ensure stable sample conditions, the temperatures should not go above -130°C. This condition must be ensured otherwise the direct contact with liquid nitrogen is more stable, safer and recommended for long period storage. Several freezing, sperm bank management protocols (Mortimer 2004; Wolf 1995) and cryoprotectants are available commercially. The WHO laboratory manual for the examination and processing of human semen details a home-made protocol of cryopreservation, storage and thawing of human spermatozoa for normozoospermic samples, oligozoospermic samples and surgically retrieved spermatozoa (WHO, 2010). The cryoprotectant used is glycerol-egg-yolk-citrate.

In the freezing procedure the cryoprotectant is added in a proportion 1/2 to semen at 37°C. Successively, the mixture is incubated at 30-35°C for 5 minutes and filled in 0.5 ml plastic sterile straws or in cryovials. The straws are sealed. The cooling procedure can be performed in programmable freezer or manually. The common cooling program is to cool the straws at 1.5°C per minute from 20°C to -6°C and then at 6°C per minute to -100°C. The chamber is than hold at -100°C for 30 minutes to allow the straws to be transferred to liquid nitrogen. In the manual method, the straws are placed at -20°C for 30 minutes, then placed at -70-79°C for 30 minutes and finally in liquid nitrogen (-196°C).

The straws are placed in plastic storage tubes (mini-goblets) and inserted in large storage goblets within the bank in liquid nitrogen. At this stage, the straws can be transported in appropriate tanks and stable conditions of temperature. At the present time there is no limit of time for the storage of frozen sample.

In the thawing procedure, the straws are removed from liquid nitrogen and placed at room temperature. Within 10 minutes, the straws (or cryovials) are opened and emptied. The post-thaw spermatozoa motility is valuated. The cryoprotectant is removed by washing procedures and the motile spermatozoa are available for clinical use.

In case of oligozoospermic samples and surgically retrieved spermatozoa, the few motile spermatozoa can be frozen for subsequent ICSI previous centrifugation at 1500g to concentrate the few motile spermatozoa.

Several samples can be frozen per patient, depending on the quality of the sample and the indication for sperm cryopreservation. As in the other procedures of ART, the identity and updated sierology of the patient must be confirmed at the beginning of each freezing set-up.

In recent studies, Agarwal *et al.* (2004) reported the outcomes of ART according to the invasivity of the technique with thawed sperm in male cancer survivors. A total of 87 cycles were performed with the respective pregnancy rates: 7% after IUI, 23% after IVF and 37%

after ICSI. On the same way, Schmith *et al.* (2004) reported 14.8% after IUI and 38.6% after ICSI.

Furthermore, there is no significant difference in quality between fresh and frozen-thawed epididymal or testicular spermatozoa in patients with obstructive azoospermia (Griffiths *et al.* 2004). The pregnancy rate from fresh and frozen-thawed spermatozoa extracted from the epididymis and testicular are similar among them (Nicopoullos *et al.* 2004b).

5. ART and genetic male infertility

In cases of male infertility due to severe non obstructive azoospermia or severe oligoastheteratozoospermia, a search for the karyotype for peripheral blood and microdeletions of AZF gene on Yp11 region should be performed.

In infertile men, the Klineferter syndrome (47,XXY) is the most common genetic abnormality, which occurs in 1 of 500 live male births and is present in 13% of azoospermic pazients (Rucker *et al.* 1998). In these patients, spermatozoa can easily be found from surgically intervention and good fertilization rates have been reported (Staessen *et al.* 2003). Oligozoospermic patients can present autosomal chromosomal aberrations such as Robertsonian and reciprocal translocations (Yoshida *et al.* 1997).

The prevalence of Y-chromosome microdeletions is 8% in infertile patients (Pagani *et al.* 2002). These microdeletions are rare in patients with a spermatozoa concentration higher than 5 millions per ml. The male children of patients with microdeletions will carry the Y defect and it has been reported an association with Turner's stigmata and sexual ambiguity (Patsalis *et al.* 2002).

In patients with congenital bilateral absence of the vas deferens (CBAVD), mutations in the cystic fibrosis membrane conductance regulator gene (CFTR) should be evaluated. Cystic Fibrosis (CF) is the most common autosomal recessive disease in Caucasians with an incidence of 1 in 2500 and a carrier rate of 1 in 25. CF mutations is associated with CBAVD in 72% of the patients, and with Congenital Unilateral Absence of the Vas Deferens (CUAVD) and epididymal obstruction in respectively 30 and 34% of the patients (Mak *et al.* 1999). In case of male carrier for CF mutations, the female patients must be screened prior to attempted ICSI and an appropriate genetic counseling must be given to the couple.

Normally, fewer than 30 CAG repeats are present in the exon 1 of androgen receptor gene. The abnormal expansion of repeats would be due to failure in DNA to repair and lead to a severe neurodegenerative syndrome called Kennedy's syndrome (Mak and Jarvi, 1996). Several studies have evidenced an increase of CAG repeats in normal men with idiopathic azoospermic (Yoshida *et al.* 1999) and in testicular tissue of infertile men (Maduro *et al.* 2003). Consequently, the future generations may be concerned by accelerated expansion of instable DNA such as CAG repeats.

The preimplantation genetic diagnosis (PGD) allows the couple at risk in the transmission of genetic defects such as chromosomal rearrangements (inherited chromosomal abnormalities), aneuploidy, X-linked diseases, autosomal single-gene disorders such as cystic fibrosis, haemoglobinopathies, Tay-Sachs disease to have an healthy child avoiding therapeutic abortion. Alternatives applications of PGD are for human leukocyte antigen (HLA) typing, nonmedical sex selection, genetic diseases with late onset. The principle of PGD is the genetic analysis of a minimum of one embryo cells that should reflect the genetic embryonic inheritance. Only unaffected embryos are transferred *in utero*. PGD was applied clinically for the first time in 1990 (Handyside *et al.* 1990) and nowadays the ESHRE PGD Consortium gives updated data of PGD clinical application around the world (Harper *et al.* 2010).

Imprinting of gene by methylation is an epigenetic phenomenon that regulates the gene expression. Cystidines located within dinucleotide CG repeated sequences are methyled into CpG islands lying outside the genes'coding regions. Imprinting occurs at different loci during gametogenesis and induces a gender-defined pattern of gene expression. At fertilization time, each gamete brings methylation patterns that are maintained in the offspring. If a failure of imprinting occurs during gametogenesis, two male or two female methylation pattern will be present at fertilization. This event is associated with spedific disease syndrome. In a recent study (Pacheco *et al.* 2011), CpG methylation profiles and mRNA alterations have been associated with low sperm motility.

The frequency of imprinting disorders such as Beckwith-Wiedemann syndrome and Angelman syndrome are higher in children born after ICSI (Cox *et al.* 2002; De Baun *et al.* 2003). The absolute risk is estimated at 1/3 000 for Beckwith-Wiedemann syndrome and 1/20 000 for Angelman syndrome. This data remains too low to be routinely screened of all ART children born (De Rycke, 2001).

6. Conclusion

A couple is considered infertile if no pregnancy is obtained after one year of unprotected intercourse. Infertility affects 15% of the couples. In 30% of the cases, pure female or pure male factor are the causes of infertility with an equal proportion. On a general point of view, the male factor is involved in half of the cases.

In the treatment of couple infertility, it has been understood very early that ART would give a big help in reaching the pregnancy of an healthy child. Nowadays it is nearly impossible to calculate how many millions of children were born after assisted reproduction around the world.

In the last decades, huge progresses have been made in helping the infertile male to become father, even in cases of very severe oligoteratoasthenozoospermia, azoospermia and carrying the risk of transmission of defective genetic trait. The sperm banking combined with ART plays a fundamental role in the preservation of male fertility for cancer patients.

In any assisted reproductive technique proposed to the couple to resolve their infertility problem, the patients must be informed on medical procedure and all risks linked to the procedure. The most common risks are hyperstimulation (1-4% patients) and multiple pregnancies. Around 29% of all IVF and ICSI cycles results in twin gestation, and 5% results in three or more fetus (SART, 2004). Furthermore, an increasing rate of major congenital malformation has been observed after IVF and ICSI, mainly due to the causes of infertility.

In the European Community, the donation, procurement, testing, processing, preservation, storage and distribution of reproductive cells and embryos are regulated in a view to guarantee the quality and the safety of their use and distribution (The European Parliament and the Council of the European Union, 2004)

7. References

Aboulghar MA, Mansour RT, Serour GI *et al.* (1997) Fertilization and pregnancy rates after intracytoplasmic sperm injection using ejaculated semen and surgically retrieved sperm. *Fertility and Sterility*, 68, 109-111

Agarwal A, Ranganathan P, Kattal N *et al.* (2004) Fertility after cancer: a prospective review of assisted reproductive outcome with banked semen specimens. *Fertility and Sterility*, 81, 342-348

Amann RP and Katz DF (2004) Reflections on CASA after 25 years. *Journal of Andrology*, 25, 317-325

Andersen AN, Goosens V, Gianaroli L *et al.* (2007) Assisted reproductive technology in Europe, 2003. Results generated from European registrers by ESHRE. *Human Reproduction*, 22, 1513-1525

Anger JT, Gilbert BR and Goldstein M (2003) Cryopreservation of sperm: indications methods and results. *Journal of Urology*, 170, 1079-1084

Balaban B, Yakin K, Alatas *et al.* (2011) Clinical outcome of intracytoplasmic injection of spermatozoa morphologically selected under high magnification: a prospective randomized study, *Reproductive BioMedicine Online*, 22, 472-476

Berkovitz A, Eltes F, Paul M *et al.* (2007) The chance of having a healthy normal child following intracytoplasmic morphologically-select sperm injection (IMSI) treatment is higher compared to conventional IVF-ICSI treatment. *Fertility and Sterility*, 88, S20

Berkovitz A, Eltes F, Yaari S *et al.* (2005) The morphological normalcy of the sperm nucleus and pregnancy rate of intracytoplasmic injection with morphologically selected sperm. *Human Reproduction* 20,185–190.

Bartoov B, Berkovitz A, Eltes F, Kogosowski A, Menezo Y and Baraik Y (2002) Real-time fine morphology of motile human sperm cells is associated with IVF-ICSI outcomes, *Journal of Andrology*, 23(1), 1-8

Bonduelle M, Camus M, De Vos A *et al.* (1999) Seven years of intracytoplasmic sperm injection and follow-up of 1987 subsequent children. *Human Reproduction*, 14(suppl 1), 243-264

Bonduelle M, Van Assche E, Joris H *et al.* (2002) Prenatal testing in ICSI pregnancies: incidence of chromosomal anomalies in 1586 karyotypes and relation to sperm parameters. *Human Reproduction*, 17, 2600-2614

Burr RW, Siegberg R, Flaherty SP, Wang XJ, Matthews CD (1996) The influence of sperm morphology and the number of motile sperm inseminated on the outcome of intrauterine insemination combined with mild ovarian stimulation. *Fertility and Sterility*, 65, 127-132

Chemes HE, Rawe YV (2003) Sperm pathology: a step beyond descriptive morphology. Origin, characterization and fertility potential and abnormal sperm phenotypes in infertile men. *Human Reproduction Update*, 9, 405-428

Clarke GN *et al.* (2006) Recovery of human sperm motility and ability to interact with the human zona pellucida after more than 28 years of storage in liquid nitrogen. *Fertility and Sterility*, 86, 721-722

Cohen J, Malter H, Whright G *et al.* (1989) Partial zona dissection of human oocytes when failure of zona pellucid penetration is anticipated. *Human Reproduction*, 4(4), 435-442

Calogero AE (2003) Absolute polymorphic teratozoospermia in patients with oligo-asthenozoospermia is associated with an elevated sperm aneuploidy rate. *Journal of Andrology* 24, 598–603

Carrll DT, Emery BR, Wilcox AL *et al.* (2004) Sperm chromosome aneuploidy as related to male factor infertility and some ultrastructure defects. *Archives of Andrology* 50, 181–185

Correa-Perez *et al.* (2004) Clinical management of men producing ejaculates characterized by high levels of dead sperm and altered seminal plasma factors consistent with epididymal necrospermia. *Fertility and Sterility*, 81, 1148-1150

Cox GF, Burger J, Lip V *et al.* (2002) Intracytoplasmic sperm injection may increase the risk if imprinting defects. *American Journal of Human Genetics*, 71, 162-164

De Baun MR, Niemitz EL and Feinberg AP (2003) Association of in vitro fertilization with Beckwith-Wiedemann syndrome and epigenetic alteration of LIT1 and H19. *American Journal of Human Genetics*, 72, 150-160

De Rycke M (2001) Epigenetics and ART. Infertility and assisted reproduction, *Cambridge University Press*, p677-683

De Sutter P, Veldeman L, Kok P *et al.* (2005) Comparison of outcome of pregnancy after intra-uterine insemination (IUI) and IVF. *Human Reproduction*, 20, 1642-1646

De Vos A, Van De Velde H. Joris H *et al.* (2003) Influence of individual sperm morphology on fertilization, embryo morphology, and pregnancy outcome of intracytoplasmic sperm injection, *Fertility and Sterility*, 79, 42-8

Devroey P, Godoy H, Smitz J *et al.* (1996) Female age predicts embryonic implantation after ICSI: a case controlled study. *Human Reproduction*, 11, 1324-1327

European Society of Human Reproduction and Embryology (ESHRE) (2006) Three million babies born using assisted reproductive technologies. Press release at the 2006 Annual Meeting

Feldschuh J *et al.* (2005) Successful sperm storage for 28 years. *Fertility and Sterility*, 84, 1017

Franco JG, Baruffi RLR, Mauri AL *et al.* (2008) Significance of large nuclear vacuoles in human spermatozoa: implications for ICSI, *Reproductive BioMedicine Online*, 17(1), 42-45

Gillin-Smith C. *et al.* (2006) HIV and reproductive care – a review of current practice. *British Journal of Gynaecology*, 113, 869-878

Gomez E, Perez-Cano I, Amorocho B *et al.* (2000) Effects of injected spermatozoa morphology on the outcome of intracytoplasmic sperm injection in humans. *Fertility and Sterility*, 74, 842-843

Griffiths M, Kennedy CR, Rai J *et al.* (2004) Should cryopreserved epididymal or testicular sperm be recovered from obstructive azoospermic men for ICSI? *BJOG*, 111, 1289-1293

Hammadeh ME, Al-Hasani S, Stieber M *et al.* (1996) The effect of chromatin condensation (Aniline Blue staining) and morphology (strict criteria) of human spermatozoa on fertilization, cleavage and pregnancy rated in an intracytoplasmic sperm injection programme. *Human Reproduction*, 11, 2468-2471

Handyside AH, Kontogianni EH, hardy K and Winston RM (1990) Pregnancies from biopsied human preimplantation embryos sexed by Y-specific DNA amplification, *Nature*, 344(6268), 768-770

Hansen M, Bower C, Milne E *et al.* (2005) Assisted reproductive technologies and the risk of birth defects-a systematic review. *Human Reproduction*, 20(2), 328-338

Harper JC, Coonen E, De Rycke M (2010) ESHRE PGD consortium data collection X: cycles from January to December 2007 with pregnancy followup, to October 2008, Human Reproduction, Vol.25, No.11 pp. 2685–2707

Hazout A, Dumont-Hassan M, Junca AM *et al.* (2006) High-magnification ICSI overcomes paternal effect resistant to conventional ICSI. *Reproductive BioMedicine Online* 12, 19–25.

Helmerhost FM, Perquin DA, Donker D *et al.* (2004) Perinatal outcome of singletons and twins after assisted conception: a systematic review of controlled studies. *BMJ*, 328(7434), 261.

Hirsh AV, Mills C, Bekir J *et al.* (1994) Factors iinfluencing the outcome of in vitro fertilization with epididymal spermatozoa in irreversible obstructive azoospermia. *Human Reproduction*, 9, 1710-1716

Holden CA, Fuscaldo GF, Jackson P *et al.* (1997) Frozen.thawed epididymal spermatozoa for intracytoplasmic sperm injection. *Fertility and Sterility*, 67, 81-87

Human Fertilization and Embryology Authority (HFEA) (2005) The patient's guide. London: HFEA

Jackson RA, Gibson KA, Wu YW *et al.* (2004) Perinatal outcomes in singletons following in vitro fertilization: a meta-analysis. *Obstetricts and Gynecology*, 103(3), 551-563

Jouannet P. *et al.* (1988) Male factors and the likelihood of pregnancy in infertile couples. I. Study of sperm characteristics. *International Journal of Andrology*, 11:379-394

Kamischke A *et al.* (2004) Cryopreservation of sperm from adolescents and adults with malignancies. *Journal of Andrology*, 25, 586-592

Larsen L *et al.* (2000) Computeur-assisted semen analysis parameters as predictors for fertility of men from the general population. The Danish First Pregnancy Planner Study Team. *Human Reproduction*, 15: 1562-1567

Larson K, DeJonge C, Barnes A *et al.* (2000) Relationship of assisted reproductive technique (ART) outcomes with sperm chromatin integrity and maturity as measured by the sperm chromatin structure assay (SCSA). *Human Reproduction* 15, 1717–1722.

Laws-King A, Trounson A, Sathananthan H *et al.* (1987) Fertilization of human oocytes by microinjection of single spermatozoa under the zona pellucida. *Fertility and Sterility*, 48(4), 637-642

Le Lannou D and Lansac J (1993) Artificial procreation with frozen donor semen: the French experience of CECOS. In: Barratt CLR, Cooke ID, eds. Donor insemination. *Cambridge, Cambridge University Press*: 152-169

LudwigAK, Sutcliffe AG ,Dietrich K, Ludwig M (2006) Post-neonatal health and development of children born after assisted reproduction: a systematic review of controlled studies. *European Journal of Obstetric Gynecology Reproductive Biology* , 127(1), 3-25

Maduro MR, Casella R, Kim E *et al.* (2003) Microsatellite instability and defects in mismatch repair proteins: a new aetiology for Sertoli-cell-only syndrome. *Molecular Human Reproduction*, 9, 61-68

Mansour RT, Aboulghar MA, Serour GI *et al.* (1996) Intracytoplasmic sperm injection using microsurgically retrieved epididymal and testicular sperm. *Fertility and Sterility*, 65(3), 566-572

Mak V and Jarvi KA (1996) The genetics of male infertility. *Journal of Urology*, 156, 1245-1256

Mak V, Zielenski J, Tsui LC *et al.* (1999) Proportion of cystic fibrosis gene mutations not detected by routine testing in men with obstructive azoospermia. *JAMA*, 281, 2217-2224

Montanaro Gauci M, Kruger TF, Coetzee K *et al.* (2001) Stepwise regression analysis to study male and female factors impacting on pregnancy rate in an uterine insemination programme. *Andrologia*,33, 135-141

Mortimer D (1994) Practical Laboratory Andrology. New York, NY: Oxford University Press.

Mortimer D (2004) Current and future concepts and practices in human sperm cryobanking. *Reproductive BioMedicine Online*, 9, 134-151

Nadalini M, Tarozzi N, Distratis V, Scaravelli G and Borini A (2009) Impact of intracytoplasmic morpholocically selected sperm injection on assisted reproduction outcome: a review. *Reproductive BioMedicine Online*, 19(3), 45-55

Nagy ZP, Liu J, Joris H *et al.* (1995) The results of intracytoplasmic sperm injection is not related to any of the three basic sperm parameters. *Human Reproduction*, 10(5), 1123-1129

Nicopoullos JDM, Gilling-Smith C and Ramsay JWA (2004a) Does the cause of obstructive azoospermia affect the outcome of intracytoplasmic sperm injection: a meta-analysis. *BJU Int*, 93, 1282-1286

Nicopoullos JDM, Gilling-Smith C, Almeida PA *et al.* (2004b) Use of chirurgical sperm retrieval in azoospermic men: meta-analysis. *Fertility and Sterility*, 82, 691-701

Ombelet W, Vandeput H, Van de Putte G *et al.* (1997) Intrauterine insemination after ovarian stimulation with clomiphene citrate: predictive potential of inseminating motile count and sperm morphology, *Human Reproduction*, 12, 1458-1465

Oehninger S, Acost AA, Morshedi M *et al.* (1988) Corrective measures and pregnancy outcome in in vitro fertilization in patients with severe sperm morphology abnormalities. *Fertility and Sterility*, 50, 283-287

Oehninger S, Veeck L, Lanzendorf S *et al.* (1995) Intracytoplasmic sperm injection: Achievement of high pregnancy rates in couples with severe male factor infertility is dependent primarily upon female and not male factors. *Fertility and Sterility*, 64, 977-981

Pacheco SE, Andres Houseman E, Christensen BC, *et al.* (2011) Integrative DNA methylation and gene expression analyses identify DNA packaging and epigenetic regulatory genes associated with low motility sper. *PLoS ONE*, 6(6), e20280

Pagani R, Brugh VMIII, Lamb DJ (2002) Chromosome and male infertility. *The Urologic Clinics of North America*, 29, 745-753

Palermo G, Joris H, Devroey P *et al.* (1992) Pregnancies after intracytoplasmic sperm injection of single spermatozoa into an oocyte. *Lancet*, 340, 17-18

Palermo G, Joris H, Derde MP *et al.* (1993) Sperm characteristics and outcome of human assisted fertilization by subzonal insemination and intracytoplasmic sperm injection. *Fertility and Sterility*, 63, 1231-1240

Palermo GD, Alikani M, Bertoli M *et al.* (1996) Oolemma characteristics in relation to survival and fertilization patterns of oocytes treated by intracytoplasmic sperm injection. *Human Reproduction*, 11(1), 172-176

Patrizio P (2000) Cryopreservation of epidydimal sperm. *Molecular and Cellular Endocrinology*, 27, 11-14

Patsalis PC, Sismani C, Quintana-Murci L *et al.* (2002) Effects of transmission of Y chromosome AZFc deletions. *Lancet*, 360, 1222-4

Polge C, Smith A and Parkes A (1949) Revival of spermatozoa after vitrification and dehydration at low temperature. *Nature*, 164, 666

Ramos L, Wetzels AM, Hendriks JC *et al.* (2004) Percutaneous epididymal sperm aspiration: a diagnostic tool for the prediction of complete spermatogenesis. *Reproductive BioMedicine Online*, 8, 657-663

Ranganathan P, Mahran AM, Hallak J and Agarwal A (2002) Sperm cryopreservation for men with nonmalignant, systemic diseases : a descriptive stidy. *Journal of Andrology*, 23, 71-75

Rimm AA, Katayama AC, Diaz M *et al.* (2004) A meta-analysis of controlled studies comparing major malformation rates in IVF and ICSI infants with naturally conceived children. *Journal of Assisted Reproduction and Genetics*, 21(12), 437-443

Rucker GB, Mielnik A, King P *et al.* (1998) Preoperative screening for genetic abnormalities in men with nonobstructive azoospermia before testicular sperm extraction. *Journal of Urology*, 160, 2068-2071

Ryu HM, Lin WW, Lamb DJ *et al.* (2004) Increaesed chromosome X, Y, and 18 nondisjunction in sperm from infertile patients that were identified as normal by strict morphology: implication for intracytoplasmic sperm injection. *Fertility and Sterility*, 76, 879-883

Sacks PC and Simon JA (1991) Infectious complications of intrauterine insemination: a case report and literature review. *International Journal of Fertility*, 36, 331-339

Savasi V. *et al.* (2007) Safety of sperm washing and ART outcome in 741 HIV-1-serodiscordant couples. *Human Reproduction*, 22, 772-777

Sbracia M, Grasso J, Stronk J and Huszar G (1997) Hyaluronic acid substantially increases the retention of motility in cryopreserved/thawed human spermatozoa. *Human Reproduction*, 12, 1949-1054

Schlegel PN, Su LM and Li PS (1998) Gonadal sperm retrieval: potential for testicular damage in non-obstructive azoospermia. In Fillicori & C. Flamigni, eds. *Treatment of Infertility: The new frontiers.* New Jercy, NJ: Communications Media for Education, 383-392

Schlegel PN (1999) Testicular sperm extraction; micro dissection improves sperm yield with minimal tissue excision. *Human Reproduction*, 14, 131-135

Schyosman R, Vanderzwalmen P, Nijs M *et al.* (1993) Successful fertilization by testicular spermatozoa in an in vitro fertilization programme. *Human Reproduction*, 8(8), 1339-1340

Schmith KL, Larsen E, Bangsboll S *et al.* (2004) Assisted reproduction in male cancer survivors: fertility tretmant and outcome in 67 couples. *Human Reproduction*, 19, 2806-2810

Schover LR, Brey K, Lichtin A, Lipshultz LI and Jeha S (2002) Knowledge and experience regarding cancer, infertility, and sperm banking in younger male survivors. *Journal of Clinical Oncology*, 20, 1880-1889

Schroeder-Printzen I, Zumbé J, Bispink L (2000) Microsurgical epididymal sperm aspiration: aspirate analysis and straws available after cryopreservation in patients with non-reconstructable obstructive azoospermia. *Human Reproduction*, 15, 2531-2535

Sherman JK (1963) Improved methods of preservation of human spermatozoa by freezing and freeze-dying. *Fertility and Sterility*, 14, 49-64

Sherman JK and Bunge RG (1953) Observation of preservation of human spermatozoa at low temperatures. *Preceedings of the Society for Experimental Biology and Medicine. Society for Experimental Biology and Medicine*,82, 686-688

Shin D, Lo KC and Lipshultz LI (2005) Treatment options for infertile male with cancer. *Journal of the National Cancer Institute Monographs*, 34, 48-50

Silber S, Ord T, Balmaceda J, Patrizio P and Asch RH (1990) Congenital absence of the vas deferens: studies on the fertilizing capacity of the human epididymal sperm. *New England Jurnal of Medicine*, 323, 1788-1792

Silber S.J, Nagy ZP, Liu J *et al.* (1994) Conventional in vitro fertilization versus intracytoplasmic sperm injection for patients requiring microsurgical sperm aspiration. *Human Reproduction*, 9(9) 1705-1709

Silber S.J, Van Steirteghem AC, Liu J *et al.* (1995) High fertilization and pregnancy rate after intracytoplasmic sperm injection with spermatozoa obtained from testicular biopsy. *Human Reproduction*, 10(1), 148-152

Society for Assisted Reproductive Technology and Centers for Disease Control and Prevention (2004) ART success rates: national summary and fertility clinic reports. www.cdc.gov/reproductivehealth

Staessen C and Van Steirteghem AC (1997) The chromosomal constitution of embryos developing from abnormal fertilized oocytes after intracytoplasmic sperm injection and conventional in vitro fertilization. *Human Reproduction*, 12(2), 321-327

Staessen C, Tournaye H, Van Aasche E *et al.* (2003) PGD in 47,XXY Klineferter's syndrome patients. *Human Reproduction Update*, 9, 319-330

Steptoe PC and Edwards EG (1978) Birth after the re-implanted of a human embryo. *Lancet*, 2, 366

Svalander P, Jakobsson AH, Forsberg AS, Bengtsson AC, Wikland M (1996) The outcome of intracytoplasmic sperm injection is unrelated to "strict criteria" sperm morphology. *Human Reproduction*, 11, 1019-1022

The European Parliament and the Council of the European Union (2004) DIRECTIVE 2004/23/EC OF THE EUROPEAN PARLIAMENT AND OF THE COUNCIL of 31 March 2004 on setting standards of quality and safety for the donation, procurement, testing, processing, preservation, storage and distribution of human tissues and cells, *Official Journal of the European Union*, L 102/48-58

Tournaye H, Devroey P, Liu J *et al.* (1994) Microsurgical epididymal sperm aspiration and intracytoplasmic sperm injection : a new effective approach to infertility as a result of congenital bilateral absence of the vas deferens. *Fertility and Sterility*, 61(6), 1045-1051

Tournaye H, Liu J, Nagy Z *et al.* (1996) The use of testicular sperm for intracytoplasmic sperm injection in patients with necrozoospermia. *Fertility and Sterility*, 66(2), 331-334

Van Steirteghem AC, Liu J, Nagy Z *et al.* (1993a) Higher success rate by intracytoplasmic sperm injection than by subzonal insemination: report of a second series of 300 consecutive treatment cycles. *Human Reproduction*, 8(7), 1055-1066

Van Steirteghem AC, Nagy Z, Joris H *et al.* (1993b) High fertilization and implantation rates after intracytoplasmic sperm injection. *Human Reproduction*, 8(7), 1061-1066

Van Steirteghem AC (2007) Assisted Fertilization. In vitro fertilization, a practical approach. Eds Informal Healtcare USA, Inc.

Van Waart J, Kruger TF, Lombard CJ, Ombelet W (2001). Predictive value of normal sperm morphology in intrauterine insemination (IUI): a structural literature review. *Human Reproduction Update*, 7, 495-500

Vanderzwalmen P, Hiemer A, Rubner P *et al.* (2008) Blastocyst development after sperm selection at high magnification is associated with size and number of nuclear vacuoles. *Reproductive BioMedicine Online*, 17(5), 617-627

Wennerholm UB and Bergh C (2004) what is the most relevant standard of success in assisted reproduction? Singleton live births should also include preterm births. *Human Reproduction*, 19(9), 1943-1945

Wilton LJ *et al.* (1988) Human male infertility caused by degeneration and deaths of sperms in the epididymis. *Fertility and Sterility*, 49, 1051-1058

Wolf DP (1995) Semen cryopreservation. In: Keye WR *et al.*, eds. *Infertility evaluation and treatment*. Philadelphia, WB Saunders, 686-695

World Healt Organization (1987) WHO Laboratory Manual for the Examination of Human Semen and Sperm-Cervical Mucus Interaction. Cambridge University Press, Second edition. Cambridge.

World Healt Organization (1992) WHO Laboratory Manual for the Examination of Human Semen and Sperm-Cervical Mucus Interaction. Cambridge University Press, Third edition. Cambridge.

World Healt Organization (2010) WHO Laboratory Manual for the Examination and Processing of Human Semen. Cambridge University Press, Fifth edition. Cambridge.

Yalti S, Gurbuz B, Sezer H, Celik S (2004) Effects of semen characteristics on IUI combined with mild ovarian stimulation, *Arch Androl*, 50(4), 239-246

Yeung CH, Cooper TG, Nieschlag E (1997) A technique for standardization and quality control of subjective sperm motility assessment in semen analysis, *Fertility and Sterility*, 67, 1156-1158

Yoshida A, Miura K, Shirai M (1997) Cytogenetic survey of 1007 infertilt males. *International Journal of Urology*, 58, 166-76

Yoshida KI, Yano M, Chiba K , Honda M, Kitahara S (1999) CAG repeat length in the androgen receoptor gene is enhanced in patients with idiopathic azoospermia, *Urology*, 54, 1078-1081

Zinaman MJ *et al.* (2000) Semen quality and human fertility: a prospective study with healthy couples. *Journal of Andrology*, 21: 145-153

6

Makings of the Best Spermatozoa: Molecular Determinants of High Fertility

Erdogan Memili et al.*
Mississippi State University, Animal and Dairy Sciences, MS, USA

1. Introduction

What is the significance of sperm in reproduction? Recent studies have demonstrated surprising clues that have changed the answers to this question. In addition to providing half of the genome of a mammalian organism, sperm also contributes other molecules such as mRNA, microRNAs (miRNA), proteins, and metabolites that are vitally important for fertility (Feugang et al., 2009, 2010; Peddinti et al., 2008). Furthermore, molecular health of the sperm chromatin and DNA quality also play major roles in sperm viability. Put together, these recent advances have produced a wealth of new knowledge that can provide a systems biology point of view for fertility. These findings highlight the fact that changes in sperm DNA and expressed gene products provide information on the effects of environment on development and disease.

There is a comprehensive database of bull fertility records from thousands of artificial inseminations, which allow cattle producers to draw conclusions about fertility. Additionally, *in vitro* fertilization (IVF) in cattle is well established allowing us to exploit a method to study the molecular basis of sperm quality assessing and quantifying male infertility experimentally. Moreover, cow and human genomes and reproductive physiologies are similar; which makes it possible to apply to humans some of the knowledge produced in cattle. In consequence this review will mainly use the bull as the animal model, although it will also include studies on other mammals including humans and mice.

* Sule Dogan[1], Nelida Rodriguez-Osorio[2], Xiaojun Wang[1], Rodrigo V. de Oliveira[1,3], Melissa C. Mason[1,4], Aruna Govindaraju[1], Kamilah E. Grant[1], Lauren E. Belser[1], Elizabeth Crate[1,5], Arlindo Moura[4] and Abdullah Kaya[6]
[1]*Mississippi State University; Animal and Dairy Sciencesl; MS, USA*
[2]*University of Antioquia,Colombia*
[3]*Federal University of Ceara; Department of Animal Science, Brazil*
[4]*Alcorn State University; Department of Agriculture; MS, USA*
[5]*New College of Florida; FL, USA*
[6]*Alta Genetics, Incorporated; WI, USA*
**Corresponding Authors*

Fertility variation is an essential factor limiting efficient production of cattle. There are several factors that influence sperm quality and fertility which can be divided into subcategories of compensatory (sperm viability, motility, etc.), and uncompensatory (molecular defects in the sperm) traits (Dejarnette, 2005). High fertility can be achieved for bulls suffering from compensable sperm defects by increasing the number of spermatozoa deposited in the cow's reproductive tract. Despite providing high numbers of sperm cells with normal morphology (motility and viability), bulls with non-compensable defects may never achieve adequate fertility, and the molecular mechanisms involved in these defects remain unclear. This gap in the knowledge base engenders millions of dollars of economic impact; in spite of this, there is no conventional method to adequately predict sire fertility. A thorough understanding of the mechanisms regulating bull fertility is essential for obtaining consistently high reproductive efficiency, ensuring lower costs and preventing serious time-loss for breeders.

Male infertility can be classified as pre-testicular, testicular and post-testicular, depending on its anatomic and physiologic origin. Patrizio and Broomfield have proposed a classification that includes male infertility with a single gene defect, which includes Usher's, Kallmann's and Immotile cilia syndromes; and male infertility with a chromosomal defect including Kleinfelter's, Noonan's and Prader-Will's syndromes as well as deletions on the AZF a, b or c regions of the Y chromosome. (Cram et al., 2001; De Kretser and Baker, 1999; Ferlin et al., 2007; Krausz and Giachini, 2007). Although sperm dysfunction is known to be a major cause of infertility, there is no pharmacological treatment to improve fertility. The only option for subfertile or infertile men is assisted reproductive technology (ART), which usually consists of treatments that might include intrauterine insemination (IUI), *in vitro* fertilization (IVF), or intracytoplasmic sperm injection (ICSI) depending on the severity of the dysfunction. It has been established that in men undergoing ICSI that 5% of those suffering from oligozoospermia, teratozoospermia and asthenoospermia show an abnormal karyotype compared to 20% of the ones with azoospermia. Our current limited understanding of the cellular and molecular mechanisms involved in sperm function is the main reason for the lack of clinical progress in this area.

2. Main theme summary

Male fertility, the ability of the sperm to fertilize and activate the egg and support early embryonic development is an essential factor for animal reproduction and development. Despite producing adequate numbers of sperm with normal morphology and motility, fertility of some bulls remains poor. This review summarizes molecular phenotypes of the sperm that are associated with sperm viability, methods to study these phenotypes, and implications of new biomolecular markers for improving fertility. There are several assays and tests which are utilized to predict sperm viability and potential fertility. The pitfall of these particular methods is their reliance on phenotypic data of sires which can be misleading and does not predict actual fertility. Further, no diagnostic assessment based on molecular characteristics of the sperm has been identified to accompany said analyses. Some males with normal sperm motility, morphology and cell number have been suffering from subpar fertility causing a decline in male fertility in mammals and other species (Saacke et al., 2000). Molecular mechanisms responsible for this developmental problem are currently unknown. Addressing this issue is imperative to prevent deficiency in reproduction, as well as aggressively pursuing solutions to remedy reproductive health disparities in multiple species.

2.1 Spermatogenesis

In mammals, spermatozoa are produced in the testis, subjected to maturation in the epididymis and stored in the cauda region of this organ. Upon ejaculation, gametes are mixed with accessory sex gland (ASG) secretions, starting their journey to fertilization. In this context, constituents of the sperm themselves and of fluids surrounding them potentially modulate the fertilizing capacity of these cells. In male offspring, germ cells, called prospermatogonia (De Felici, 2009) remain in mitotic arrest in the seminiferous tubules until the male reaches puberty. Morphologically three spermatogonial subtypes have been identified in human testis: type A pale spermatogonia, type A dark spermatogonia and type B spermatogonia. Type A pale spermatogonia are derived from the spermatogonial stem cells and they are maintained in the testis by mitosis as precursor cells. On the other hand, type A dark spermatogonia generate type B spermatogonia, which will undergo meiosis producing spermatocytes (Sadler, 2000). Serial cross-sections of a seminiferous tubule show that sperm cells differentiate in cycles, known as spermatogenic cycles, which are initiated by a surge in gonadotropin releasing hormone (GnRH) from the hypothalamus. Each cycle represents the time it takes for the recurrence of the same cellular stage within the same segment of the tubule. Each stage of the cycle follows in an orderly sequence along the length of the tubule. The number of stages in the spermatogenic cycle is species-specific with six stages in man (~64 days) and twelve stages in both the mouse and the bull (Phillips et al., 2010). During each spermatogenic cycle, spermatogonia proliferate by mitosis and after several stages primary spermatocytes are formed. Each primary spermatocyte will enter meiosis and through the first meiotic division will produce two secondary spermatocytes, each of which will finish meiosis becoming round haploid spermatids. The last part of the process is spermiogenesis (spermatid to spermatozoon), characterized by (*1*) formation of the acrosome; (*2*) condensation of the nucleus; (*3*) shaping of flagellum including mid-piece, and (*4*) loss of the cytoplasmic residues (Sadler, 2000). Spermatogenesis is ended by the delivery of these tailed cells (spermatozoa) into the seminiferous tubule lumen (Lie et al., 2009). Spermatozoa will then be transported into the epididymis, where they will be stored and will acquire forward motility. However, final maturation of sperm cells (sperm capacitation) is only completed in the female reproductive tract.

In contrast, mammalian oogenesis is accomplished through three developmental stages: the initiation of meiosis, the formation of a follicle around each oocyte during the perinatal period, and finally the cyclic growth of follicles and maturation of the oocytes within. Primordial germ cells in a female divide mitotically and differentiate into oogonia. The peak number of female primordial germ cells is reached at the transition from mitosis to meiosis (Gondos, 1981), but this number is drastically reduced, as a result of apoptosis, before the female is born (Hartshorne et al., 2009; Morita and Tilly, 1999). Most of them undergo mitosis whereas some are arrested in prophase of meiosis I and become primary oocytes. Near the time of birth, all primary oocytes undergo meiosis, passing through leptotene, zygotene, and pachytene stages before arresting in the diplotene stage (McLaren, 2003), which is a resting stage that is maintained by effect of oocyte maturation inhibitor (Sadler, 2000; Elsik et al. 2009). Oocytes do not complete the first meiotic division, so they remain in a meiotic arrest until the female reaches puberty. The events that coordinate the initiation of meiosis are not completely understood, however, several studies have proposed that retinoic acid (RA) is the molecular switch that determines meiotic entry in the developing ovary (Bowles et al., 2006; Koubova et al., 2006; Wang and Tilly, 2010). During each estrous or menstrual cycle, a cohort of follicles is recruited; these follicles will grow and develop an antrum or cavity therefore being known as antral follicles. From this cohort, only a subset of follicles (in polytocous species) or only one follicle (in monotocous species) is selected for dominance and ovulation becoming preovulatory follicles (McGee and Hsueh, 2000). Prior to ovulation oocytes resume meiosis, this can be recognized by dissolution of the nuclear envelope known as germinal vesicle breakdown (GVBD). However, meiosis is stopped again and oocytes are ovulated at the metaphase of the second meiotic division (MII oocytes). The final stage of meiosis will only be completed if the oocyte is fertilized; otherwise, the oocyte degenarates in 24 hr post ovulation (Sadler 2000).

Fertilization mostly occurs in the ampullary region of the Oviduct by a sperm that completes capacitation and acrosome reaction. The sperm's entrance into the oocyte triggers a release of calcium from storage sites into the ooplasm in a wave like pattern (Kline and Kline, 1992; Swann and Yu, 2008), giving rise to a set of events known as oocyte activation. This activation includes the release of cortical granules leading to the block of polyspermy known as zona reaction (Abbott and Ducibella, 2001) and the cell cycle resumption, leading to the culmination of meiosis and the extrusion of the second polar body. Within around 24 hours of fertilization, the paternal and maternal genomes are assembled into pronuclei (PNs), which replicate their DNA. Chromosomes then come together at syngamy, the last step of fertilization that culminates with the formation of the one cell embryo, the zygote followed by embryogenesis.

2.2 Chromatin structure and DNA integrity of spermatozoa

2.2.1 Sperm chromatin and condensation

Since genetic material in the sperm is essential for fertilization in mammals, DNA is tightly packaged in the sperm head for its protection. In the course of this packaging DNA would be more condensed than that of somatic cells by replacing histones, with arginine and cysteine rich protamines. Histones are first replaced by transition proteins (TPs) and then by protamines. Nucleoprotamines package DNA over ten times more efficiently than nucleohistones, bringing DNA replication or RNA transcription to a halt during sperm maturation (Shaman et al., 2007; Miller et al., 2010). In somatic cells, DNA is packaged in a structure known as a selonoid; however, sperm DNA is packed as a loop named doughnut or torus (Ward, 1993). Once mammalian sperm chromatin is packaged into protamines, DNA is tightly coiled into a compact doughnut shape, known as a protamine toroid. Protamine-DNA toroids attach to a proteinaceous nuclear matrix via matrix attachment regions (MAR) similar to those of somatic cells. Several key factors play roles in chromatin remodeling such as protamine 1 (PR1), protamine 2 (PR2), TPs and MARs (Sharma et al., 2004). Towards the end of sperm maturation, 15% of spermatozoa still have histones associated with their DNA, whereas almost 85% have replaced them with protamines (Oliva, 2006) . There are two types of protamines found in sperm; P1, which are always present in mammals and are mature proteins, and P2, which are absent in some species and are generated by precursors (Mengual et al., 2003). A reduction in protamine content in the sperm nucleus is considered to be protamine deficiency; this seems to occur when there is a decrease in P2 levels, which alters the normal P1/P2 ratio by increasing the P1 to P2 levels (Oliva, 2006). Although the results are still being debated, one theory on the altered P1/P2 ratio is that there is an abnormal processing of the P2 precursor (de Yebra et al., 1998) that would increase the P1 to P2 ratio. A second theory for protamine deficiency is that there is a malfunction in the replacement of histones for protamines during spermiogenesis (Blanchard et al., 1990).

There are three basic reasons that could explain why DNA is more compact in the sperm cells compared to that of somatic cells. The first reason for this compaction is the optimization of the sperm cells' shape that enables their movement through the female reproductive tract. Secondly, sperm nuclei are protected by super-compaction from the effects of genotoxic factors. Lastly, sperm compaction assures the "frozen" state of the paternal genome, preserving its post-fertilization epigenetic function in the developing embryo (Miller et al., 2010). Histone-packaged chromatin is more susceptible to DNA damage than the bulk, protamine-packaged DNA that has an important function in embryonic development (Aoki et al., 2006). Protamines are essential for normal fertilization as their deficiency leads to much higher levels of sperm DNA strand breakage. It was observed that abnormal chromatin packaging can affect the accuracy of paternal gene expression (Tesarik et al., 2004). The relationship between sperm chromatin packaging anomalies and sub-fertility in human was shown in terms of sperm dysfunction caused by higher levels of DNA damage (Aoki et al., 2006; Oliva, 2006). Nicks in DNA occur in toroid linkers, between protamine-toroid loops and in sperm nuclear matrix. Endogenous DNAse digestion of DNA occurs at MAR regions. Finally, from a very condensed state, sperm DNA becomes decondensed right after fertilization. It has been shown that the sperm nuclear matrix is vital for activation of the fertilized egg (Shaman et al., 2007).

2.2.2 Sperm DNA integrity

Fundamentally, DNA integrity can influence sperm quality because sperm DNA damage is clearly associated with male infertility, but only a small percentage of spermatozoa from fertile males possess detectable levels of DNA damage (Spano et al., 2000). Among the main examined factors affecting DNA are defective sperm chromatin packaging, apoptosis, and oxidative stress (Agarwal and Said, 2003).

The first cause of DNA damage in sperm is defective and/or insufficient DNA packaging during spermiogenesis. As mentioned previously, sperm chromatin is a highly organized and compact structure consisting of DNA and heterogeneous nucleoproteins. It is condensed and insoluble in nature, which are features that protect genetic integrity and facilitate transport of the paternal genome through the male and female reproductive tracts (Manicardi et al., 1998). Sperm chromatin rearrangement takes place in the later stages of spermatogenesis that involves the replacement of histones with protamines. Protamines, the major nuclear sperm proteins, are essential for sperm head condensation, DNA stabilization and paternal genome protection (Aoki and Carrell, 2003). During condensation and de-condensation, sperm's DNA is more vulnerable to environmental changes; therefore, it is believed that DNA breaks mostly occur during this transition process (Aitken et al., 2004; Sharma et al., 2004).

Secondly, apoptosis-the process of programmed cell death that occurs in multicellular organisms- is another well-known reason of DNA damage in sperm. This is a natural and beneficial process for any organism to prevent their cells from uncontrolled proliferation (Vaux and Korsmeyer, 1999). In male reproduction, apoptosis controls the overproduction of male gametes. There are two pathways that control apoptosis; the intrinsic and extrinsic pathways. In the extrinsic pathway, the Fas ligand (FasL) binds to the Fas positive cell which signals for the apoptotic death of a normal sperm cell, thus limiting the size of the germ cell population (Rodriguez et al., 1997). Infertile males have been shown to have an increase in the number of Fas positive cells. This would indicate that the correct amount of spermatozoa undergoing apoptosis is not occurring; therefore, the presence of spermatozoa that possess apoptotic markers, such as Fas positivity can indicate DNA damage and infertility (Agarwal and Said, 2003).

The last reason for DNA damage in sperm is oxidative stress caused by an imbalance between reactive oxygen species (ROS) and antioxidants. One feature of the semen of infertile males is the production of excessive levels of ROS; which can cause damages to DNA (Dizdaroglu, 1992). ROS have free radicals, which are unpaired electrons that tend to bind to other molecules and alter them. The sperm cell is highly susceptible to damage by these reactive molecules because of the lipid membrane structure covering its head and mitochondria. The sources of ROS in semen are sperm itself that generates reactive radicals as metabolites and the white blood cells found among sperm (Agarwal et al., 2003). One consequence of excessive ROS is peroxidative damage to the plasma membrane of sperm that causes spermatozoa to become dysfunctional and incapable of initiating fertilization (Irvine et al., 2000).

2.2.3 Methods to detect sperm DNA damage

The quality of sperm DNA is important in maintaining the reproductive potential of males. Damage to sperm nuclear DNA negatively affects assisted and natural fertility as well. Sperm DNA damage is significant in assisted reproductive techniques (Hartshorne et al. 2009) because these techniques by-pass the natural barriers of the reproductive tract that remove damaged sperm cells. ARTs can potentially allow genetically damaged sperm to fertilize the egg, which may cause decreased fertility in the offspring or pregnancy losses. DNA damage influences male fertility by affecting sperm functions through multiple avenues such as defective sperm chromatin packaging, apoptosis, and oxidative stress. Several assays have been developed to evaluate sperm chromatin and DNA integrity; TUNEL assay, sperm chromatin structure assay (SCSA), single-cell gel electrophoresis (SCGE: COMET) assay, the sperm chromatin dispersion (SCD) test and DNA breakage detection- fluorescent in situ hybridization (DBD-FISH) assay. There are also certain stains that can be used to detect DNA damage and chromatin abnormalities. For example, acridine orange (AOT) and Chromomycin A_3 using fluorescence microscopy whereas Toluidine blue (Gur and Breitbart) stain and Acidic aniline blue using bright field microscopy. Some of these tests can only detect DNA fragmentation induced by apoptosis such as TUNEL, whereas single- and double-stranded breaks associated with DNA damage (ss/dsDNA) can be determined by COMET assay (Collins et al., 1997). In this review only five major and commonly used assays are discussed.

2.2.3.1. Terminal deoxynucleotidyl transferase mediated dUTP nick-end-labeling (TUNEL) assay

This is the most common method of determination of DNA damage in the sperm. This method can be performed either by bright and (or) fluorescence microscopy or by flow cytometry. TUNEL assay detects either single or double fragmented DNA caused by endogenous endonucleases' activity during apoptosis and labels the 3'-hydroxyl DNA ends generated by virtue of terminal deoxyribonucleotidyl transferase (TdT) (Nagata et al., 2003).

Since nuclear DNA becomes fragmented by endogenous endonucleases during apoptosis, this assay is designed to detect DNA damages induced by apoptosis in the cell population. TUNEL assay involves fixing and permeabilizing of the cell, incubation steps with DNA labeling, and then staining and detection steps. Flow cytometry is a technique used for counting and examining microscopic particles; it uses a beam of light that is directed into a stream of fluid (containing the potentially damaged DNA), and quantifies the amount of damaged DNA from the non-damaged DNA in TUNEL assay (Anzar et al., 2002; Martin et al., 2007; Martin et al., 2004). In addition to this, in the fluorescence detection, the location of DNA damage induced by apoptosis can be determined. However, the fluorescence microscopic method is based on the microscopic observation of individual cells, and thus, flow cytometry provides more accurate data.

2.2.3.2 Sperm chromatin structure assay (SCSA)

Since abnormal sperm with damaged DNA is more vulnerable to DNA denaturation *in situ,* the SCSA measure the susceptibility of sperm nuclear DNA to induced denaturation. It is based on the ability of acridine orange (AO) to stain differently double-stranded or single-stranded DNA. For SCSA sperm is acid or heat treated to induce denaturation followed by AO staining (Agarwal and Said, 2003). Acridine orange binds to double-stranded DNA (native DNA) as a monomer, producing a green fluorescent color at 515–530 nm. On the other hand, AO intercalates single-stranded DNA (denatured DNA) as an aggregate, emitting a red fluorescence 630nm. The SCSA relies on visual interpretation of fluorescing spermatozoa under a microscope (Eggert-Kruse et al., 1996), which could cause a biased interpretation due to color confusion from individual to individual. An alternative parameter of the SCSA is the DNA fragmentation index (%DFI), which represents the population of cells with DNA damage (Evenson et al., 2002).

2.2.3.3 Single-cell gel electrophoresis COMET assay

Single cell gel electrophoresis (SCGE) also known as COMET assay is another technique to detect DNA damage in spermatozoa. In this assay, sperm cells are embedded in a slide containing an agarose matrix, and then lysed by either detergents or high salt leading to deproteinization. Afterwards, DNA is electrophoresed so that broken DNA strands migrate towards the anode, resulting in the formation of a Comet tail. At the end, two components are detected; a comet head that contains intact DNA and a comet tail that consists of damaged DNA; the higher the DNA density in the tail, the greater the extent of DNA damage. There are two types of SCGE techniques: in the neutral Comet, DNA migrates under neutral conditions, which allows for identification of double-stranded DNA breaks (DSB); in the alkaline Comet, DNA is denatured under alkaline conditions (pH>13). This technique detects both single-stranded DNA breaks (SSB) and DSB, but would not allow for differentiation between the two. Recently a two-tailed Comet assay has been developed (Enciso et al., 2009), which by revealing the total level of both SSB and DSB in individual cells, allows for a more precise and extensive analysis of the damage. However, since the technique is based on fluorescence microscopy the slides should be analyzed by an experienced observer for interpretation of the results.

2.2.3.4 DNA Breakage detection-fluorescence *in situ* hybridization (DBD-FISH)

This assay is based upon the detection of DNA breakage in cells embedded on a slide within an agarose matrix following a treatment with alkaline unwinding solution leading to the single-stranded DNA (ssDNA) motifs. These ssDNA motifs serve as the ends for hybridization of probes. The *in situ* detection of DNA breaks and structural features in the sperm chromatin can be detected by DBD–FISH. Following neutralization, protein removal and hybridization with whole genome or specific DNA probes are performed, respectively. During incubation of these probes with the ssDNA motifs, they would intercalate to the specific area in the ssDNA leading to the nuclear halo detected. The intensity of these halos derived from ssDNA breaks hybridized by specific DNA probes are then detected by fluorescence microscopy. Spermatozoa with abnormal packaged chromatin are more sensitive to denaturation by alkali treatment, which results in more intense labeling (red fluorescence) by DBD–FISH (Agarwal and Said, 2003).

2.2.3.5 Sperm chromatin dispersion (SCD) assay

This test is based on the principle that sperm with fragmented DNA fail to produce the characteristic halo when mixed with an aqueous agarose following acid denaturation and removal of nuclear proteins. In detail, undamaged DNA of spermatozoa would be dispersed following acid treatment and lysis leading to deproteinized nuclei, which would be seen as a halo around the sperm head. In contrast to spermatozoa with undamaged or nonfragmented DNA, the halo is either limited or absent in spermatozoa with damaged or fragmented DNA. Although SCD test can be performed either by light microscopy or by fluorescence microscopy, it does not require any staining for detection because dispersed and nondispersed cells can be easily determined under the light microscope. Although SCD test is simple, fast, and cost-effective, its clinical significance is limited (Agarwal and Said, 2003).

2.2.4 Apoptosis in spermatozoa

Necrosis and apoptosis are two forms of cell death. Necrosis affects groups of neighboring cells as a result of acute cellular injury. Conversely, apoptosis influences single cells due to naturally occurring processes within the cell. In contrast to apoptosis, necrosis causes cell swelling and loss of plasma membrane integrity, producing a significant inflammatory response. Under normal circumstances, apoptosis is a mechanism used to remove unnecessary or damaged cells, and contributes to the maintenance of tissue homeostasis (Marchetti et al., 2002). Moreover, there must be a balance between apoptosis, cell death, mitosis, and cell gain. Apoptosis can be classified by the presence of three distinct stages: induction, execution, and degradation; each of these three stages involves activation of the mitochondrial pathway (Martin et al., 2007). Signals for the activation of apoptotic pathways can be either extrinsic or intrinsic. Extrinsic pathways involve expression of pro-apoptotic factors, such as CD95 and TNF receptor 1, on the cell surface. Intrinsic pathways are used to initiate apoptosis from within the cell in response to cytotoxic stimuli and pro-apoptotic factors, such as cytochrome C and endonuclease G, which signal the activation of caspases (Fulda and Debatin, 2006). Induction of apoptosis causes an opening in the mitochondrial pores, resulting in decreased mitochondrial membrane potential and the release of pro-apoptotic factors (Anzar et al., 2002; Martin et al., 2007). Apoptotic cells can be distinguished by translocation of phosphatidylserine (PS) from the inner leaflet to the outer leaflet of the cell (Anzar et al., 2002; Martin et al., 2004).

Apoptosis is a vital part of normal embryonic development; it has been found that abnormal apoptotic processes will result in abnormal development (van den Eijnde et al., 1997).

Additionally, apoptosis has been identified as an important mechanism for the continual replacement of the lining of the gastrointestinal tract in mammals; balance between cell gain and cell loss is crucial in this process (Hall et al., 1994). Apoptosis also plays a role in sperm cell maturation and germ cell apoptosis during spermatogenesis is essential in the production of sperm (Anzar et al., 2002; Marchetti et al., 2002). In human testis, 5% of spermatozoa undergo apoptosis to maintain germ cell population and to reduce abnormal spermatozoa that are being produced. However, increased level of sperm apoptosis may affect male fertility resulting in production of limited numbers of healthy spermatozoa. Increased levels of apoptotic sperm have been shown to have a direct impact on poor bull fertility by decreasing sperm viability (Anzar et al., 2002; Martin et al., 2007; Martin et al., 2004). Loss of sperm viability includes a decrease in mitochondrial membrane potential, increased membrane permeability, and DNA fragmentation. It is thought that cryopreservation of sperm cells induces apoptosis by causing PS translocation, targeting the cell for programmed cell death (Anzar et al., 2002). There are many hypothesized reasons as to why cryopreservation causes PS translocation. Some of these include physical and chemical stress due to low temperature and high salt concentration as a result of crystal formation, which are thought to destabilize the sperm plasma membrane (Anzar et al., 2002).

2.2.4.1 Annexin V assay

In the course of apoptosis, phosphatidylserine (PS) is relocated from the inner plasma membrane to the outer plasma membrane in the cell. Annexin V is a calcium-dependent phospholipid-binding protein that is especially sensitive to PS located on the apoptotic cell surface. Annexin V that detects the translocation of PS across the plasma membrane is generally used with Propidium Iodide (PI) that stains DNA to detect damage. Annexin V assay can be performed using flow cytometry to obtain more accurate and quantitative results. This assay can be performed using fluorescence microscopy to detect the location of apoptotic PS-translocation including its quantification (Anzar et al., 2002; Martin et al., 2007; Martin et al., 2004). In flow cytometry, four distinct populations can be identified through Annexin-V/PI assay: viable cells, necrotic cells, apoptotic cells, and late necrotic cells. Annexin V assay is generally used with TUNEL assay that is an established method to detect nicked DNA to confirm apoptotic-induced DNA fragmentation (Anzar et al., 2002).

2.2.4.2 Apoptotic genes and caspase activation

Another indicator of apoptosis is the activity of apoptotic genes and caspases, which can be linked back to the Fas model and nDNA apoptosis, as the Fas receptor activates caspases which can cause nDNA breaks. Expression of the pro-apoptotic gene (*bax*) (Elsik et al. 2009) and anti-apoptotic gene (*bcl-2*) can be detected using real-time RT PCR. Besides transcripts, protein expression from these two genes can be determined to assess apoptosis in the cell. Both of these proteins come from the same family, however, they each have distinctly different purposes. Bcl-2 inhibits the activation of caspase 9, which in turn would inhibit apoptosis as caspase 9 helps begin the apoptotic pathway. BAX is a pro-apoptotic protein that promotes the activation of caspases and creates pores in organelles that would help promote apoptosis. Both, Bcl-2 and BAX provide a signaling pathway that helps maintain the apoptotic balance in a cell and if this balance is disrupted it can disturb normal apoptotic levels (Fulda and Debatin, 2006).

2.3 Transcriptome of spermatozoa

2.3.1 mRNAs of spermatozoa

Spermatozoa deliver more than just the paternal genome into the egg. The newly transcribed and remnant sperm RNA from spermatogenesis are totally or partially transmitted to the oocyte (Eddy, 2002; Gur and Breitbart, 2006; Miller and Ostermeier, 2006a; Miller and Ostermeier, 2006b; Ostermeier et al., 2004). Diverse mRNAs have been found in human, rodent and bovine mature spermatozoa (Dadoune et al., 2005; Gilbert et al., 2007; Miller and Ostermeier, 2006a). Although the roles of these transcripts during embryonic and fetal development are still unclear, analysis of their profiles could serve as a diagnostic tool to assess male infertility (Bissonnette et al., 2009; Garrido et al., 2009; Lalancette et al., 2009), or it could have prognostic value for fertilization and embryo development (Boerke et al., 2007; Ostermeier et al., 2004; Sassone-Corsi, 2002).

Microarray technology has been successfully used for global gene expression profiling in human, mouse and bovine spermatozoa (Gilbert et al., 2007; He et al., 2006). However, in the case of high merit bulls, the great demand and cost of their semen 36 limit their availability for research needs. Determination of transcript abundance in mammalian spermatozoa is challenging. Several techniques including TRIZOL (Invitrogen), Guanidine Isothiocyanate and commercial kits (i.e., RNeasy from Qiagen, MirVana from Ambion) have been used to improve both the purity and the recovery rate of spermatozoal total RNA extraction (Gilbert et al., 2007; Lalancette et al., 2008b; Ostermeier et al., 2002; Ostermeier et al., 2004). Sperm RNA profiles revealed the absence or low amounts of ribosomal RNAs (28S and 18S) (Gilbert et al., 2007). These levels of ribosomal RNAs (i) correlate with the idea of low translational activity in mature spermatozoa (Boerke et al., 2007, Elsik et al. 2009) remain the principal signature of spermatozoal RNA profile compared to somatic cells (which contain both types of rRNAs).

Although the presence of RNAs within the spermatozoa is well-documented, both the identity and the role of these transcripts remain largely uncharacterized. It has been proposed that sperm RNA could play an important role in the developmental success of the early embryo. Sperm RNA population includes transcripts involved in a wide variety of cellular functions. The absence of genes associated with cell cycle regulation in the spermatozoon could indicate that the mature gamete does not require the cell cycle machinery. Considering the limited capacity of the spermatozoon to store RNA relatively to the oocyte, a specific role of sperm RNAs for early embryonic development could imply the targeting of particular pathways by the accumulation of specific transcripts during the later stages of spermatogenesis (Gilbert et al., 2007).

2.3.2 Small non coding RNAs (snc-RNAs) of spermatozoa

Highly specialized gene regulation is necessary for the expression of spermatogenic genes during the complex developmental processes leading to mature sperm formation. Different small non-coding RNAs, microRNAs (miRNA), small interfering RNAs (siRNAs), and Piwi-interacting RNAs (piRNAs) are noted for their germline expression. The following section briefly describes how these small non-coding RNAs (sncRNAs) function at the molecular level.

MicroRNAs are negative regulators of mRNA translation and stability. They regulate gene expression by binding to the 3′ untranslated region of specific mRNA containing complementary sequences to those within the seed region of miRNAs. MicroRNAs are found in various tissues and, especially in the testis, they are important for proliferation and early differentiation of spermatogenic stem cells (Hayashi et al., 2008). PiwiRNAs protect the germline from invading transposons. PiRNAs are germ line specific and found abundantly during spermiogenesis where they are involved in the repression of retrotransposons during spermatogenesis (Frost et al., 2010).

Piwi proteins and their variants, MIWI and MILI are regulatory proteins playing essential roles in spermatogenesis. These proteins rely upon their interaction with miRNA and piRNA to influence gene regulation. Spermatogenic arrest in MIWI deficient testis implies the importance of small non-coding RNA mediated gene regulation with the help of other RNA processing molecules. MILI is shown to be an essential factor for meiotic differentiation during spermatogenesis. In MILI null mice spermatogenesis was blocked at the early prophase stage of first meiosis (Kuramochi-Miyagawa et al., 2004)

So far, 22 testis-preferential and 6 testis-specific miRNAs have been identified in male germ and Sertoli cells in mouse (Ro et al., 2007). Specifically, Mir122a is predominately expressed in post-meiotic germ cells, and it suppresses the transcription of transition protein 2, a testis-specific protein involved in chromatin remodeling during mouse spermatogenesis (Yu et al., 2005). Mirn34b is highly expressed in adult testis compared to the prepubertal testis, indicating its potential role in the differentiation of male germ cells (Barad et al., 2004). Compared to adult testis, 14 miRNAs are upregulated and 5 miRNAs are downregulated in immature testis. Characteristic miRNA signatures for testis and ovary are elucidated in mouse providing an insight into the sex-based functional roles of miRNA (Mishima et al., 2008).

MiRNAs are initially transcribed as pri-miRNA where the miRNA portion pair up to form dsRNA. A dsRNA specific ribonuclease, Drosha converts the pri-mRNA into precursor miRNA (pre-miRNA) in the nucleus. Exportin-5 transports pre-miRNA from the nucleus to cytoplasm. Dicer, a member of the RNase III superfamily cleaves pre-miRNA to yield 19-22 bp dsRNA with 1-4 bp 3′ overhang at either end. The single stranded mature miRNA which gets incorporated into RNA-induced silencing complex (RISC) controls the target mRNA expression. Identification of miRNA expression is the first step towards understanding their biological role and the pathway involved. Array based methods and real-time PCR are used for miRNA profiling (Barad et al., 2004). Besides, bioinformatics tools have been designed to scan mRNA sequences for binding sites of known and registered miRNAs (Rusinov et al., 2005). Several novel miRNAs have been identified in germ cells. MiRNAs belonging to miR-17-92 cluster and are found to be highly expressed in primordial germ cells (PGCs). The Mir-290-295 cluster is preferentially expressed in PGCs, and the expression is notably reduced in differentiated cells indicating its role in the pluripotency of embryonic stem (ES) cells (Hayashi et al., 2008). Comparison of miRNA expression patterns between immature and mature mouse testes revealed significant differences. From the miRNA microarray data, a range of miRNAs in immature testis showed higher expression levels compared to the mature testes. Through computational search for putative targets, mammalian developmental and spermatogonial genes are found to be potential targets for differentially expressed miRNAs. Among those are Brd2, a gene highly expressed in diplotene spermatocytes and round spermatids and expressed at low levels in spermatogonia being targeted by mmu-miR-127, Usp42, a gene expressed during spermatogenesis and embryogenesis in mouse being targeted by mmu-miR-411 and mmu-miR-29b. Also, several other genes exhibiting germ cell-specific expression are predicted to be the targets for identified miRNAs (Yan et al., 2007). This explains the need for recruiting specific miRNAs in adult testis to regulate spermatogenesis. Further, miRNAs such as Mirn-24-1, Mirn-25 were identified from sperm derived samples which excluded cytosolic materials but retained nuclear and perinuclear components, mimicking the actual sperm components entering the oocyte during fertilization. However, those miRNAs are found to play a limited role only in fertilization, postulating that sperm-borne miRNAs are majorly directed towards spermatogenic regulation (Amanai et al., 2006).

Recently, a testis specific miRNA, miR-34c was identified. TGIF2 (TGFβ-induced factor homeobox 2) and NOTCH2 (Neurogenic locus notch homolog protein 2) are identified to be its direct targets indicating the possibility that these pathways are involved in regulation. TGIF2 is an inhibitor of the TGFβ pathway which plays a major role during spermatogenesis. NOTCH signaling pathway controls inhibition of cell differentiation, proliferation control, and stem cell count (Bouhallier et al., 2010). These two key pathways requiring miRNA mediated regulation reinforces the essential role of miRNA in spermatogenesis. Dgcr8 is a gene encoding an RNA-binding protein specifically required for miRNA processing. Dgcr8-deficient oocytes matured normally and produced healthy-appearing offspring, even though miRNA levels were reduced. The mRNA profiles of wild-type and Dgcr8 null oocytes are identical, whereas Dicer null oocytes showed hundreds of misregulated transcripts. These findings show that miRNA function is globally suppressed during oocyte maturation and preimplantation development where siRNA instead of miRNA, obviating the Dgcr8 requirement take up the regulatory role. This possibly explains the abnormalities of Dicer null oocytes (Suh et al., 2010). In addition, a recent study showed a reprogramming of major small RNA class from siRNA/piRNA to zygotically derived miRNA during pre-implantation development (Ohnishi et al., 2010), thus, manifesting the indispensable role of miRNA regulation in the shaping up of early embryo. Although maternally derived small RNAs decrease as fertilization proceeds, a class of small RNA called L1 functions till the 8–16-cell stage of embryo. Zygotically derived siRNAs and piRNAs also participate in regulating early development. The potential involvement of these small RNAs in pre-implantation development is confirmed by Dicer knock down studies resulting in reduced expression of N-myc, a component associated with pluripotency in embryo. In general, both maternal and zygotic small RNAs are involved in preventing retrotransposon invasion of the genome. MiRNAs are the most predominant small RNAs found in the inner cell mass of blastocyst (Ohnishi et al., 2010).

Transcripts for the RNA-induced silencing complex (RISC) catalytic components- EIF2C2, EIF2C3, and EIF2C4 are found to be up-regulated during preimplantation development in the mouse. RISC incorporates miRNA to function; hence, miRNA plays a role in early preimplantation as well. Similarly, gene knockout of Dicer renders the embryo non-viable due to unsuccessful preimplantation differentiation (Amanai et al., 2006). Several distinct miRNAs have been identified and characterized from the bovine. The miRNA candidates are found by homology searching and partially verified by cloning from small cattle RNA library where distinct and homologous miRNAs are identified (Long and Chen, 2009). The

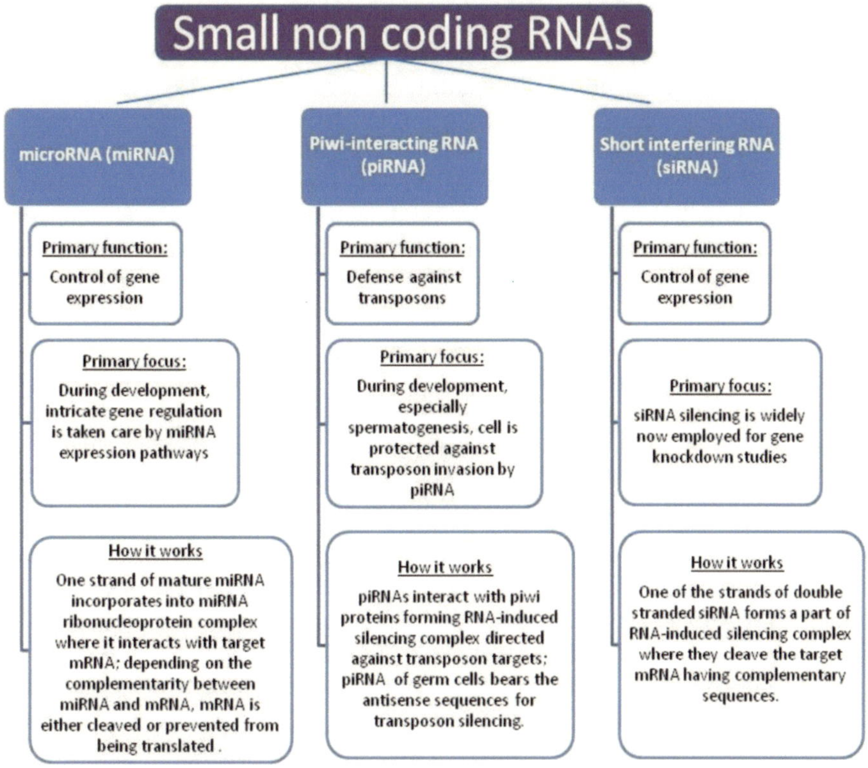

Fig. 1. Diversity of snc-RNAs

cattle genome sequence provides the resource for *in silico* miRNA and target prediction (Elsik et al., 2009). The bovine miRNA genes have been annotated based on the sequence similarity with other species miRNA (Strozzi et al., 2009). The miRNA expression pattern among 11 tissues revealed that most miRNAs are ubiquitously expressed while few are tissue specific (Jin et al., 2009). The role of miRNAs has been elucidated to understand the developmental processes and gene regulation, for example, miR-133 plays a role in the development and physiology of the rumen (Gu et al., 2007). Embryonic tissues also have a distinct profile of miRNA expression including miR-122a and miR-199a as embryo-specific miRNAs (Coutinho et al., 2007). Further, miRNAs were mapped to find how they are clustered in the chromosome (Jin et al., 2009). Depending on miRNA clustering and functionality they may serve as potential molecular markers. Finally, the study on miRNA expression in cattle is important because it serves as a mammalian model organism and their functional genomics are comparative. Conserved miRNAs among mammalian species are expected to have similar evolutionary roles.

All these seminal studies indicate the need to unravel the indispensable role of small non coding RNAs, especially miRNAs and piRNAs in regulating the germ cell development and beyond. With the increasing association of male infertility with genetic and epigenetic factors, exploring the regulatory events towards spermatogenesis and following fertilization will be worthwhile.

2.3.3 Long non coding RNAs (lnc-RNAs) of spermatozoa

In the diverse RNA species, a small number of long RNA transcripts are assigned with functions other than protein coding. This family of RNA is called long non-coding RNAs (lncRNAs). From the genome, these RNAs are transcribed as interlaced and overlapping transcripts that are greater than 200 nt in length (Carninci et al., 2005). Although it is doubtful whether the long non-coding RNAs are biologically meaningful or merely transcriptional "noise", few long ncRNAs have been functionally characterized. Experimental observations suggest that these ncRNAs contribute to the complex networks of gene regulation involved in cell functions (Mattick, 2001). Mercer et al have identified 849 long transcripts with little or no protein-coding potential that were transcribed in the adult mouse brain. They are observed to be posttranscriptionally modified and exhibit highly specific expression, suggesting that these transcripts are functional and are likely to play a role in cell function (Mercer et al., 2008). Dosage compensation in mammals involves X-chromosome inactivation (XCI) mediated by Xist, a lncRNA (Penny et al., 1996). Xist mediated transcriptional inactivation of one X chromosome is the result of stable high level Xist expression in inactive X chromosome (Panning et al., 1997).

The non-coding RNAs which take up either housekeeping or regulatory role are evolutionarily conserved. Analyses of 3,122 long ncRNAs from the mouse showed a proportion of conservation in their sequence which comparable to the density of exons within protein-coding transcripts (Ponjavic et al., 2007). Two long ncRNAs associated with trimethylated H3K4 histones and histone methyltransferase MLL1 in mouse embryonic stem cell are shown to be developmentally regulated, contributing to the pluripotency of the cell (Dinger et al., 2008). Quantitative real-time RT–PCR analysis of 15 long, conserved non-coding transcripts was performed in different normal human tissue and in breast and ovarian cancers. The results showed altered expression of many of these non-coding transcripts in both cancer types. This study indicates that lncRNAs may play an important

lncRNA	Organism	Function	Protein partner	References
steroid receptor activator RNA (SRA)	Mammals	NR co-activator	SRC-1, SLIRP, SHARP, SKIP, and others	(Lanz et al., 1999)
Evf-2	Mouse	Activator of DLX-5/6 enhancer	Dlx-2	(Feng et al., 2006)
7SK small nuclear RNA	Human cell lines	Suppressor of P-TEFb (general transcription inhibition)	HEXIM-1	(Yik et al., 2003)
B2 RNA	Mouse	General transcription inhibitor	RNA polymerase II	(Espinoza et al., 2004)
6S RNA	Bacteria	General transcription inhibitor	Bacterial RNA polymerase	(Trotochaud and Wassarman, 2005)
heat shock RNA-1 (HSR1)	Mammals	Activator of HSF1 (master regulator of heat shock genes)	eEF1A	(Shamovsky et al., 2006)

Table 1. Few long non-coding RNAs and their roles in transcription regulation. Adapted from Shamovsky and Nudler, 2006

function in both normal cells and in cancer development (Perez et al., 2008). Owing to the functions of lncRNA in cellular regulation and development, Lee et al has suggested that lncRNA may also play a role in male germ cell development (Lee et al., 2009). Recently, a novel non-coding RNA has been identified in the rat epididymis, named HongrES2. It is a 1.6 kb mRNA-like precursor that gives rise to a new microRNA-like small RNA. Upon over-expression of this small RNA in the cauda epididymis, a reduced expression of CES7 protein is observed. CES7 is a carboxylesterase with cholesterol esterase activity, which is necessary during sperm capacitation process. Also, tyrosine phosphorylation of the sperm protein during capacitation was affected by high expression of this microRNA-like small RNA indicating the requisite of low level expression for normal sperm maturation process in epididymis (Ni et al., 2011). In summary, although there exist significant numbers of lncRNAs in the body, their expression dynamics and functions in sperm are not well studied.

2.4 Methylome of sperm DNA

Epigenetics is the study of changes in gene expression without causing a change in the structure of DNA. Genes may be over or under-expressed which could be beneficial or detrimental to the organism depending on what genes are being activated or silenced. Epigenetics can shed some light on how non-genetic factors such as environment and nutrition can influence gene expression. There are several mechanisms involved in epigenetics; such as chromatin re-modeling, and the most studied epigenetic phenomenon, DNA methylation. In the following section, DNA methylation in sperm and its impacts on fertility will be described.

Cytosine methylation is the most common covalent modification of DNA in eukaryotes. DNA methylation is essential for normal development and is associated with a number of key processes including genomic imprinting and X-chromosome inactivation. In the course of gametogenesis, imprinting of parental (paternal and maternal) allele or alleles occurs, which is closely associated with the methylation of cytidines. DNA methylation involves the addition of a methyl group to the cytosine, which occurs in the CpG islands, regions composed of cytosine and guanine. DNA methylation often leads to transcriptional silencing of a gene (Zilberman and Henikoff, 2007). Either the loss or gain of methylation at specific genes can lead to developmental abnormalities (Gehring and Henikoff, 2007). Despite the clear importance of DNA methylation, the extent to which changes in DNA methylation are involved in mammalian gene regulation is unclear (Goll and Bestor, 2005). There have been a number of studies done on DNA methylation, varying from the mechanism of methylation itself to its different methods of study and the analysis of the methylation results. The role of DNA methylation in the regulation of mouse and human insulin gene expression was examined (Kuroda et al., 2009). These findings suggested that insulin promoter demethylation may play a crucial role in beta cell maturation and tissue specific insulin gene expression. A high correlation between DNA methylation and chronological age has been described; and interestingly, these highly correlated associations take place close to genes involved in the DNA binding and transcription process (Hernandez et al., 2011).

Although differential DNA methylation has been demonstrated in human and chimp sperm, associations of specific DNA methylation patterns with male fertility have not been adequately investigated. De novo methylation is known to occur during germ cell maturation and spermatogenesis and this creates hypomethylated regions in the male germ line that are associated with promoters; especially sperm-specific promoter regions that are associated with germ cell functions at distinct stages of spermiogenesis (Houshdaran et al., 2007). With the use of immunostaining, the connection between DNA methylation and fertility was attempted, however, no association was found between sperm DNA methylation and fertilization rate or embryo quality (Benchaib et al., 2005). Houshdaran et al. (2007) suggest that if erasing the initial methylation pattern in epigenetic reprogramming does not occur correctly, that there is a possibility of epigenetic defects in the sperm that would ultimately affect male fertility. Additionally, Henckel et al. (2009) suggest that there is a mechanistic link between DNA methylation and histone methylation in which H3.3 is required for DNA methylation. Brykcznska et al. (2010) suggest that molecular genetic experiments will be needed to explain the extent and functional significance of methylation at specific histone loci.

Generation of genome-scale DNA methylation profiles at nucleotide resolution in mammalian cells has become as a powerful technology for epigenetic profiling of cell populations (Meissner et al., 2008). There are three different methods for studying DNA methylation; bisulfite conversion, methylation-sensitive restriction enzymes, and affinity purification. It is known that methylated cytosines and unmethylated cytosines have similar characteristics and it is hard to discern which is which with standard sequencing (Zilberman and Henikoff, 2007). In order to overcome this obstacle, the bisulfite conversion test can be performed on the sperm by treating the DNA with bisulfite which converts non-methylated cytosine residues to uracil, but leaves methylated cytosine residues unaffected. PCR amplification of converted DNA replaces the uracil with thymine and analysis of the PCR product can be used to quantify the extent of methylation at each cytosine (Eckhardt et al., 2006). A second method for studying DNA methylation is by by the use of methylation-sensitive restriction enzymes. This method cleaves DNA at specific methylated-cytosine residues in CpG islands which have lost their methyl group, leaving only hypermethylated DNA intact (Yegnasubramanian et al., 2006). Digestion is followed by amplification of the products, and they can be detected when digestion of the products are inhibited by presence of methylation. The third method of study is the affinity purification and is the most recently discovered. This method takes advantage of the methyl-binding domain (MBD) that binds to the methylated CpG sites. A MBD that has been attached to a CG site can be expressed in *E. coli* and affinity purified and then methylated DNA can be purified (Zhang et al., 2006).

2.5 Proteome of spermatozoa

Proteins and their cofactors, located both in the cytoplasm and on the membrane play important roles at different stages of gametogenesis, fertilization and embryonic development. Cell-cell interaction is the main function of membrane proteins during fertilization. The participation of such proteins in sperm, especially cytoplasm proteins injected into the occytes, are required for egg activation and subsequently early embryonic development. An area of focus for some key players is that of sperm-egg fusion. The integrin, a disintegrin and metalloprotease (ADAM) and Protein Kinase C (PKC) families are principal groups of proteins significant for fertilization and its succeeding steps. Current knowledge and understanding of molecular mechanisms of the proteomics during sperm egg fusion as well as the complicated networks of these proteins throughout embryonic development is still at the dawn of investigative process. Pioneering experiments have however been able to classify some specific proteins as potential molecular markers of fertility. Among them are Fertilin α and β. Both Fertilin α (ADAM1) and Fertilin β (ADAM2) are members of the ADAM family and together form a heterodimer. Fertilin β was initially discovered through initial implications of being the antigen to the antibody PH30 that prevented the fertilization of Guinea pig oocytes (Primakoff et al., 1987). There are a total of five members of the ADAM family that have been discovered. All of which are localized in the testis in the mouse (Heinlein et al., 1994; Wolfsberg et al., 1995). These proteins have been implicated as essential contributors during sperm egg fusion. Results of experiments conducted by Cohen et al. (2008) showed appearance of CRISP1 involvement in the first step of sperm binding to the zona pellucida. They also observed that sperm testicular CRISP2 is also able to bind to the egg surface which is indicative of its necessity in gamete fusion.

Massive changes in transcription and translation occur during spermatogenesis (Alcivar et al., 1990; Hake et al., 1990; Hecht, 1988). Considering the limited contents in the sperm, proteins that exist in the spermatozoa are speculated to have importance in sperm maturation and fertilization. Jmjd1a, for example, is a regulator of histone modification through demethylation in the testes, and its deficiency induced many infertile symptoms, indicating the essential role in spermatogenesis (Liu et al., 2010). In spermatids, Kinesin family member C 1 (KIFC1) motor which is a member of the Kinesin-14 subfamily associates with nucleoporin-containing complex and is postulated to be involved in acrosome elongation and motility (Yang et al., 2006; Yang and Sperry, 2003). TLRR is a leucine-rich repeat protein which interacts with KIFC1 (Wang and Sperry, 2008). Associating with the manchette, TLRR binds with testis specific isoform of protein phosphatase-1 (PP1) and was suggested to take part in cytoskeleton modulation (Wang and Sperry, 2008) Izumo was identified through the production of monoclonal antibody that inhibited sperm–egg fusion (Okabe et al., 1987; Rubinstein et al., 2006). The expression of Izumo was found to be testis-specific and was not detectable on the surface of fresh sperm but only became apparent after initiation of the acrosome reaction (Rubinstein et al., 2006)

In addition, a number of enzymes mediating the process of spermatogenesis have also been discovered. The Testis Specific Serine Kinases (TSSKs) are a collection of kinases in germ cells or in testis, which include TSSK1, TSSK2, TSSK3 and others (Bielke et al., 1994; Blaschke et al., 1994; Kueng et al., 1997; Zuercher et al., 2000). Since Specific Serine Kinases are only synthesized postmeiotically in spermatogenesis, they were proposed to act during sperm maturation, capacitation and fertilization. Sosnik et al. demonstrated Tssk6's essential role in maintaining sperm structural integrity and suggested its function to regulate actin dynamics (Sosnik et al., 2009). Trypsin is another enzyme that is active during spermatogenesis. In addition to being secreted into the intestine to digest proteins, trypsin also functions in the initiation of meiosis, spermiogenesis, and fertilization (Miura et al., 2009). Miura et al. also implicated the involvement of trypsin in the entry site of the meiosis cycle. The proteins mentioned here are sperm specific for involvement in the fertilization process. Their continuous investigation further proves the complexity of the multifaceted fertilization process on a molecular level. Moreover, it rationalizes the necessity for incessant investigation into the mounting issues of subfertility in males across species.

2.5.2 Approaches for the study of sperm proteomes

To date there are several popular and accepted techniques utilized in proteomic studies to investigate sperm proteomes related to sperm functions such as motility, oocyte-sperm fusion, and fertilization. Since sperm is transcriptionally silent, proteomic approaches provide precious information on sperm proteins coded during spermatogenesis. The most common method SDS-PAGE, the precursor to 2D-DIGE, produces the direct and global two dimensional views of several hundred proteins from a sample. Its combination with dyes and software achieves the precise and fast process of an image. Western Blotting and Immunocytochemistry are primarily used to detect the quantity and localization of the target proteins, respectively. Elemental composition of proteins can be determined by mass spectrometry techniques. It is well documented that many sperm proteins that remain as remnants in spermatozoa are critical for fertilization and embryo development. Collectively these techniques have aided in the advancement of sperm-specific protein identification as well as provided an enhanced understanding of protein function in motility, capacitation, acrosome reaction and fertilization (du Plessis et al., 2011).

2.5.2.1 SDS-PAGE electrophoresis

Sodium dodecyl sulfate polyacrylamide gel electrophoresis (SDS-PAGE) is a proteomic approach in biochemical experiments to separate proteins. SDS-PAGE was first published as a method in 1970 (Laemmli, 1970). The principle of SDS-PAGE relies on the same attachment of SDS in each unit of peptic length, which induces the same charge per mass unit. Proteins are denatured by SDS, which is an anion detergent and rounded with negative charge. Therefore, the charge of protein is relative with its size which enables researchers to separate proteins according to their molecular weight. The negatively-charged proteins migrate across the gel towards the anode in the electric field. The running system is determined by the concentration and size of the gel and molecular weight of protein samples. Following electrophoresis, Coomassie Brilliant Blue R-250 is commonly used to stain and visualize the proteins on the gel. The molecular weight of target proteins can be approximated in the gel by markers whose molecular weights have already been determined. The amount and purity of protein samples can be viewed according to the densities and numbers of the bands using software. The blotting application in addition to SDS-PAGE expands its usage. However, unlike native electrophoresis, SDS-PAGE cannot be applied to keep protein's native state due to the presence of the detergent. A limitation of this technique is the inability of proteins with similar or same molecular weight to be differentially separated; in addition SDS-PAGE is not a suitable method for the detection of low-molecular weight proteins. Despite minimal shortcomings, SDS-PAGE is a useful and critical tool for proteomics as a result of its broad application in protein size modification, protein identification, purity examination and protein quantification.

2.5.2.2 Two-dimensional differential in gel electrophoresis (2D- DIGE)

Using the same fundamental principles of SDS-PAGE, two-dimensional differential in-gel electrophoresis (2D-DIGE) was developed to separate proteins by molecular weight as well as isoelectric point (PI). The 2D-DIGE technique was not described in literature until 1975 (O'Farrell, 1975). In 1997, 2D-DIGE was developed to run more than one sample by pre-labeling samples with fluorescent cyanine dyes (Unlu et al., 1997). Trichloroacetic Acid in Acetone Protocol (TCA precipitation) or Bio-Rad protein assay is carried out to extract proteins. Accuracy during quantification in experiments possessing more samples is better determined by use of an internal control. A linear or nonlinear (Bjellqvist et al., 1993) program is run following the loading of samples onto the IPG strips. The first dimension will separate the proteins according to their PI. In the second dimensional step, IPG strips are loaded on the SDS-PAGE where proteins will be separated again by their charge or molecular weight. To visualize the protein spots, both Coomassie Brilliant Blue and silver staining (Merril et al., 1981; Oakley et al., 1980) are utilized. However, neither stain possesses the quality or sensitivity of detection methods that rely on fluorescent compounds and radiolabeling of proteins (Gorg et al., 2004). The diluted protein samples and internal controls are pre-labeled with the fluorescent cyanine dyes (CyDye, Cy2, Cy3, and Cy5 separately) before being loaded onto the IPG strips so that groups of samples can be visualized individually at different wavelengths.

The length of IPG strip varies from 7-24 cm and its pH range is between 2.5 and 12. More than 5,000 proteins can be resolved in the gel and this technique can detect as little as 1 ng of protein per spot (Gorg et al., 2004). This is the only technique to parallel large sets of protein mixtures. The protein expression level, isoforms or modification can be reflected from the protein mapping. Since the dyes cannot bind to the proteins without lysine, 2D-DIGE has varying sensitivity towards proteins too few or too many lysine.

2.5.2.3 Western blotting (also known as immunoblotting)

Protein signals can be detected through antibody specific binding in Western Blotting. The antibodies bind to target proteins which work as antigens on a membrane and emit signals by the conjugated enzymes. SDS-PAGE electrophoresis in addition to a positive control is needed so that the proteins can be separated on the gel and later transferred to a membrane. The positive control works as a marker to confirm the existence of target protein. The transfer process can be monitored by reversible staining or Ponceau S staining of the membrane. Transfer of proteins from the gel onto the membrane can be developed on several apparatuses. Wet transfer is less likely to possess background due to the drying of the membrane. It has been suggested that large proteins (>100 kDa) are transferred more effectively during wet transfer. By utilizing the semi-dry transfer, transfer time can be reduced to an hour or less and is currently the most widely used method. Dry transfer takes approximately eight minutes or less, however, the application is restricted by its transfer efficiency. Nitrocellulose and Polyvinylidene fluoride (PDVF) are the most popular membranes in Western blotting. Fixing or staining of gels will lower the efficiency of transfer, especially for the proteins more than 50 kDa (Perides et al., 1986). Post transfer staining might be applied by using compatible reversible stains such as Ponceau-S Red, CPTS (Copper Phthalocyanine Tetrasulfonic Acid) amido Black and Spyro Ruby (need laser to visualize) or non-compatible stains like Coomassie Brilliant Blue and Colloidal Gold (known to block some epitopes) (Millipore). In order to prevent non-specific binding and to decrease the occurrence of background noise during development, the membrane is incubated in blocking buffer at room temperature. Traditional blocking buffer is usually produced by adding blocking agent (0.5% casein, 5% nonfat milk and 5% Bovine serum albumin) in TBS (50 mM Tris.HCl, pH 7.4 and 150 mM NaCl). Followed by three rounds of washing, the membrane is then incubated with primary antibody, which binds to the target protein. Following washing, secondary antibodies conjugated with horseradish peroxidase or alkaline phosphatases are added to the membrane. The horseradish peroxidase or alkaline phosphatase enzymes react with substrates and emit light or other detectable signal. Final signals can be detected and visualized by X-ray film or digital images.

Therefore, electrophoretic separation of proteins cannot be examined by staining the gel until completion of the transfer step. The capacity of analyzing and identifying target proteins has led to the popularity of Western Blotting. Protein concentration can be quantified by implementing this technique according and calculation of subsequent signal intensity. However, it cannot show the localization of this protein in the cell, which can be performed by immunocytochemistry. Although Western Blotting has been widely utilized, its reliability is reduced by its nonspecificity and possible degradation of target protein causing visualization of multiple bands.

2.5.2.4 Immunocytochemistry

Immunocytochemistry is used to visualize the presence and localization specific proteins and other molecules within the cell. It is further also utilized for the investigation of protein processing and interaction. The application of immunocytochemistry is expanded by combination with other techniques, such as Formaldehyde-Induced Fluorescence, Autoradiography and Microinjection. However, since the immune system is adjustable and flexible, immunocytochemistry is questioned for its specificity. Secondly, immunocytochemistry cannot characterize the charge, size or hydrophobicity of the molecules (Larsson and Sjoquist, 1988). Compared to other immunoassays, it is expensive and difficult to quantify the signals to determine the amounts of proteins expressed.

2.5.2.5 Mass spectrometry

Mass spectrometry (MS) is a powerful technique used to ionize and determine elemental composition regarding mass-to-change ratio. An ion source, mass-selective analyzer, and an ion detector are the three chief modules in a MS instrument. The procedures in this analytical technique generally include five steps. First, a sample is vaporized prior to an ion source. Secondly, the ion source converts gas phase sample molecules into positively charged ions. Then the magnetic field in the instrument accelerates all the ions. The high speed ions are finally separated based on various masses. Lastly, the detector collects the data for analysis.

Tandem mass spectrometry is the main MS employed to identify proteins. Electrospray ionization (Elsik et al. 2009) and matrix assisted laser desorption ionization (MALDI) are two other major developed methods of MS, which are able to analyze molecules of very high molecular weight. The importance of mass spectrometry is not limited to protein identification but rather expands to its wide application in isotope dating, atom probe, protein characterization and so on. Mass spectrometry is a high throughput technique coupled with other techniques, such as SDS-PAGE and 2D-DIGE. The combination of MS and liquid chromatography (LC) enhances protein separation and identification of more than 1,000 proteins simultaneously (Liu et al., 2004; Peng et al., 2003; Sadygov et al., 2004; Washburn et al., 2001). However, MALDI has its limitation of protein quantification due to its nonlinear signal intensity and ESI-MS/MS has a high requirement of high purity protein samples and poor tolerance for electrolytes and detergents (Barnidge et al., 1999).

2.6 Proteome of seminal fluid

As mentioned previously, sperm proteins (D'Amours et al., 2010), DNA integrity (Ward, 2010) and mRNA profile (Lalancette et al., 2008a) are some of the sperm components that influence male fertility, and the seminal plasma is the principal medium enclosing the sperm. Seminal fluid contains a diverse cohort of proteins, including chaperones, proteins with redox activity, ion and phospholipid-binding proteins, carriers of lipophilic substances, glycosidases, proteases and protease inhibitors, among others, which in turn modulate numerous functions, from sperm protection, capacitation and acrosome reaction to sperm-oocyte interaction and fertilization. Knowledge of seminal plasma composition is more advanced for the bovine than for other farm animals and, for this reason, the present review will focus on the bovine, unless otherwise specified.

Proteins acting to prevent oxidative stress and immune reactions are expressed in the seminal plasma. Sperm usually produce reactive oxygen species (ROS) as part of their normal physiology (Aitken et al., 2004) but, if in excess, ROS have detrimental effects on spermatozoa. Thus, antioxidant systems must be present in the reproductive fluids to control these effects. Proteins participating in such systems include albumin, acidic seminal fluid protein (aSFP), glutathione peroxidase and transferring, among others. Albumin is present in both cauda epididymal and accessory sex gland (ASG) secretions of the bovine (Moura et al., 2007b; Moura et al., 2010) and its protective effect on sperm comes from its ability to absorb lipid 22 peroxides (Alvarez and Storey, 1995). Bovine aSFP is a typical component of the ASG fluid (Moura et al., 2007b; Wempe et al., 1992), although evidence exists that it is expressed in the cauda epididymal fluid as well (Moura et al., 2010). aSFP has redox activity superior to that of glutathione peroxidase (Einspanier et al., 1993; Schoneck et al., 1996), binds to ejaculated bovine sperm (Dostalova et al., 1994) and inhibits sperm motility in a reversible manner (Schoneck et al., 1996). Thus, aSFP protects sperm against oxidative stress in both pre- and post-ejaculation media and its inhibition of motility may be of importance during sperm storage in the cauda epididymis. Besides reactive oxygen species, transitional metal ions, like iron, can generate lipid peroxide radicals, with potential damage to sperm integrity (Agarwal et al., 2005; Wakabayashi et al., 1999). As a consequence, the expression of transferrin in the seminal fluid is a strategy to deal with excessive iron. Moreover, through its ability to bind iron, an essential ion for bacterial growth, transferrin represents a line of defense against pathogenic microorganisms (Farnaud and Evans, 2003). Most studies classically define transferrin as an epididymal protein (Belleannee et al., 2011; Moura et al., 2010) but it has also been detected in the seminal vesicle fluid of rams (Souza et al., 2011). Clusterin is another seminal protein designated to protect sperm and appears as multiple isoforms in the bovine cauda epididymal (Moura et al., 2010) and accessory sex gland fluid (Moura et al., 2007b). It prevents oxidative damage to cells (Reyes-Moreno et al., 2002), agglutinates abnormal spermatozoa in bulls (Ibrahim et al., 1999) and acts like a chaperone, protecting sperm from the toxic effects of protein precipitation (Humphreys et al., 1999). Clusterin has the ability to inhibit complement-induced sperm lysis (Ibrahim et al., 1999; O'Bryan et al., 1990), another form to preserve sperm cell integrity.

Proteins of the seminal fluid play important roles in capacitation, one of the early events occurring after sperm comes in contact with ASG secretions. In the bovine, Binder of Sperm Proteins (BSP) represents the most abundant group of seminal fluid proteins (Manjunath et al., 2009; Moura et al., 2007b). BSPs are characterized by two tandemly-arranged, fibronectin type II domains, which bind to membrane phospholipds (Kim et al., 2010) and induces cholesterol efflux, a crucial step in capacitation (Manjunath and Therien, 2002). Moreover, bovine BSPs mediates the interaction between sperm and the oviductal epithelium and contributes to sperm survival in that region of the female tract (Gwathmey et al., 2006). Interestingly, homologues of BSPs also represent the major constituents of seminal plasma from other ungulates, such as *Bos indicus* bulls (Moura et al., 2010), and rams (Rego et al., 2011). Albumin is another seminal fluid protein that affects sperm capacitation through its ability to modulate membrane efflux of cholesterol (Go and Wolf, 1985; Visconti and Kopf, 1998).

Phospholipase A_2 (PLA_2) and osteopontin (OPN) are two of seminal plasma proteins participating in acrosome reaction and fertilization-related events. PLA2 exists as a secreted form in the seminal plasma (Moura et al., 2007a; Soubeyrand et al., 1997) and in membrane extracts from bull sperm (Ronkko et al., 1991). Sperm-anchored PLA_2 synthesizes arachidonic acid, which is converted to prostaglandin E_2, a step leading to acrosome reaction. Sperm PLA_2 is also implicated in sperm-egg fusion (Yuan et al., 2003) and secreted PLA_2 stimulates cytokine release by immune cells (Granata et al., 2005), exerting antimicrobial action in the seminal plasma (Bourgeon et al., 2004; Weinrauch et al., 1996). Osteopontin is typically involved in cell adhesion, tissue remodeling and activation of intracellular signaling (Denhardt, 2004; Mazzali et al., 2002). OPN comes mainly from accessory sex glands (Cancel et al., 1999) and binds to sperm at ejaculation, as observed for the BSPs (Souza et al., 2008). Information about OPN roles in male reproduction has been demonstrated by experiments using in vitro fertilization (IVF). In this regard, incubation of bovine oocytes with OPN or fertilization of oocytes with sperm previously treated with OPN enhanced fertilization, cleavage rates and blastocyst development at days 8 and 11 (Goncalves et al., 2008; Monaco et al., 2009). Following this same conception, studies conducted with the swine species confirmed that OPN, when added to IVF media, also increased fertilization and embryo survival (Hao et al., 2006). These results indicate that OPN works during sperm-oocyte interaction and even influences post-fertilization events, although by mechanisms not yet completely understood. Given OPN´s biochemical features, it is plausible that OPN adheres to sperm and this complex binds to the oocyte, facilitating sperm penetration, fusion and fertilization, as suggested before (Souza et al., 2008). Also, interaction of sperm OPN with integrins and/or CD44 receptors in the oocyte could trigger intracellular signaling and affect early embryo development (Souza et al., 2008).

Several proteases and glycolytic enzymes are present in the seminal plasma and reportedly take part in remodeling of sperm membrane components during epididymal transit and capacitation. Proteases and constituents of the seminal plasma that interact with the extracellular matrix act during mammalian fertilization as well, when sperm contacts and crosses barriers formed by cumulus cells and the zona pellucida. Proteins belonging to these categories include enolase, fucosidases, glucosaminidases, galactosidases, leucine aminopeptidase, dipeptidyl peptidase, matrix metalloproteinase 2, angiotensin-converting enzyme, plasma glutamate carboxipeptidase, arylsulfatase A, cathepsins, among others. As expected, activity of these enzymes needs to be modulated to avoid undesirable cleavages and protect tissue integrity, and protease inhibitors are in fact secreted by the seminal plasma, such as tissue inhibitor of metalloproteinase 2, alpha 2 macroglobulin, serine protease inhibitors and cystatin (Kelly et al., 2006; Moura et al., 2007b; Moura et al., 2010).

As a typical fluid, the seminal plasma contains proteins with affinity to lipophilic substances, such as apolipoprotein A1 (Apo-A1), epididymal secretory protein E1 (also known as cholesterol transfer protein) and prostaglandin D-synthase (PGDS). Apo-A1 is part of the high-density lipoprotein complex (Rader, 2006) and interacts with ejaculated sperm. HDL present in the female reproductive tract is involved in sperm capacitation (Therien et al., 1997) but it is still unknown if Apo-A1 directly contributes to that event. Epididymal secretory protein E1, the second most abundant protein in the bovine cauda epididymal fluid (Moura et al., 2010) , binds to sperm (Kirchhoff et al., 1996) and alters the ratio of cholesterol and phospholipids of membranes, which occurs during sperm capacitation (Manjunath and Therien, 2002). PGDS, in turn, is a typical component of the epididymis and distinctively binds to the upper region of acrosome of both epididymal and ejaculated bull sperm. PGDS may act as a transporter of retinol and other lipophilic substances in the epididymis and semen (Leone et al., 2002) but how this putative role exactly affects sperm function is still unclear.

2.6.1 Approaches for the study of seminal proteome

Usually, approaches to analyze the seminal fluid proteome include 2-D electrophoresis (2-D SDS-PAGE) and/or chromatography, allied with mass spectrometry. Availability of several options of "strips" with immobilized pH and with different sizes (from 7 to 24 cm, in most cases) practically allows endless combinations of methods for electrofocalization of the majority of seminal proteins. For the second dimension, choices of gel mashes separate proteins based on their mass, especially those between 10 and 150 kDa. Typically, 2-D gels of bovine seminal plasma obtained with 18- or 24-cm "strips", within the 3-10 pH range, show at least 400 spots. Higher rates of spot detection are possible using strips with narrow pH intervals for electrical focalization, among other alternatives. Sensitive stains, such as SyproRuby (Bio Rad, USA), help detection of more spots in 2-D gels of seminal proteins but silver-staining has limitations. Silver stains are not saturable and thus, as it stains low abundance proteins, it will also increase the size of the BSP spots, reaching a point where these spots overshadow large sections of the gels. Despite the valuable pieces of information generated by 2-D SDS-PAGE, this method still limits the detection of low abundance proteins expressed in complex samples, such as the seminal plasma, or those that are too acidic or too basic, or with kDa values below or above 10 and 200, respectively. The gel-based method provides a quantitative "snapshot" of protein expression that can be analyzed and compared among different samples by imaging software (Gorg et al., 2004). The capacity of measuring this relative abundance has been improved with the development of two-dimensional differential in-gel electrophoresis, which allows distinct samples to be separated within a single map (Unlu et al., 1997). This method reportedly reduces the between-gel variability and allows more precise comparisons between samples related to contrasting phenotypes or treatments. Chromatography is another method for protein separation, using matrices such as ion-exchange, gel-filtration, affinity and multidimensional (Stroink et al., 2005). Given the complexity of seminal plasma, pre-separation of samples by chromatography enhances the detection of components during proteome-based studies. For instance, separation of seminal proteins in a gel-filtration column enhances spot detection in 2-D gels, given that a "zoon" is formed at different kDa ranges. This strategy isolates the BSP proteins in specific sections of the gels, allowing detection of low abundance proteins in others. The seminal constituents can also be divided based on biochemical attributes, such as heparin- and gelatin-biding capacity. After separation of proteins, either by 2-D SDS-PAGE alone or coupled with chromatography, identification of spots is mandatory and today mass spectrometry remains the cost effective technique for this purpose. N-terminal can be used to corroborate results from that method. In conclusion, several approaches are available for separation of proteins into comprehensive maps, relative quantification, and identification of such components, which are the foundations to establish the seminal plasma proteome.

3. Conclusion and future directions

Conventional evaluation of sperm biophysical characteristics has a large number of limitations which have not been successful to identify sub fertile or high fertile semen so far. While differences in lifetime fertility among males is the biggest concern, the day to day variation in semen quality causes major economic losses to animal breeding companies when expensive semen must be discarded. Identification of molecular determinants of fertile spermatozoa has great potential for enhancing the economic well-being of animal breeding companies and human IVF laboratories. In animal agriculture, these molecular fingerprints will allow us to assess semen quality which is more powerful than any previous sperm selection criteria, and should provide a foundation for early identification and selection of animals with superior genetics in the animal breeding and for male factor human infertility. Implementation of new approaches is crucial to reduce the cost of male fertility prediction, increase sire fertility and increase the overall financial margins in the dairy industry.

Chromatin structure and integrity of spermatozoa DNA is associated with sperm viability and thus fertility. Development of reliable molecular tests that provide quantitative measures of abnormalities in chromatin structure and DNA damage is expected to be a significant advance in predicting fertility. Diverse sets of transcripts in human and livestock spermatozoa have been well documented. Due to the low amount of transcription and translation in the spermatozoa, the "meaning" of these transcripts remains a mystery. These transcripts might play important roles during spermatogenesis, in egg activation and/or sustaining early embryonic development. Regardless of the significance of these transcripts in mature spermatozoa, there is a potential for spermatozoa transcripts to be used as predictors of sperm viability.

DNA methylation has been speculated for many years to have a close association with reproduction and fertility. Benchaib et al. (2005) attempted to determine the relationship between sperm DNA methylation level and fertilization and pregnancy rates. It was found that DNA methylation level in human sperm could represent a new approach to study the ability of sperm to lead to pregnancy. Jammes et al. (2011) proposed that in humans, abnormal epigenetic programming, via DNA methylation, is a possible mechanism compromising male fertility. Another study with Houshdaran et al. (2007) proposed that abnormal epigenetic programming of the germline is a possible mechanism compromising spermatogenesis of some men currently diagnosed with infertility (Houshdaran et al., 2007). Additional studies are necessary to clearly define the roles of DNA methylation in fertility.

A number of spermatozoa proteins have been identified using proteomics approaches followed by reductionist methods. Researchers have determined differentially expressed proteins in sperm from males with high and low fertility; enabling a list of proteins to be used as potential markers to predict fertility. Further validation of these proteins as well as posttranslational modifications of these proteins is important for considering these as reliable biomolecular markers. Because seminal plasma proteins play vital roles in sperm physiology and fertilization, studies have evaluated empirical associations between semen criteria, such as sperm motility of fresh or frozen semen, and seminal constituents as well. A classic study published in 1993 (Killian et al., 1993) showed that fertility of Holstein bulls was related to the relative abundance of four protein spots depicted in seminal plasma 2-D gels, two of which were identified as osteopontin (OPN) and prostaglandin D-synthase (Cancel et al., 1997; Gerena et al., 1998). This study was conducted with 35 bulls and later on, the evaluation of accessory sex fluid proteome from other 37 Holstein bulls confirmed that OPN had greater expression in high fertility than in low fertility sires. In contrast to BSP 30 kDa (now named BSP 5) and PLA_2, spermadhesin Z13 is inversely related to fertility. Similar results were obtained in the swine species (Hao et al., 2006). Other studies have identified a seminal fluid, 30-kDA heparin-binding protein as a marker of bull fertility. This protein binds to sperm and was first named "Fertility Associate Antigen" and later identified as a DNAse I like protein (Bellin et al., 1996; Bellin et al., 1998).

In conclusion, sperm viability is surely determined by multifactor mechanisms, from those inherent to the cells to constituents of seminal proteins. Because fertility is a complex trait with low inheritance rate, studies on both genetic and epigenetic aspects of sperm viability are crucial in understanding the nature and mechanisms regulating male fertility. The molecular attributes of the spermatozoa and the methods including the *"omics"* approaches reviewed in this chapter are certainly testaments for great progresses. However, much needs to be accomplished to fully understand the complexity of male fertility and develop ways by which to diagnose and prevent infertility. For example, there is a need for systems physiology of sperm where all components of sperm viability, i.e., spermatozoal proteins, transcripts, small molecules, and chromatin dynamics should be all considered to determine "the best spermatozoa". It would then be possible to include all of these biomolecular markers in a comprehensive evaluation scheme to define potential male fertility.

4. References

Abbott, A. L. and Ducibella, T. (2001). Calcium and the control of mammalian cortical granule exocytosis. *Front Biosci* 6, D792-806.

Agarwal, A. and Said, T. M. (2003). Role of sperm chromatin abnormalities and DNA damage in male infertility. *Hum Reprod Update* 9, 331-45.

Agarwal, A., Prabakaran, S. A. and Said, T. M. (2005). Prevention of oxidative stress injury to sperm. *J Androl* 26, 654-60.

Agarwal, A., Saleh, R. A. and Bedaiwy, M. A. (2003). Role of reactive oxygen species in the pathophysiology of human reproduction. *Fertil Steril* 79, 829-43.

Aitken, R. J., Ryan, A. L., Baker, M. A. and McLaughlin, E. A. (2004). Redox activity associated with the maturation and capacitation of mammalian spermatozoa. *Free Radic Biol Med* 36, 994-1010.

Alcivar, A. A., Hake, L. E., Hardy, M. P. and Hecht, N. B. (1990). Increased levels of junB and c-jun mRNAs in male germ cells following testicular cell dissociation. Maximal stimulation in prepuberal animals. *J Biol Chem* 265, 20160-5.

Alvarez, J. G. and Storey, B. T. (1995). Differential incorporation of fatty acids into and peroxidative loss of fatty acids from phospholipids of human spermatozoa. *Mol Reprod Dev* 42, 334-46.

Amanai, M., Brahmajosyula, M. and Perry, A. C. (2006). A restricted role for sperm-borne microRNAs in mammalian fertilization. *Biol Reprod* 75, 877-84.

Anzar, M., He, L., Buhr, M. M., Kroetsch, T. G. and Pauls, K. P. (2002). Sperm apoptosis in fresh and cryopreserved bull semen detected by flow cytometry and its relationship with fertility. *Biol Reprod* 66, 354-60.

Aoki, V. W. and Carrell, D. T. (2003). Human protamines and the developing spermatid: their structure, function, expression and relationship with male infertility. *Asian J Androl* 5, 315-24.

Aoki, V. W., Liu, L., Jones, K. P., Hatasaka, H. H., Gibson, M., Peterson, C. M. and Carrell, D. T. (2006). Sperm protamine 1/protamine 2 ratios are related to in vitro fertilization pregnancy rates and predictive of fertilization ability. *Fertil Steril* 86, 1408-15.

Barad, O., Meiri, E., Avniel, A., Aharonov, R., Barzilai, A., Bentwich, I., Einav, U., Gilad, S., Hurban, P., Karov, Y. et al. (2004). MicroRNA expression detected by oligonucleotide microarrays: system establishment and expression profiling in human tissues. *Genome Res* 14, 2486-94.

Barnidge, D. R., Dratz, E. A., Jesaitis, A. J. and Sunner, J. (1999). Extraction method for analysis of detergent-solubilized bacteriorhodopsin and hydrophobic peptides by electrospray ionization mass spectrometry. *Anal Biochem* 269, 1-9.

Belleannee, C., Labas, V., Teixeira-Gomes, A. P., Gatti, J. L., Dacheux, J. L. and Dacheux, F. (2011). Identification of luminal and secreted proteins in bull epididymis. *J Proteomics* 74, 59-78.

Bellin, M. E., Hawkins, H. E., Oyarzo, J. N., Vanderboom, R. J. and Ax, R. L. (1996). Monoclonal antibody detection of heparin-binding proteins on sperm corresponds to increased fertility of bulls. *J Anim Sci* 74, 173-82.

Bellin, M. E., Oyarzo, J. N., Hawkins, H. E., Zhang, H., Smith, R. G., Forrest, D. W., Sprott, L. R. and Ax, R. L. (1998). Fertility-associated antigen on bull sperm indicates fertility potential. *J Anim Sci* 76, 2032-9.

Benchaib, M., Braun, V., Ressnikof, D., Lornage, J., Durand, P., Niveleau, A. and Guerin, J. F. (2005). Influence of global sperm DNA methylation on IVF results. *Hum Reprod* 20, 768-73.

Bielke, W., Blaschke, R. J., Miescher, G. C., Zurcher, G., Andres, A. C. and Ziemiecki, A. (1994). Characterization of a novel murine testis-specific serine/threonine kinase. *Gene* 139, 235-9.

Bissonnette, N., Levesque-Sergerie, J. P., Thibault, C. and Boissonneault, G. (2009). Spermatozoal transcriptome profiling for bull sperm motility: a potential tool to evaluate semen quality. *Reproduction* 138, 65-80.

Bjellqvist, B., Pasquali, C., Ravier, F., Sanchez, J. C. and Hochstrasser, D. (1993). A nonlinear wide-range immobilized pH gradient for two-dimensional electrophoresis and its definition in a relevant pH scale. *Electrophoresis* 14, 1357-65.

Blanchard, Y., Lescoat, D. and Le Lannou, D. (1990). Anomalous distribution of nuclear basic proteins in round-headed human spermatozoa. *Andrologia* 22, 549-55.

Blaschke, R. J., Howlett, A. R., Desprez, P. Y., Petersen, O. W. and Bissell, M. J. (1994). Cell differentiation by extracellular matrix components. *Methods Enzymol* 245, 535-56.

Boerke, A., Dieleman, S. J. and Gadella, B. M. (2007). A possible role for sperm RNA in early embryo development. *Theriogenology* 68, S147-S155.

Bouhallier, F., Allioli, N., Lavial, F., Chalmel, F., Perrard, M. H., Durand, P., Samarut, J., Pain, B. and Rouault, J. P. (2010) Role of miR-34c microRNA in the late steps of spermatogenesis. RNA 16, 720-31.

Bourgeon, F., Evrard, B., Brillard-Bourdet, M., Colleu, D., Jegou, B. and Pineau, C. (2004). Involvement of semenogelin-derived peptides in the antibacterial activity of human seminal plasma. *Biol Reprod* 70, 768-74.

Bowles, J., Knight, D., Smith, C., Wilhelm, D., Richman, J., Mamiya, S., Yashiro, K., Chawengsaksophak, K., Wilson, M. J., Rossant, J. et al. (2006). Retinoid signaling determines germ cell fate in mice. *Science* 312, 596-600.

Brykczynska, U., Hisano, M., Erkek, S., Ramos, L., Oakeley, E., Roloff, T., Beisel, C., Schubeler, D., Stadler, M. and Peters, A. (2010). Repressive and active histone methylation mark distinct promoters in human and mouse spermatozoa. Nature 17, 679-88.

Cancel, A. M., Chapman, D. A. and Killian, G. J. (1997). Osteopontin is the 55-kilodalton fertility-associated protein in Holstein bull seminal plasma. *Biol Reprod* 57, 1293-301.

Cancel, A. M., Chapman, D. A. and Killian, G. J. (1999). Osteopontin localization in the Holstein bull reproductive tract. *Biol Reprod* 60, 454-60.

Carninci, P. Kasukawa, T. Katayama, S. Gough, J. Frith, M. C. Maeda, N. Oyama, R. Ravasi, T. Lenhard, B. Wells, C. et al. (2005). The transcriptional landscape of the mammalian genome. *Science* 309, 1559-63.

Cohen, D. J., Busso, D., Da Ros, V., Ellerman, D. A., Maldera, J. A., Goldweic, N. and Cuasnicu, P. S. (2008). Participation of cysteine-rich secretory proteins (CRISP) in mammalian sperm-egg interaction. *Int J Dev Biol* 52, 737-42.

Collins, A. R., Dobson, V. L., Dusinska, M., Kennedy, G. and Stetina, R. (1997). The comet assay: what can it really tell us? *Mutat Res* 375, 183-93.

Coutinho, L. L., Matukumalli, L. K., Sonstegard, T. S., Van Tassell, C. P., Gasbarre, L. C., Capuco, A. V. and Smith, T. P. (2007). Discovery and profiling of bovine microRNAs from immune-related and embryonic tissues. *Physiol Genomics* 29, 35-43.

Cram, D. S., O'Bryan, M. K. and de Kretser, D. M. (2001). Male infertility genetics--the future. *Journal of Andrology* 22, 738-746.

Dadoune, J. P., Pawlak, A., Alfonsi, M. F. and Siffroi, J. P. (2005). Identification of transcripts by macroarrays, RT-PCR and in situ hybridization in human ejaculate spermatozoa. *Molecular Human Reproduction* 11, 133-140.

D'Amours, O., Frenette, G., Fortier, M., Leclerc, P. and Sullivan, R. (2010). Proteomic comparison of detergent-extracted sperm proteins from bulls with different fertility indexes. *Reproduction* 139, 545-56.

De Felici, M. (2009). Primordial germ cell biology at the beginning of the XXI century. *Int J Dev Biol* 53, 891-4.

De Kretser, D. M. and Baker, H. W. (1999). Infertility in men: recent advances and continuing controversies. *J Clin Endocrinol Metab* 84, 3443-50.

de Yebra, L., Ballesca, J. L., Vanrell, J. A., Corzett, M., Balhorn, R. and Oliva, R. (1998). Detection of P2 precursors in the sperm cells of infertile patients who have reduced protamine P2 levels. *Fertil Steril* 69, 755-9.

Dejarnette, J. M. (2005). The effect of semen quality on reproductive efficiency. *Vet Clin North Am Food Anim Pract* 21, 409-18.

Denhardt, D. T. (2004). The third international conference on osteopontin and related proteins, San Antonio, Texas, May 10-12, 2002. *Calcif Tissue Int* 74, 213-9.

Dinger, M. E., Amaral, P. P., Mercer, T. R., Pang, K. C., Bruce, S. J., Gardiner, B. B., Askarian-Amiri, M. E., Ru, K., Solda, G., Simons, C. et al. (2008). Long noncoding RNAs in mouse embryonic stem cell pluripotency and differentiation. *Genome Res* 18, 1433-45.

Dizdaroglu, M. (1992). Oxidative damage to DNA in mammalian chromatin. *Mutat Res* 275, 331-42.

Dostalova, Z., Calvete, J. J., Sanz, L., Hettel, C., Riedel, D., Schoneck, C., Einspanier, R. and Topfer-Petersen, E. (1994). Immunolocalization and quantitation of acidic seminal fluid protein (aSFP) in ejaculated, swim-up, and capacitated bull spermatozoa. *Biol Chem Hoppe Seyler* 375, 457-61.

du Plessis, S. S., Kashou, A. H., Benjamin, D. J., Yadav, S. P. and Agarwal, A. (2011) Proteomics: a subcellular look at spermatozoa. Reprod Biol Endocrinol 9, 36.

Eckhardt, F., Lewin, J., Cortese, R., Rakyan, V. K., Attwood, J., Burger, M., Burton, J., Cox, T. V., Davies, R., Down, T. A. et al. (2006). DNA methylation profiling of human chromosomes 6, 20 and 22. *Nat Genet* 38, 1378-85.

Eddy, E. M. (2002). Male Germ Cell Gene Expression. *Recent Progress in Hormone Research* 57, 103-128.

Eggert-Kruse, W., Rohr, G., Kerbel, H., Schwalbach, B., Demirakca, T., Klinga, K., Tilgen, W. and Runnebaum, B. (1996). The Acridine Orange test: a clinically relevant screening method for sperm quality during infertility investigation? *Hum Reprod* 11, 784-9.

Einspanier, R., Amselgruber, W., Sinowatz, F., Henle, T., Ropke, R. and Schams, D. (1993). Localization and concentration of a new bioactive acetic seminal fluid protein (aSFP) in bulls (Bos taurus). *J Reprod Fertil* 98, 241-4.

Elsik, C. G. Tellam, R. L. Worley, K. C. Gibbs, R. A. Muzny, D. M. Weinstock, G. M. Adelson, D. L. Eichler, E. E. Elnitski, L. Guigo, R. et al. (2009). The genome sequence of taurine cattle: a window to ruminant biology and evolution. *Science* 324, 522-8.

Enciso, M., Sarasa, J., Agarwal, A., Fernandez, J. L. and Gosalvez, J. (2009). A two-tailed Comet assay for assessing DNA damage in spermatozoa. *Reprod Biomed Online* 18, 609-16.

Espinoza, C. A., Allen, T. A., Hieb, A. R., Kugel, J. F. and Goodrich, J. A. (2004). B2 RNA binds directly to RNA polymerase II to repress transcript synthesis. *Nat Struct Mol Biol* 11, 822-9.

Evenson, D. P., Larson, K. L. and Jost, L. K. (2002). Sperm chromatin structure assay: its clinical use for detecting sperm DNA fragmentation in male infertility and comparisons with other techniques. *J Androl* 23, 25-43.

Farnaud, S. and Evans, R. W. (2003). Lactoferrin--a multifunctional protein with antimicrobial properties. *Mol Immunol* 40, 395-405.

Feng, J., Bi, C., Clark, B. S., Mady, R., Shah, P. and Kohtz, J. D. (2006). The Evf-2 noncoding RNA is transcribed from the Dlx-5/6 ultraconserved region and functions as a Dlx-2 transcriptional coactivator. *Genes Dev* 20, 1470-84.

Ferlin, A., Raicu, F., Gatta, V., Zuccarello, D., Palka, G. and Foresta, C. (2007). Male infertility: role of genetic background. *Reproductive BioMedicine Online* 14, 734-745.

Feugang, J. M., Kaya, A., Page, G. P., Chen, L., Mehta, T., Hirani, K., Nazareth, L., Topper, E., Gibbs, R. and Memili, E. (2009). Two-stage genome-wide association study identifies integrin beta 5 as having potential role in bull fertility. *BMC Genomics* 10, 176.

Feugang, J. M., Rodriguez-Osorio, N., Kaya, A., Wang, H., Page, G., Ostermeier, G. C., Topper, E. K. and Memili, E. (2010) Transcriptome analysis of bull spermatozoa: implications for male fertility. Reprod Biomed Online 21, 312-24.

Frost, R. J., Hamra, F. K., Richardson, J. A., Qi, X., Bassel-Duby, R. and Olson, E. N. (2010) MOV10L1 is necessary for protection of spermatocytes against retrotransposons by Piwi-interacting RNAs. Proc Natl Acad Sci U S A 107, 11847-52.

Fulda, S. and Debatin, K. M. (2006). Extrinsic versus intrinsic apoptosis pathways in anticancer chemotherapy. *Oncogene* 25, 4798-811.

Garrido, N., Martinez-Conejero, J. A., Jauregui, J., Horcajadas, J. A., Simon, C., Remohi, J. and Meseguer, M. (2009). Microarray analysis in sperm from fertile and infertile men without basic sperm analysis abnormalities reveals a significantly different transcriptome. *Fertil Steril* 91, 1307-10.

Gehring, M. and Henikoff, S. (2007). DNA methylation dynamics in plant genomes. *Biochim Biophys Acta* 1769, 276-86.

Gerena, R. L., Irikura, D., Urade, Y., Eguchi, N., Chapman, D. A. and Killian, G. J. (1998). Identification of a fertility-associated protein in bull seminal plasma as lipocalin-type prostaglandin D synthase. *Biol Reprod* 58, 826-33.

Gilbert, L., Bissonnette, N., G., Vallee, M., Robert, C. (2007) A molecular analyses of the population of mRNA in bovine spermatozoa. Reproduction 133, 1073-1086

Go, K. J. and Wolf, D. P. (1985). Albumin-mediated changes in sperm sterol content during capacitation. *Biol Reprod* 32, 145-53.

Goll, M. G. and Bestor, T. H. (2005). Eukaryotic cytosine methyltransferases. *Annu Rev Biochem* 74, 481-514.

Goncalves, R. F., Staros, A. L. and Killian, G. J. (2008). Oviductal fluid proteins associated with the bovine zona pellucida and the effect on in vitro sperm-egg binding, fertilization and embryo development. *Reprod Domest Anim* 43, 720-9.

Gondos, B. (1981). Cellular interrelationships in the human fetal ovary and testis. *Prog Clin Biol Res* 59B, 373-81.

Gorg, A., Weiss, W. and Dunn, M. J. (2004). Current two-dimensional electrophoresis technology for proteomics. *Proteomics* 4, 3665-85.

Granata, F., Petraroli, A., Boilard, E., Bezzine, S., Bollinger, J., Del Vecchio, L., Gelb, M. H., Lambeau, G., Marone, G. and Triggiani, M. (2005). Activation of cytokine production by secreted phospholipase A2 in human lung macrophages expressing the M-type receptor. *J Immunol* 174, 464-74.

Gu, Z., Eleswarapu, S. and Jiang, H. (2007). Identification and characterization of microRNAs from the bovine adipose tissue and mammary gland. *FEBS Lett* 581, 981-8.

Gur, Y. and Breitbart, H. (2006). Mammalian sperm translate nuclear-encoded proteins by mitochondrial-type ribosomes. *Genes and Development* 20, 411-416.

Gwathmey, T. M., Ignotz, G. G., Mueller, J. L., Manjunath, P. and Suarez, S. S. (2006). Bovine seminal plasma proteins PDC-109, BSP-A3, and BSP-30-kDa share functional roles in storing sperm in the oviduct. *Biol Reprod* 75, 501-7.

Hake, L. E., Alcivar, A. A. and Hecht, N. B. (1990). Changes in mRNA length accompany translational regulation of the somatic and testis-specific cytochrome c genes during spermatogenesis in the mouse. *Development* 110, 249-57.

Hall, P. A., Coates, P. J., Ansari, B. and Hopwood, D. (1994). Regulation of cell number in the mammalian gastrointestinal tract: the importance of apoptosis. *J Cell Sci* 107 (Pt 12), 3569-77.

Hao, Y., Mathialagan, N., Walters, E., Mao, J., Lai, L., Becker, D., Li, W., Critser, J. and Prather, R. S. (2006). Osteopontin reduces polyspermy during in vitro fertilization of porcine oocytes. *Biol Reprod* 75, 726-33.

Hartshorne, G. M., Lyrakou, S., Hamoda, H., Oloto, E. and Ghafari, F. (2009). Oogenesis and cell death in human prenatal ovaries: what are the criteria for oocyte selection? *Mol Hum Reprod* 15, 805-19.

Hayashi, K., Chuva de Sousa Lopes, S. M., Kaneda, M., Tang, F., Hajkova, P., Lao, K., O'Carroll, D., Das, P. P., Tarakhovsky, A., Miska, E. A. et al. (2008). MicroRNA biogenesis is required for mouse primordial germ cell development and spermatogenesis. *PLoS One* 3, e1738.

He, Z., Chan, W.-Y. and Dym, M. (2006). Microarray technology offers a novel tool for the diagnosis and identification of therapeutic targets for male infertility. *Reproduction* 132, 11-19.

Hecht, N. B. (1988). Post-meiotic gene expression during spermatogenesis. *Prog Clin Biol Res* 267, 291-313.

Heinlein, M., Brattig, T. and Kunze, R. (1994). In vivo aggregation of maize Activator (Ac) transposase in nuclei of maize endosperm and Petunia protoplasts. *Plant J* 5, 705-14.

Henckel, A., Nakabayashi, K., Sanz, L., Feil, R., Hata, K. and Arnaud, P. (2009). Histone methylation is mechanistically linked to DNA methylation at imprinting control regions in mammals. Human Molecular Genetics 18, 3375-83.

Hernandez, D. G., Nalls, M. A., Gibbs, J. R., Arepalli, S., van der Brug, M., Chong, S., Moore, M., Longo, D. L., Cookson, M. R., Traynor, B. J. et al. (2011) Distinct DNA methylation changes highly correlated with chronological age in the human brain. Hum Mol 41 Genet 20, 1164-72.

Houshdaran, S., Cortessis, V. K., Siegmund, K., Yang, A., Laird, P. W. and Sokol, R. Z. (2007). Widespread epigenetic abnormalities suggest a broad DNA methylation erasure defect in abnormal human sperm. *PLoS One* 2, e1289.

Humphreys, D. T., Carver, J. A., Easterbrook-Smith, S. B. and Wilson, M. R. (1999). Clusterin has chaperone-like activity similar to that of small heat shock proteins. *J Biol Chem* 274, 6875-81.

Ibrahim, N. M., Troedsson, M. H., Foster, D. N., Loseth, K. J., Farris, J. A., Blaschuk, O. and Crabo, B. G. (1999). Reproductive tract secretions and bull spermatozoa contain different clusterin isoforms that cluster cells and inhibit complement-induced cytolysis. *J Androl* 20, 230-40.

Irvine, D. S., Twigg, J. P., Gordon, E. L., Fulton, N., Milne, P. A. and Aitken, R. J. (2000). DNA integrity in human spermatozoa: relationships with semen quality. *J Androl* 21, 33-44.

Jammes, H., Junien, C. and Chavatte-Palmer, P. Epigenetic control of development and expression of quantitative traits. *Reprod Fertil Dev* 23, 64-74.

Jin, W., Grant, J. R., Stothard, P., Moore, S. S. and Guan, L. L. (2009). Characterization of bovine miRNAs by sequencing and bioinformatics analysis. *BMC Mol Biol* 10, 90.

Kelly, V. C., Kuy, S., Palmer, D. J., Xu, Z., Davis, S. R. and Cooper, G. J. (2006). Characterization of bovine seminal plasma by proteomics. *Proteomics* 6, 5826-33.

Killian, G. J., Chapman, D. A. and Rogowski, L. A. (1993). Fertility-associated proteins in Holstein bull seminal plasma. *Biol Reprod* 49, 1202-7.

Kim, H. J., Choi, M. Y. and Llinas, M. (2010). Conformational dynamics and ligand binding in the multi-domain protein PDC109. *PLoS One* 5, e9180.

Kirchhoff, C., Osterhoff, C. and Young, L. (1996). Molecular cloning and characterization of HE1, a major secretory protein of the human epididymis. *Biol Reprod* 54, 847-56.

Kline, D. and Kline, J. T. (1992). Repetitive calcium transients and the role of calcium in exocytosis and cell cycle activation in the mouse egg. *Dev Biol* 149, 80-9.

Koubova, J., Menke, D. B., Zhou, Q., Capel, B., Griswold, M. D. and Page, D. C. (2006). Retinoic acid regulates sex-specific timing of meiotic initiation in mice. *Proc Natl Acad Sci U S A* 103, 2474-9.

Krausz, C. and Giachini, C. (2007). Genetic Risk Factors in Male Infertility. *Archives of Andrology* 53, 125-133.

Kueng, P., Nikolova, Z., Djonov, V., Hemphill, A., Rohrbach, V., Boehlen, D., Zuercher, G., Andres, A. C. and Ziemiecki, A. (1997). A novel family of serine/threonine kinases participating in spermiogenesis. *J Cell Biol* 139, 1851-9.

Kuramochi-Miyagawa, S., Kimura, T., Ijiri, T. W., Isobe, T., Asada, N., Fujita, Y., Ikawa, M., Iwai, N., Okabe, M., Deng, W. et al. (2004). Mili, a mammalian member of piwi family gene, is essential for spermatogenesis. *Development* 131, 839-49.

Kuroda, A., Rauch, T. A., Todorov, I., Ku, H. T., Al-Abdullah, I. H., Kandeel, F., Mullen, Y., Pfeifer, G. P. and Ferreri, K. (2009). Insulin gene expression is regulated by DNA methylation. *PLoS One* 4, e6953.

Laemmli, U. K. (1970). Cleavage of structural proteins during the assembly of the head of bacteriophage T4. *Nature* 227, 680-5.

Lalancette, C., Miller, D., Li, Y. and Krawetz, S. A. (2008a). Paternal contributions: new functional insights for spermatozoal RNA. *J Cell Biochem* 104, 1570-9.

Lalancette, C., Platts, A. E., Johnson, G. D., Emery, B. R., Carrell, D. T. and Krawetz, S. A. (2009). Identification of human sperm transcripts as candidate markers of male fertility. *J Mol Med* 87, 735-48.

Lalancette, C., Thibault, C., Bachand, I., Caron, N. and Bissonnette, N. (2008b). Transcriptome analysis of bull semen with extreme nonreturn rate: use of suppression-subtractive hybridization to identify functional markers for fertility. *Biol Reprod* 78, 618-35.

Lanz, R. B., McKenna, N. J., Onate, S. A., Albrecht, U., Wong, J., Tsai, S. Y., Tsai, M. J. and O'Malley, B. W. (1999). A steroid receptor coactivator, SRA, functions as an RNA and is present in an SRC-1 complex. *Cell* 97, 17-27.

Larsson, A. and Sjoquist, J. (1988). Chicken antibodies: a tool to avoid false positive results by rheumatoid factor in latex fixation tests. *J Immunol Methods* 108, 205-8.

Lee, T. L., Pang, A. L., Rennert, O. M. and Chan, W. Y. (2009). Genomic landscape of developing male germ cells. *Birth Defects Res C Embryo Today* 87, 43-63.

Leone, M. G., Haq, H. A. and Saso, L. (2002). Lipocalin type prostaglandin D-synthase: which role in male fertility? *Contraception* 65, 293-5.

Lie, P. P., Cheng, C. Y. and Mruk, D. D. (2009). Coordinating cellular events during spermatogenesis: a biochemical model. *Trends Biochem Sci* 34, 366-73.

Liu, H., Sadygov, R. G. and Yates, J. R., 3rd. (2004). A model for random sampling and estimation of relative protein abundance in shotgun proteomics. *Anal Chem* 76, 4193-201.

Liu, Z., Zhou, S., Liao, L., Chen, X., Meistrich, M. and Xu, J. (2010). Jmjd1a demethylase-regulated histone modification is essential for cAMP-response element modulator-regulated gene expression and spermatogenesis. *J Biol Chem* 285, 2758-70.

Long, J. E. and Chen, H. X. (2009). Identification and characteristics of cattle microRNAs by homology searching and small RNA cloning. *Biochem Genet* 47, 329-43.

Manicardi, G. C., Tombacco, A., Bizzaro, D., Bianchi, U., Bianchi, P. G. and Sakkas, D. (1998). DNA strand breaks in ejaculated human spermatozoa: comparison of susceptibility to the nick translation and terminal transferase assays. *Histochem J* 30, 33-9.

Manjunath, P. and Therien, I. (2002). Role of seminal plasma phospholipid-binding proteins in sperm membrane lipid modification that occurs during capacitation. *J Reprod Immunol* 53, 109-19.

Manjunath, P., Lefebvre, J., Jois, P. S., Fan, J. and Wright, M. W. (2009). New nomenclature for mammalian BSP genes. *Biol Reprod* 80, 394-7.

Marchetti, C., Obert, G., Deffosez, A., Formstecher, P. and Marchetti, P. (2002). Study of mitochondrial membrane potential, reactive oxygen species, DNA fragmentation and cell viability by flow cytometry in human sperm. *Hum Reprod* 17, 1257-65.

Martin, G., Cagnon, N., Sabido, O., Sion, B., Grizard, G., Durand, P. and Levy, R. (2007). Kinetics of occurrence of some features of apoptosis during the cryopreservation process of bovine spermatozoa. *Hum Reprod* 22, 380-8.

Martin, G., Sabido, O., Durand, P. and Levy, R. (2004). Cryopreservation induces an apoptosis-like mechanism in bull sperm. *Biol Reprod* 71, 28-37.

Mattick, J. S. (2001). Non-coding RNAs: the architects of eukaryotic complexity. *EMBO Rep* 2, 986-91.

Mazzali, M., Kipari, T., Ophascharoensuk, V., Wesson, J. A., Johnson, R. and Hughes, J. (2002). Osteopontin--a molecule for all seasons. *QJM* 95, 3-13.

McGee, E. A. and Hsueh, A. J. (2000). Initial and cyclic recruitment of ovarian follicles. *Endocr Rev* 21, 200-14.

McLaren, A. (2003). Primordial germ cells in the mouse. *Dev Biol* 262, 1-15.

Meissner, A., Mikkelsen, T. S., Gu, H., Wernig, M., Hanna, J., Sivachenko, A., Zhang, X., Bernstein, B. E., Nusbaum, C., Jaffe, D. B. et al. (2008). Genome-scale DNA methylation maps of pluripotent and differentiated cells. *Nature* 454, 766-70.

Mengual, L., Ballesca, J. L., Ascaso, C. and Oliva, R. (2003). Marked differences in protamine content and P1/P2 ratios in sperm cells from percoll fractions between patients and controls. *J Androl* 24, 438-47.

Mercer, T. R., Dinger, M. E., Sunkin, S. M., Mehler, M. F. and Mattick, J. S. (2008). Specific expression of long noncoding RNAs in the mouse brain. *Proc Natl Acad Sci U S A* 105, 716-21.

Merril, C. R., Dunau, M. L. and Goldman, D. (1981). A rapid sensitive silver stain for polypeptides in polyacrylamide gels. *Anal Biochem* 110, 201-7.

Miller, D. and Ostermeier, G. C. (2006a). Spermatozoal RNA: why is it there and what does it do? *Gynecologie Obstetrique & Fertilite* 34, 840-846.

Miller, D. and Ostermeier, G. C. (2006b). Towards a better understanding of RNA carriage by ejaculate spermatozoa. *Human Reproduction Update* 12, 757-767.

Miller, D., Brinkworth, M. and Iles, D. (2010) Paternal DNA packaging in spermatozoa: more than the sum of its parts? DNA, histones, protamines and epigenetics. Reproduction 139, 287-301.

Mishima, T., Takizawa, T., Luo, S. S., Ishibashi, O., Kawahigashi, Y., Mizuguchi, Y., Ishikawa, T., Mori, M., Kanda, T. and Goto, T. (2008). MicroRNA (miRNA) cloning analysis reveals sex differences in miRNA expression profiles between adult mouse testis and ovary. *Reproduction* 136, 811-22.

Miura, C., Ohta, T., Ozaki, Y., Tanaka, H. and Miura, T. (2009). Trypsin is a multifunctional factor in spermatogenesis. *Proc Natl Acad Sci U S A* 106, 20972-7.

Monaco, E., Gasparrini, B., Boccia, L., De Rosa, A., Attanasio, L., Zicarelli, L. and Killian, G. (2009). Effect of osteopontin (OPN) on in vitro embryo development in cattle. *Theriogenology* 71, 450-7.

Morita, Y. and Tilly, J. L. (1999). Oocyte apoptosis: like sand through an hourglass. *Dev Biol* 213, 1-17.

Moura, A. A., Chapman, D. A. and Killian, G. J. (2007a). Proteins of the accessory sex glands associated with the oocyte-penetrating capacity of cauda epididymal sperm from holstein bulls of documented fertility. *Mol Reprod Dev* 74, 214-22.

Moura, A. A., Chapman, D. A., Koc, H. and Killian, G. J. (2007b). A comprehensive proteomic analysis of the accessory sex gland fluid from mature Holstein bulls. *Anim Reprod Sci* 98, 169-88.

Moura, A. A., Souza, C. E., Stanley, B. A., Chapman, D. A. and Killian, G. J. (2010). Proteomics of cauda epididymal fluid from mature Holstein bulls. *J Proteomics* 73, 2006-20.

Nagata, S., Nagase, H., Kawane, K., Mukae, N. and Fukuyama, H. (2003). Degradation of chromosomal DNA during apoptosis. *Cell Death Differ* 10, 108-16.

Ni, M. J., Hu, Z. H., Liu, Q., Liu, M. F., Lu, M. H., Zhang, J. S., Zhang, L. and Zhang, Y. L. (2011) Identification and characterization of a novel non-coding RNA involved in sperm maturation. PLoS One 6, e26053.

Oakley, B. R., Kirsch, D. R. and Morris, N. R. (1980). A simplified ultrasensitive silver stain for detecting proteins in polyacrylamide gels. *Anal Biochem* 105, 361-3.

O'Bryan, M. K., Baker, H. W., Saunders, J. R., Kirszbaum, L., Walker, I. D., Hudson, P., Liu, D. Y., Glew, M. D., d'Apice, A. J. and Murphy, B. F. (1990). Human seminal clusterin (SP-40,40). Isolation and characterization. *J Clin Invest* 85, 1477-86.

O'Farrell, P. H. (1975). High resolution two-dimensional electrophoresis of proteins. *J Biol Chem* 250, 4007-21.

Ohnishi, Y., Totoki, Y., Toyoda, A., Watanabe, T., Yamamoto, Y., Tokunaga, K., Sakaki, Y., Sasaki, H. and Hohjoh, H. (2010) Small RNA class transition from siRNA/piRNA to miRNA during pre-implantation mouse development. Nucleic Acids Res 38, 5141-51.

Okabe, M., Adachi, T., Takada, K., Oda, H., Yagasaki, M., Kohama, Y. and Mimura, T. (1987). Capacitation-related changes in antigen distribution on mouse sperm heads and its relation to fertilization rate in vitro. *J Reprod Immunol* 11, 91-100.

Oliva, R. (2006). Protamines and male infertility. *Hum Reprod Update* 12, 417-35.

Ostermeier, G. C., Miller, D., Huntriss, J. D., Diamond, M. P. and Krawetz, S. A. (2004). Reproductive biology Delivering spermatozoan RNA to the oocyte. *Nature* 429, 154-154.

Panning, B., Dausman, J. and Jaenisch, R. (1997). X chromosome inactivation is mediated by Xist RNA stabilization. *Cell* 90, 907-16.

Patrizio P, Broomfield D. The genetic basis of male infertility. In: Glover TD, Barratt CLR, editors. Male fertility and infertility. Cambridge: Cambridge University; 1999, p 163- 76.

Peddinti, D., Nanduri, B., Kaya, A., Feugang, J. M., Burgess, S. C. and Memili, E. (2008). Comprehensive proteomic analysis of bovine spermatozoa of varying fertility rates and identification of biomarkers associated with fertility. *BMC Syst Biol* 2, 19.

Peng, J., Elias, J. E., Thoreen, C. C., Licklider, L. J. and Gygi, S. P. (2003). Evaluation of multidimensional chromatography coupled with tandem mass spectrometry (LC/LC-MS/MS) for large-scale protein analysis: the yeast proteome. *J Proteome Res* 2, 43-50.

Penny, G. D., Kay, G. F., Sheardown, S. A., Rastan, S. and Brockdorff, N. (1996). Requirement for Xist in X chromosome inactivation. *Nature* 379, 131-7.

Perez, D. S., Hoage, T. R., Pritchett, J. R., Ducharme-Smith, A. L., Halling, M. L., Ganapathiraju, S. C., Streng, P. S. and Smith, D. I. (2008). Long, abundantly expressed non-coding transcripts are altered in cancer. *Hum Mol Genet* 17, 642-55.

Perides, G., Plagens, U. and Traub, P. (1986). Protein transfer from fixed, stained, and dried polyacrylamide gels and immunoblot with protein A-gold. *Anal Biochem* 152, 94-9.

Phillips, B. T., Gassei, K. and Orwig, K. E. (2010). Spermatogonial stem cell regulation and spermatogenesis. *Philos Trans R Soc Lond B Biol Sci* 365, 1663-78.

Ponjavic, J., Ponting, C. P. and Lunter, G. (2007). Functionality or transcriptional noise? Evidence for selection within long noncoding RNAs. *Genome Res* 17, 556-65.

Primakoff, P., Hyatt, H. and Tredick-Kline, J. (1987). Identification and purification of a sperm surface protein with a potential role in sperm-egg membrane fusion. *J Cell Biol* 104, 141-9.

Rader, D. J. (2006). Molecular regulation of HDL metabolism and function: implications for novel therapies. *J Clin Invest* 116, 3090-100.

Rego, J. P., Souza, C. E., Oliveira, J. T., Domont, G., Gozzo, F. C. and Moura, A. A. (2011). WITHDRAWN: Major proteins from the seminal plasma of adult Santa Ines rams. *Anim Reprod Sci*.

Reyes-Moreno, C., Boilard, M., Sullivan, R. and Sirard, M. A. (2002). Characterization of secretory proteins from cultured cauda epididymal cells that significantly sustain bovine sperm motility in vitro. *Mol Reprod Dev* 63, 500-9.

Ro, S., Park, C., Sanders, K. M., McCarrey, J. R. and Yan, W. (2007). Cloning and expression profiling of testis-expressed microRNAs. *Dev Biol* 311, 592-602.

Rodriguez, I., Ody, C., Araki, K., Garcia, I. and Vassalli, P. (1997). An early and massive wave of germinal cell apoptosis is required for the development of functional spermatogenesis. *EMBO J* 16, 2262-70.

Ronkko, S., Lahtinen, R. and Vanha-Perttula, T. (1991). Phospholipases A2 in the reproductive system of the bull. *Int J Biochem* 23, 595-603.

Rubinstein, E., Ziyyat, A., Wolf, J. P., Le Naour, F. and Boucheix, C. (2006). The molecular players of sperm-egg fusion in mammals. *Semin Cell Dev Biol* 17, 254-63.

Rusinov, V., Baev, V., Minkov, I. N. and Tabler, M. (2005). MicroInspector: a web tool for detection of miRNA binding sites in an RNA sequence. *Nucleic Acids Res* 33, W696-700.

Saacke, R. G., Dalton, J. C., Nadir, S., Nebel, R. L. and Bame, J. H. (2000). Relationship of seminal traits and insemination time to fertilization rate and embryo quality. *Anim Reprod Sci* 60-61, 663-77.

Sadler, T.W. (2000). Langman's medical embryology eight edition, Lippincott Williams & Wilkins. Page 24-34.

Sadygov, R. G., Liu, H. and Yates, J. R. (2004). Statistical models for protein validation using tandem mass spectral data and protein amino acid sequence databases. *Anal Chem* 76, 1664-71.

Sassone-Corsi, P. (2002). Unique Chromatin Remodeling and Transcriptional Regulation in Spermatogenesis. *Science* 296, 2176-2178.

Schoneck, C., Braun, J. and Einspanier, R. (1996). Sperm viability is influenced in vitro by the bovine seminal protein aSFP: effects on motility, mitochondrial activity and lipid peroxidation. *Theriogenology* 45, 633-42.

Shaman, J. A., Yamauchi, Y. and Ward, W. S. (2007). Function of the sperm nuclear matrix. *Arch Androl* 53, 135-40.

Shamovsky, I. and Nudler, E. (2006). Gene control by large noncoding RNAs. *Sci STKE* 2006, pe40.

Shamovsky, I., Ivannikov, M., Kandel, E. S., Gershon, D. and Nudler, E. (2006). RNA-mediated response to heat shock in mammalian cells. *Nature* 440, 556-60.

Sharma, R. K., Said, T. and Agarwal, A. (2004). Sperm DNA damage and its clinical relevance in assessing reproductive outcome. *Asian J Androl* 6, 139-48.

Sosnik, J., Miranda, P. V., Spiridonov, N. A., Yoon, S. Y., Fissore, R. A., Johnson, G. R. and Visconti, P. E. (2009). Tssk6 is required for Izumo relocalization and gamete fusion in the mouse. *J Cell Sci* 122, 2741-9.

Soubeyrand, S., Khadir, A., Brindle, Y. and Manjunath, P. (1997). Purification of a novel phospholipase A2 from bovine seminal plasma. *J Biol Chem* 272, 222-7.

Souza, C. E., Moura, A. A., Monaco, E. and Killian, G. J. (2008). Binding patterns of bovine seminal plasma proteins A1/A2, 30 kDa and osteopontin on ejaculated sperm before and after incubation with isthmic and ampullary oviductal fluid. *Anim Reprod Sci* 105, 72-89.

Souza, C., Rego, J., Fioramonte, M., Gozzo, F., Oliveira, J. and Moura, A. (2011). Proteomic Identification of the Cauda Epididymal and Vesicular Gland Fluids of Brazilian Hairy Rams. *Journal of Andrology*, 78-79.

Spano, M., Bonde, J. P., Hjollund, H. I., Kolstad, H. A., Cordelli, E. and Leter, G. (2000). Sperm chromatin damage impairs human fertility. The Danish First Pregnancy Planner Study Team. *Fertil Steril* 73, 43-50.

Stroink, T., Ortiz, M. C., Bult, A., Lingeman, H., de Jong, G. J. and Underberg, W. J. (2005). On-line multidimensional liquid chromatography and capillary electrophoresis systems for peptides and proteins. *J Chromatogr B Analyt Technol Biomed Life Sci* 817, 49-66.

Strozzi, F., Mazza, R., Malinverni, R. and Williams, J. L. (2009). Annotation of 390 bovine miRNA genes by sequence similarity with other species. *Anim Genet* 40, 125.

Suh, N., Baehner, L., Moltzahn, F., Melton, C., Shenoy, A., Chen, J. and Blelloch, R. (2010) MicroRNA function is globally suppressed in mouse oocytes and early embryos. Curr Biol 20, 271-7.

Swann, K. and Yu, Y. (2008). The dynamics of calcium oscillations that activate mammalian eggs. *Int J Dev Biol* 52, 585-94.

Tesarik, J., Greco, E. and Mendoza, C. (2004). Late, but not early, paternal effect on human embryo development is related to sperm DNA fragmentation. *Hum Reprod* 19, 611-5.

Therien, I., Soubeyrand, S. and Manjunath, P. (1997). Major proteins of bovine seminal plasma modulate sperm capacitation by high-density lipoprotein. *Biol Reprod* 57, 1080-8.

Trotochaud, A. E. and Wassarman, K. M. (2005). A highly conserved 6S RNA structure is required for regulation of transcription. *Nat Struct Mol Biol* 12, 313-9.

Unlu, M., Morgan, M. E. and Minden, J. S. (1997). Difference gel electrophoresis: a single gel method for detecting changes in protein extracts. *Electrophoresis* 18, 2071-7.

van den Eijnde, S. M., Luijsterburg, A. J., Boshart, L., De Zeeuw, C. I., van Dierendonck, J. H., Reutelingsperger, C. P. and Vermeij-Keers, C. (1997). In situ detection of apoptosis during embryogenesis with annexin V: from whole mount to ultrastructure. *Cytometry* 29, 313-20.

Vaux, D. L. and Korsmeyer, S. J. (1999). Cell death in development. *Cell* 96, 245-54.

Visconti, P. E. and Kopf, G. S. (1998). Regulation of protein phosphorylation during sperm capacitation. *Biol Reprod* 59, 1-6.

Wakabayashi, H., Matsumoto, H., Hashimoto, K., Teraguchi, S., Takase, M. and Hayasawa, H. (1999). Inhibition of iron/ascorbate-induced lipid peroxidation by an N-terminal peptide of bovine lactoferrin and its acylated derivatives. *Biosci Biotechnol Biochem* 63, 955-7.

Wang, N. and Tilly, J. L. (2010). Epigenetic status determines germ cell meiotic commitment in embryonic and postnatal mammalian gonads. *Cell Cycle* 9, 339-49.

Wang, R. and Sperry, A. O. (2008). Identification of a novel Leucine-rich repeat protein and candidate PP1 regulatory subunit expressed in developing spermatids. *BMC Cell Biol* 9, 9.

Ward, W. S. (1993). Deoxyribonucleic acid loop domain tertiary structure in mammalian spermatozoa. *Biol Reprod* 48, 1193-201.

Ward, W. S. (2010). Function of sperm chromatin structural elements in fertilization and development. *Mol Hum Reprod* 16, 30-6.

Washburn, M. P., Wolters, D. and Yates, J. R., 3rd. (2001). Large-scale analysis of the yeast proteome by multidimensional protein identification technology. *Nat Biotechnol* 19, 242-7.

Weinrauch, Y., Elsbach, P., Madsen, L. M., Foreman, A. and Weiss, J. (1996). The potent anti-Staphylococcus aureus activity of a sterile rabbit inflammatory fluid is due to a 14-kD phospholipase A2. *J Clin Invest* 97, 250-7.

Wempe, F., Einspanier, R. and Scheit, K. H. (1992). Characterization by cDNA cloning of the mRNA of a new growth factor from bovine seminal plasma: acidic seminal fluid protein. *Biochem Biophys Res Commun* 183, 232-7.

Wolfsberg, T. G., Straight, P. D., Gerena, R. L., Huovila, A. P., Primakoff, P., Myles, D. G. and White, J. M. (1995). ADAM, a widely distributed and developmentally regulated gene family encoding membrane proteins with a disintegrin and metalloprotease domain. *Dev Biol* 169, 378-83.

Yan, N., Lu, Y., Sun, H., Tao, D., Zhang, S., Liu, W. and Ma, Y. (2007). A microarray for microRNA profiling in mouse testis tissues. *Reproduction* 134, 73-9.

Yang, W. X. and Sperry, A. O. (2003). C-terminal kinesin motor KIFC1 participates in acrosome biogenesis and vesicle transport. *Biol Reprod* 69, 1719-29.

Yang, W. X., Jefferson, H. and Sperry, A. O. (2006). The molecular motor KIFC1 associates with a complex containing nucleoporin NUP62 that is regulated during development and by the small GTPase RAN. *Biol Reprod* 74, 684-90.

Yegnasubramanian, S., Lin, X., Haffner, M. C., DeMarzo, A. M. and Nelson, W. G. (2006). Combination of methylated-DNA precipitation and methylation-sensitive restriction enzymes (COMPARE-MS) for the rapid, sensitive and quantitative detection of DNA methylation. *Nucleic Acids Res* 34, e19.

Yik, J. H., Chen, R., Nishimura, R., Jennings, J. L., Link, A. J. and Zhou, Q. (2003). Inhibition of P-TEFb (CDK9/Cyclin T) kinase and RNA polymerase II transcription by the coordinated actions of HEXIM1 and 7SK snRNA. *Mol Cell* 12, 971-82.

Yu, B., Yang, Z., Li, J., Minakhina, S., Yang, M., Padgett, R. W., Steward, R. and Chen, X. (2005). Methylation as a crucial step in plant microRNA biogenesis. *Science* 307, 932-5.

Yuan, Y. Y., Chen, W. Y., Shi, Q. X., Mao, L. Z., Yu, S. Q., Fang, X. and Roldan, E. R. (2003). Zona pellucida induces activation of phospholipase A2 during acrosomal exocytosis in guinea pig spermatozoa. *Biol Reprod* 68, 904-13.

Zhang, X., Yazaki, J., Sundaresan, A., Cokus, S., Chan, S. W., Chen, H., Henderson, I. R., Shinn, P., Pellegrini, M., Jacobsen, S. E. et al. (2006). Genome-wide high-resolution mapping and functional analysis of DNA methylation in arabidopsis. *Cell* 126, 1189-201.

Zilberman, D. and Henikoff, S. (2007). Genome-wide analysis of DNA methylation patterns. *Development* 134, 3959-65.

Zuercher, G., Rohrbach, V., Andres, A. C. and Ziemiecki, A. (2000). A novel member of the testis specific serine kinase family, tssk-3, expressed in the Leydig cells of sexually mature mice. *Mech Dev* 93, 175-7.

7

A Systems Biology Approach to Understanding Male Infertility

Nicola Bernabò, Mauro Mattioli and Barbara Barboni
University of Teramo
Italy

1. Introduction

Once ejaculated, mammalian spermatozoa have undergone spermatogenesis and spermiogenesis but are still unable to fertilize the oocyte. In many species, including human, male gametes become able to fertilize only upon they reside in the female genital tract for a finite period, ranging from hours to days. During this window of time important physical-chemical modifications, collectively known as "capacitation", occur, involving all the sperm biochemical machinery and conferring to male gametes the ability to fertilize. During capacitation, in one hand, spermatozoa gradually lose the decapacitating factors of epididimal origin and, on the other hand, progressively interact with regulating (either inhibiting and activating) factors present in oviductal fluid and with the tubal epithelium. Capacitation is completed when the sperm cells can successfully recognise the oocyte and extrude the acrosomal vescicle content (acrosome reaction, AR), thus penetrating the zona pellucida (ZP) and reaching the oocyte membrane.

During capacitation spermatozoa undergo important biochemical and structural modifications involving sperm head as well as sperm tail. In particular, at the head level, the membranes markedly change their architecture, tanks to their highly dynamical structure. In fact, differently from what has been believed until about ten years ago, the sperm membrane organization differs from the classical fluid mosaic model that predict a random lateral diffusion of lipids and proteins (Abou-haila & Tulsiani, 2009; Nixon & Aitken, 2009). The data from several Laboratories converge in depicting the sperm membranes as highly asymmetrical structures, either in longitudinal (membrane domains and sub-domains) (Bruckbauer et al., 2010; Gadella et al.,2008; Kotwicka et al. 2011; Venditti & Bean, 2009) and transversal (inner and outer leaflet) direction (Gadella & Harrison 2000, 2002; Harrison & Gadella 2005). Particularly in the head plasma membrane (PM) it is possible to recognize different domains, with different chemical-physical and functional proprieties: the apical ridge area, the pre-equatorial area, the equatorial area and the post-equatorial area. The apical ridge is involved in sperm-ZP binding and contains specific zona binding proteins (O'Rand & Fischer, 1987). The pre-equatorial surface is the site where the fusion between PM and outer acrosome membrane (OAM) takes place during AR, while the equatorial surface area of sperm head does not participate to the AR, but it is characterized by the presence of a hairpin like structure that is involved in the fusion of sperm and oocyte membranes at the moment of fertilization (for review see Yanagimachi, 1994 and Gadella et al., 2008). Each domain, in turn, contains specialized areas, known as microdomains. These microdomains could be isolated from the membrane, by using 0.1% Triton X-100 or similar detergent at 4°C in a discontinuous density gradient, as detergent resistant membrane (DRM). DRMs are small lipid ordered portions of membrane that contain larger amounts of cholesterol, sphingomyelin, gangliosides, phospholipids with saturated long-chain acyl chains, and proteins such as GPI anchored proteins, caveolin and flotillin. During capacitation their organization changes, leading the association and activation of proteins involved in signal transduction, such as CB1R, TRPV1, (Botto et al., 2010) and in membrane fusion (Asano et al., 2010) (see Brewis & Gadella 2010 for review).

In addition, as in others mammalian cell types, the different composition of inner and outer leaflets is different (Gadella et al., 2008; Hickey & Buhr 2011; Müller et al., 1996). Particularly the aminophospholipids phosphatidylserine (PS) and phosphatidylethanolamine (PE) are concentrated in the inner leaflet and the choline phospholipids sphingomyelin (SM) and phosphatidylcholine (PC) in the outer leaflet. This asymmetry is established and maintained by the action of several translocating enzymes with differing phospholipid specificities (for review, see Bevers et al., 1998). For instance aminophospholipid translocase (also known as flippase), is responsible for transfer of PS and PE from the outer to the inner lipid leaflet, 'floppase' transfers phospholipids from inner to outer leaflet and scramblase acts as a bi-directional carrier with little specificity, simply moving all four phospholipid species in both directions (inward and outward) across the membrane lipid bilayer, thus reducing phospholipid asymmetry ('lipid scrambling'). This last event plays a key role in the acquisition of PM and OAM tendency to fuse each other (fusogenicity), increasing their fluidity.

Lipid remodeling of sperm membranes is controlled by an integrate dialogue between activating and inhibiting stimuli. In particular after ejaculation, before the seminal plasma is completely removed, the endocannabinoids concentration is high, the phospholipid scrambling is blocked and cholesterol has a wide-spread lateral localization in the sperm head PM. After the complete removal of seminal plasma and with the contact with female genital tract secretion, the concentration of endocannabionoids gradually decreases while the bicarbonate increases. As a consequence soluble adenylate cyclase (sAC) is activated in the sperm head and cAMP/PKA pathway becames effective stimulating phospholipid scrambling in the apical plasma membrane of the sperm head (Gadella & Harrison 2000). This process enable the extracellular protein to extract cholesterol, thus the membranes can complete its reorganization with the increase of the PM and OAM fusogenicity, which is the necessary prerequisite for AR.

This dynamical evolution of membranes is paralleled by a massive reorganization of other cellular components, in particular of head cytoskeleton. In fact in spermatozoa the cytosol is virtually absent, thus the PM is in direct contact with the diverse underlying cytoskeleton structures, which are highly organized and whose architecture changes during capacitation. It is believed that actin cytoskeleton may have a structural role during capacitation and AR: when fusogenicity of PM and OAM increases, a network of actin develops acting as a diaphragm between the two membranes avoiding their premature fusion. Once the capacitation was completely achieved and the physiological stimulus (ZP proteins) was detected, the ZP-induced calcium peak causes the fast depolymerisation of actin structure, thus allowing fusion of PM and OAM and, ultimately, AR (Breitbart et al., 2005; Breitbart & , Etkovitz, 2011).

In sperm tail the most evident changes are related to the motility pattern. When stored in epididymis spermatozoa are completely immotile or weakly motile, while immediately after ejaculation, they begin to swim with a species-specific pattern. Once exposed to capacitating condition, either in physiological context or in an artificial environment, male gametes gradually express a new pattern of motion, the hyperactivated motility. This process was first decribed in 1969 by Yanagimachi (Yanagimachi, 1969), who reported that the spermatozoa able to fertilize the oocyte showed a different and more vigorous swimming pattern than those functionally immature. In human, the flagella of hyperactivated spermatozoa beat less symmetrical than flagella of ejaculated spermatozoa and, as a result, they tend to swim vigorously in circles. It was proposed that the acquisition of this motility pattern is functional to allow spermatozoa to penetrate the oviductal mucus, the cumuls-oocyte complex extracellular matrix and, finally, the ZP (Chang & Suarez, 2010; Suarez 2008).

The onset of hyperactivated motility is due to the activation of a complex biochemical pathway, still under investigation (see Suarez 2008 for review). At present it is known that the interaction with female environment stimulates a signaling cascade that leads to the increase in intracellaular concentration of second messengers, in particular of Ca^{2+} and cAMP. Specifically the phospholipase C (PLC) is activated through a heterotrimeric G protein (Gq/11)-coupled receptor (R1) and produces IP3. Binding of IP3 to its receptors (IP3R) causes an increase in cytoplasmic Ca^{2+}. The activation of membrane-associated adenylyl cyclase (AC) through high cytoplasmic Ca^{2+}, G proteins and membrane potential increases intracellular cAMP. In parallel the bicarbonate may also cause an increase in cAMP by activating the soluble form of adenylyl cyclase (sAC) directly. The increase in cAMP concentration activates cyclic nucleotide-gated channels (CNG) thus promoting the Ca^{2+} influx. In addition increased cAMP activates protein kinase A (PKA) to phosphorylate axonemal or fibrous sheath proteins and results in flagellar beating. It is thought that high cytoplasmic Ca^{2+} and Ca^{2+}–calmodulin complex are responsible for asymmetrical bending of flagella that is characteristic of hyperactivation.

Anyway at the end of capacitation, of the millions of sperm normally ejaculated, only thousands reach the isthmus of the oviduct and only a few reach the ampulla, where the fertilization takes place. During this process two important functional events are accomplished: only the more motile spermatozoa are selected, thus increasing the success rate of fertilization and decreasing the risk of polyspermy, and their fertilizing ability is maintained for a relatively long period, until the oocyte is ovulated.

Because of its important implications both for basic (developmental biology, endocrinology, biochemistry) and applied science (andrology, male infertility, contraception) these events are under the attention of Researcher starting from the pionieristic works of Austin (Austin, 1951) and Chang (Chang, 1951), that, contemporaneously and independently, proposed the concept of capacitation in the far 1951. During last 60 years a myriad of molecular data was obtained and the knowledge of biochemical aspects of capacitation was markedly increased but, despite the large amount of literature and the amazing diffusion of reproduction biotechnologies, many aspects of these events are still unsatisfactory known. In particular, this deficiency is made evident by the impossibility to *a priori* identify a capacitated spermatozoon. At present the only available tests in andrology are able to *ex post* evaluate the ability of spermatozoa to acquire a particular staining pattern (CTC) or to respond to different physiological stimuli (induction of AR, IVF). The laboratory tests usually carried out in andrology laboratories are:

- assessment of chlortetracycline staining pattern. The chlortetracycline (CTC), a UV fluorescent antibiotic, yields different patterns of distribution on the sperm surface depending on the time and conditions of the sperm incubation. These different patterns were first described in the mouse by Saling and Storey (1979), and the correlation of these patterns with the capacitation status of the sperm was subsequently empirically defined by different Authors in several species including Human (Perry et al., 1995), mice (Fraser & Herod, 1990), bull (Fraser et al., 1995), boar (Mattioli et al., 1996), etc ... The advantage of this method is that it seems to relate with the capacitation status of the sperm independently of the acrosome reaction. The disadvantage is that the mechanism by which CTC yields the different patterns is not clearly understood, and the biochemical events involved in capacitation that give rise to these patterns are completely unknown. It has been suggested that changes in the distribution of Ca^{2+}-CTC complexes bound to phospholipids in the plasma membrane are responsible for the different patterns observed, thus any compound that interferes whit this event without affecting the acquisition of spermatozoa fertilizing ability, could potentially be interpreted as changing the sperm capacitation state. In addition it was found that spermatozoa treated with cytochalasin D, a specific actin polymerization inhibitor, that display a capacitation-related pattern of fluorescence, were unable to undergo AR, when tested by induction of acrosome reaction by homologous ZP (Bernabò et al., 2011). This finding suggests the idea that CTC could changes as a consequence of the membrane lipid remodeling occurring during capacitation rather than depending on the real capacitation status of male gametes.
- induction of the Acrosome Reaction. The capacitation could be defined as the ability of a spermatozoon to undergo AR when stimulated by more or less physiologically relevant agent, such as the calcium ionophore A23187, homologous ZP or progesteron. A problem with these assays is that compounds that are able to stimulate or inhibit the acrosome reaction cannot be assumed to do so by stimulating or inhibiting capacitation. In other words, acrosome reactions might be able to occur in uncapacitated sperm when the cells are treated with compounds that bypass capacitation.
- zona-free hamster oocyte penetration test: this test is aimed to provides information on the fusinogenic nature of capacitated sperm head membranes. The fusion of human spermatozoa with the hamster oocyte is functionally the same as that with the human vitelline membrane, since it is initiated by the plasma membrane overlying the equatorial segment of acrosome-reacted human spermatozoa (World Health Organization [WHO], 2010). Unfortunately, this test may result in two types of criticism: 1) it differs from the physiological situation in that the ZP is present; 2) the results of conventional hamster oocyte test depends on the occurrence of spontaneous acrosome reactions in populations of spermatozoa incubated for prolonged periods in vitro. Since this procedure is less efficient than the biological process and may involve different mechanisms, false-negative results (men whose spermatozoa fail in the hamster oocyte test but successfully fertilize human oocytes in vitro or in vivo) have frequently been recorded (WHO,1986).
- in vitro fertilization (IVF). The most reliable way to assess capacitation is to perform *in vitro* fertilization assays. In this case also, it cannot be assumed that if a specific

compound/incubation condition inhibits *in vitro* fertilization it really inhibits capacitation, since fertilization is a multistep process that involves various aspects of sperm physiology (e.g., motility, acrosome reaction) as well as the interaction with the oocyte (e.g., ZP binding, plasma membrane binding, and/or fusion). Moreover, the concentration of sperm used in the *in vitro* fertilization assays may dramatically impact interpretation of results since these assays normally use a much higher sperm/egg ratio than is normally encountered *in vivo*. It is also time-consuming and expensive to perform and, finally, has evident ethical limitation in Humans.

From these consideration it is evident that, at the present, a reliable *a priori* marker of capacitation is unavailable. Thus, in several cases, it is impossible for clinicians and andrologists to perform an adequate diagnosis (and as a consequence a therapy and a prognosis) after seminal and clinical investigations, as it happens in the case of unexplained infertility of male origin. Recent data reported that infertility affects about 7% of all men. The etiology of this pathological condition can involve factors acting at pre-testicular, post-testicular or directly at the testicular level. Primary testicular failure accounts for about 75% of all male factor infertility. Despite the recent progress in medicine of reproduction field its etiology is still unknown in about 50% of cases, in which the only possible diagnosis is "idiopathic infertility" (Krausz, 2011).

In our opinion the inability to perform a diagnosis is not due to the insufficient amount of knowledge about sperm physiopathology. During last 60 years the data concerning lipids, proteins, glycids and ions involved capacitation are amazingly grown. Each year new molecules and new function of already known molecules are discovered thanks to the adoption of continuously evolving analytical technology (2D electrophoresis, proteomic techniques, knock-out animals, development of in vitro systems,…). The reason of this failure must be sought in the approach until now adopted, that could be considered reductionist. From a philosophical point of view, the Reductionism is a way to understand the nature of complex things, such as living beings, by reducing them to the interactions of their parts, or to simpler or more fundamental things (http://en.wikipedia.org/wiki/Reductionism). Thus a "reductionist believes that a complex system is nothing but the sum of its parts. An account of it can be reduced to accounts of individual constituents". (Interdisciplinary Encyclopaedia of Religion and Science, http://www.disf.org/en/Voci/104.asp). Until now scientists simply have studied all the molecules involved in spermatozoa post-ejaculatory maturation separately: their attention has been paid to the study of single molecular determinants. Unfortunately the knowledge arising from the so obtained data fails to give information about the whole phenomenon. This could be due to the fact that spermatozoa, as well as all other cells and all living beings, behave as complex systems, i.e. as systems constituted by a network of heterogeneous components that interact nonlinearly, to give rise to emergent behaviour. In particular, as physics theory of complexity says, in a complex system the whole system is more than the sum of its single components. This concept is well highlighted by the etymology of the word "complexity": it derives from Latin *cum* = together and *plecto* (that in turn derives from the ancient Greek πλέκω) = plait, weave, braid, twist, turn; thus giving the idea of interconnected and not separable things. For instance it is noteworthy the difference of meaning between "complex" and "complicated". "Complicated" derives from the Latin *cum* and *plicare* (to fold); the solution of a complicated problem is the explication (from Latin *explicare* = to unfold), on the contrary it is impossible to "unfold" the complexity. Complex systems have some defined and peculiar features:

- the components of a complex system may themselves be complex systems. For example, an organism is made up of tissues, which are made up of cells, which are in turn made up of organelles and macromolecular complexes - all of which are complex systems;
- relationships are non-linear. This implies that a small perturbation may cause dramatic effects (see butterfly effect), proportional effects, or even no effect at all;
- relationships may contain feedback loops: both negative (damping) and positive (amplifying) feedback are found in complex systems. The effects of each element is fed back to others, in such a way that the element itself can be altered;
- complex systems may exhibit behaviors that emerge depending on the order of magnitude of descriptor point of view. It means that the study of system basic constituents can fail to give information about the behavior of whole system, that can only be studied at a higher level: for instance the description of human physiology, biochemistry and biological development (that are at one level of analysis) fail to explain human society dynamics. This is because it is a property that emerges from the collection of Humans and needs to be analyzed at a different level.

From that it is evident that the intrinsic nature of complex systems implies many difficulties with their formal modelling and simulation. In recent years a new branch of mathematics, the science of networks, was adopted to this aim representing and studying them as graphs.

2. From the Köenigsberg bridges to the genome analysis passing trough WWW

The idea to use a model, and in particular a set of nodes connected by links (a graph), is actually no new, dating back to the 1736, when Leonhard Euler used this approach to solve the Seven Bridges of Königsberg problem. The city of Königsberg in Prussia (now Kaliningrad, Russia) was set on both sides of the Pregel River, and included two islands connected to each other and to the mainland by seven bridges. The problem was to find a walk through the city that would cross each bridge once and only once. The islands could not be reached by any route other than the bridges, and every bridge must have been crossed completely every time. Euler for the first time represented the mainland and the islands as nodes and the bridges as edges connecting them. Using this modeling strategy provided the evidence that the problem had no solution.

More than two hundred and fifty years later, the science of networks was used to explore several different phenomena, from the WWW architecture (Barabási et al., 2000; Barabási 2001) to the physical connection of computers through the world (Yook et al., 2002), from the actors collaboration chains to the company market (Barabási, 2003), pointing out as some similar features seem to be shared by the most of them. Obviously one of the research fields that have benefit more from this approach was the biology. In fact the modern technologies offer to Biologists an amazing amount of data, unimaginable until a few years ago, that are increasingly difficult to interpret because of their complexity.

In particular systems biology is the discipline that aims to collect and interpret the data from high throughput techniques, viewing at the organism as an integrated network of interacting molecules. These interactions are liked to be ultimately responsible for the organism form and functions. As R. Albert recently stated "transcription factors can activate or inhibit the transcription of genes to give mRNAs. Since transcription factors are themselves products of genes, the ultimate effect is that genes regulate each other's expression as part of gene regulatory networks. Similarly, proteins can participate in diverse post-translational interactions that lead to modified protein functions or to formation of protein complexes that have new roles; the totality of these processes is called a protein-protein interaction network. The biochemical reactions in cellular metabolism can likewise be integrated into a metabolic network whose fluxes are regulated by enzymes catalyzing the reactions. In many cases these different levels of interaction are integrated - for example, when the presence of an external signal triggers a cascade of interactions that involves both biochemical reactions and transcriptional regulation"(Albert, 2005). Aimed to provide a strategy able to study the complexity of these phenomena, systems biology brings together biology, physics, statistic and computer science, opening new perspectives in virtually all the branch of the study of life. For instance it was adopted to investigate the organization of metabolic networks, comparing the data from several organisms belonging to the three domains of life, showing as they share a common topography and similar proprieties (Jeong et al., 2000). At the same time the description of yeast proteome, carried out with the same approach, pointed out as the correlation between the connectivity and indispensability of proteins confirms that, despite the importance of individual biochemical function and genetic redundancy, the robustness against mutations is derived from the organization of interactions and the topological architecture of the network (Wagner, 2000). More recently the network representing disorders and disease genes linked by known disorder–gene associations was realized, thus offering a platform to explore all known phenotype and disease gene associations, indicating the common genetic origin of many diseases (Goh et al., 2007).

3. Systems biology of spermatozoa: The realization of a computational model

In 2010 our group, for the first time, started to apply a systems biology-based approach to the study of capacitation (Bernabò et al., 2010a). As first the human spermatozoa post-ejaculatory maturation has been modelised as a biological network (see Figure 1). To this aim, since at present a database containing the information about the molecular events occurring during this process does not exist, a new database has been realized using Microsoft Office Excel 2003. The data were obtained from peer-reviewed papers published in latest 10 years on PubMed (www.ncbi.nlm.nih.gov/pubmed/) concerning human spermatozoa. When the data are lacking or to fill incomplete pathways the data from other mammals, such as mouse, horse, pig, bull, etc.. were used, only if confirmed by a large consensus. The freely available and diffusible molecules such as H_2O, CO_2, P_i, H^+,O_2 were omitted, when not necessary and, in some cases, the record did not represent a single molecule but complex events, such as "membrane fusion" or "protein tyrosine phosphorylation" because all the single molecular determinants of the phenomenon are still unknown. The fields of the database were:

Source molecule: i.e. the molecule source of interaction.
Interaction: i.e. the nature of interaction (activation, inhibition, ...).
Target molecule: i.e. the molecule target of the interaction.
Biological function: i.e. the functional meaning or the contest of interaction (glycolysis, lipid remodelling, oxidative phosphorylation, …).
Reference: i.e. the bibliographic source of information.
Notes: i.e. all the notation such as the presence of synonyms or the explanation of complex cellular events.

These data were used to build the capacitation network by the Cytoscape 2.6.3 software (http://www.cytoscape.org). The network was spatially represented using the Cytoscape Orthogonal Layout. The node size was proportional to the connection number and the node color gradient was dependent from the closeness centrality. This parameter is computed as: $C_c(n) = 1/avg(L(n, m))$, were L (n, m) is the length of the shortest path between two nodes *n* and *m*. The closeness centrality of each node ranges from 0 to 1 and it is a measure of how fast information spreads from a given node to the others nodes. The statistical and topological analyses of networks were carried out considering the networks as directed by the Cytoscape plugin Network Analyzer (http://med.bioinf.mpi-inf.mpg.de/netanalyzer/help/2.6.1/index.html).

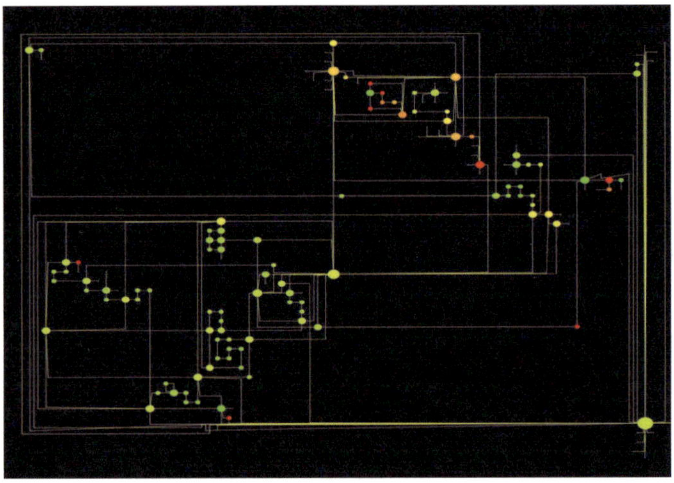

Fig. 1. Diagram showing the structure of the human spermatozoa capacitation network (see text for explanation).

Once the network was created a statistical analysis was carried out to measure the network most relevant topological proprieties (see Table 1).

The distribution of node linkages followed a power law, represented by the generic equation:

$$y = a\,x^{-b}$$

The r, R^2 and b coefficients of IN and OUT network were tabulated in Table 2.

The clustering coefficient distribution does not follow a power law, as demonstrated by the results of power law fitting of clustering coefficient distribution ($r = 0.183$, $R^2 = 0.217$).

	capacitation
N° nodes	151
N° edges	202
Clustering coefficient	0.028
Diameter	20
Averaged n° neighbours	2.662
Char. path length	6.546

Table 1. Main topological parameters of capacitation network.

The number of nodes represent the total number of molecules involved, the number of edges represents the total number of interaction found, the clustering coefficient is calculated as CI = 2nI/k(k-1),where nI is the number of links connecting the kI neighbours of node I to each other, the network diameter is the largest distance between two nodes, the Averaged n° neighbours represent the mean number of connection of each node, the Char. path length gives the expected distance between two connected nodes.

	capacitation	
	in	out
r	0.988	0.997
R^2	0.890	0.828
b	-1.542	-1.993

Table 2. Result of power law fitting of IN and OUT capacitation network.

As it is known, the analysis of networks topology made possible to recognize different architecture typologies (Barabási & Oltvai, 2004). The simpler is that of random networks, described by the Erdös-Rényi (ER) model. In this case the network has N nodes connected with probability *p*, which creates a graph with approximately $pN(N-1)/2$ randomly placed links. The node degrees follow a Poisson distribution, which indicates that most nodes have approximately the same number of links, close to the average degree, that define the scale of the network. The tail (high *k* region) of the degree distribution $P(k)$ decreases exponentially, thus indicating that the nodes that significantly deviate from the average are extremely rare. The clustering coefficient is independent of a node degree, and the mean path length is proportional to the logarithm of the network size, $l \sim \log N$.

Scale-free networks, following the Barabási-Albert (BA) model, are characterized by a power-law degree distribution, thus the probability that a node has *k* links follows $P(k) \sim k^{-\gamma}$, where γ is the degree exponent. In other word, the probability that a node is highly connected is statistically more significant than in a random graph. This imply that the network properties are strongly determined by a relatively small number of highly connected nodes (the hubs) and that a "typical" node does not exist (scale free topology). These network do not have an inherent modularity, i.e. $C(k)$ is independent of *k*. In addition scale-free networks have the average path length following $l \sim \log \log N$, which is significantly shorter than log N that characterizes random networks.

Modularity, local clustering and scale-free topology coexist in hierarchical networks, that integrate a scale-free topology with an inherent modular structure. The most important feature of hierarchical modularity is the scaling of the clustering coefficient, and the hierarchical architecture implies that sparsely connected nodes are part of highly clustered areas, with communication between the different highly clustered neighborhoods maintained by a few hubs.

From our results it was evident that capacitation network follows the BA model (scale free network) as pointed out by the power law that links the number of edges to the node frequency and the dispersion of clustering coefficient.

This particular kind of topology confers to the network some important biological characteristics. For instance, from a theoretical point of view, the marked heterogeneity in the number of links per node could justify the different consequences of the removal of differently linked nodes: if highly linked nodes will be removed, network topology will be strongly affected; on the contrary if the removal will involve the less linked ones, the network structure will undergo not significative alterations (Albert et al., 2000). To test if our model behaves as predicted, the most linked nodes ($[Ca^{2+}]_i$ and the ATP-ADP system) or two or four randomly selected nodes were eliminated from the network. In the first case, the network structure collapsed (Figure 2), in the second one the variations of network topology were minimal (data not shown).

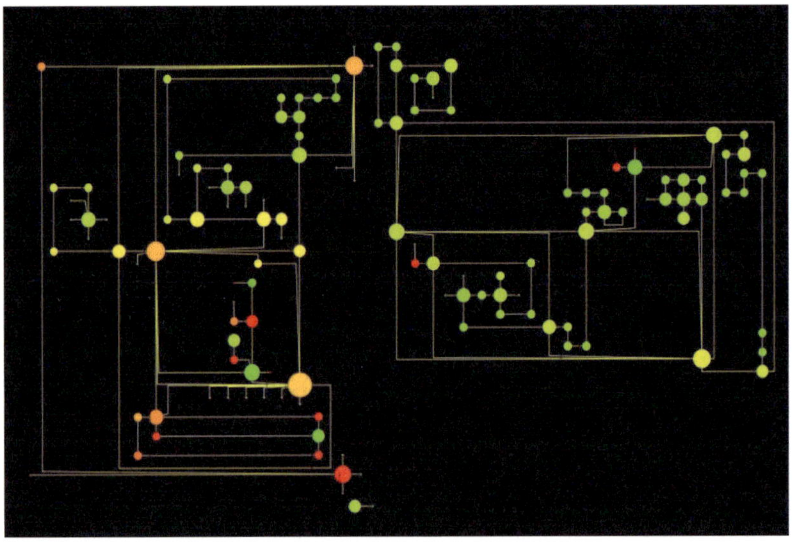

Fig. 2. Diagram showing the structure of the human spermatozoa capacitation network after [Ca2+]i and ATP/ADP nodes removal (see text for explanation).

Reasonably this particular behaviour could offer an important evolutionary advantage: the robustness against random failure. In fact a random perturbation will involve the most frequent typology of nodes, i.e. the less connected ones, with negligible consequences on network architecture, that is on whole cellular function. In our model we identified 6 hubs, thus it exist only a probability <5% (6/151) that one of them will be involved in random damages.

In detail these hubs, as shown in Table 3, are $[Ca^{2+}]_i$, ATP-ADP system, protein kynase A (PKA), Tyr phosphorylation and phospholipase D1 (PLD1).

Node	Number of links
$[Ca^{2+}]_i$	25
ATP	14
Tyr phosphorylation	13
PKA	9
ADP	8
PLD1	8

Table 3. Most connected nodes (the hubs) of capacitation and AR networks.

It is not surprising to note that in absolute the most linked node is $[Ca^{2+}]_i$. As it is well known, capacitation is a Ca^{2+}-dependent process: during this process $[Ca^{2+}]_i$ increases and the capacitation does not take place in the Ca^{2+} absence (Bretibert, 2002 ; Florman et al., 2008). Particularly the calcium homeostasis is ensured by four major Ca^{2+} clearance mechanisms, two acting on the PM and two on intracellular organelles. The PM Ca^{2+}-ATPase exports a cytoplasmic Ca^{2+} ion and imports one or two extracellular protons at the expense of ATP. When $[Ca^{2+}]_i$ is too elevated, the plasma membrane Na^{+}-Ca^{2+} exchanger operates in forward mode exporting an intracellular Ca^{2+} ion and importing approximately three Na^{+} ions at the expense of the Na^{+} gradient (Blaustein & Lederer, 1999; Fraser et al., 1993). The best characterised organellar clearance mechanisms are the sarcoplasmic-endoplasmic reticulum Ca^{2+}-ATPase (SERCA) pumps, located at the acrosomal level, and the mitochondrial Ca^{2+} uniporter (MCU), whose contribute is mainly directed to the maintenance of $[Ca^{2+}]_i$ in the midpiece of spermatozoa (Wennemuth et al., 2003). During capacitation the Ca^{2+} behaves as a second messenger converting extracelluar stimuli to chemical response in a myriad of molecular system, such as, protein kynase C (PKC), protein kynase C (PKA), actin, lipases and many others.

The ATP-ADP system is the main energetic source of spermatozoa. In fact in male gametes, the metabolic energy production is guaranteed by the glycolysis exclusively, by mitochondrial oxidative phosphorylation exclusively, or by a combination of both the pathways, depending on the species (Storey, 2008).

PKA is involved in several biochemical events, cross linking different pathways. In datail the HCO_3^- and Ca^{2+} are transported by a Na^{+}/HCO_3^- cotransporter (NBC) and a sperm-specific Ca^{2+} channel (CatSper) and stimulate, via soluble adenylyl cyclase (sAC), PKA activity. In addition this enzyme is involved in late events leading spermatozoa to acquire the hyperactivated motility. PKA activation is correlated with an increase in tyrosine phosphorylation dependent on the presence of cholesterol acceptors in the capacitation medium (Breitbart et al., 2006; Visconti, 2009).

Protein tyrosine phosphorylation pattern of spermatozoa changes during the capacitation in several species such as human, mice, cattle, pigs, hamsters and cats (Barbonetti et al., 2008; Urner & Sakkas, 2003; Visconti et al., 1995). This process appears to be a necessary prerequisite for a spermatozoon to fertilize an egg and has been demonstrated to increase either in flagellum and in sperm head. At present the molecular targets of protein tyrosine phosphorylation are still largely unknown (Naz & Rajesh, 2004).

PLD1 plays a pivotal role in actin polymerization, that is one of the most important events related with the acquisition of capacitation. In particular MAP-kinase, tyrosine kinase, and ADP-ribosylation factor are involved in PLD activation, leading to phosphatidyl-choline hydrolysis to produce phosphatidic acid, which mediates polymerization of G-actin to F-actin (Breitbart et al., 2005; Cohen et al., 2004; Gomez-Cambronero & Keire, 1998).

Other highly linked nodes are those related to terminal events (such as protein phosphorylation or membrane fusion). Reasonably this is due to the redundancy of biochemical signalling, as a safety strategy to overlap partial failure of the system.

It is of interest, also, to note that almost half of the nodes (40-45%) have two links: one in input and the other in output. This finding, together with the low value of clustering coefficient, is in agreement with the concept that the network had a signalling transduction-dedicated structure: the molecular message is carried, directionally, from the beginning to the end of the chain, avoiding the presence of loop or clusters that could to slow and to interfere with the propagation of messages.

In this context, the characteristic path length (~6.5) may have two important consequences on spermatozoa physiology. Firstly, if any molecule interacts with any other in a small number of passages, the loss of information due to the signal decrease is minimized and, consequently, the signal efficiency is maximized. Secondly, any local perturbation in signalling system could reach the whole network in a short time, thus increasing the system responsiveness to intracellular and extracellular stimuli.

It was also possible to isolate the nodes with only one link. The classical scale free model indicates that these nodes are the most peripheral and, as a consequence, less important ones. For instance in the WWW the sites with only one link are the most marginal in the network and are likely destined to disappear (Barabási, 2003). On the contrary, in sperm capacitation, the nodes with one link are often the network input terminal, These nodes are able to receive links and to interact intracellular signalling machinery with external environment (female environment, seminal fluid, artificial media in laboratory technologies, ...).

A further peculiar characteristic of this network is that the activating signals are markedly most expressed than the inhibiting ones (~95% vs. ~5%). This evidence could have two different explanations:

- it is possible that the interest to recreate in vitro sperm capacitation in the contest of Assisted Reproductive Technologies leads the Researchers to study and to describe the mainly capacitation-promoting events. Thus the activating signals are not the most expressed but the most studied and, as a consequence, the most represented in scientific literature;
- the spermatozoa are functionally disposable cells. From a teleological point of view their fate is the completion of capacitation and, after all, the AR and the fertilization. Thus, it is possible that most of the biochemical pathways are objective-oriented leading sperm cells to recognise and to bind ZP and to undergo AR.

Taken altogether these finding seem to suggest that the system biology-based approach adopted could be useful to explore the spermatozoa signalling machinery, giving us new information on its physiology. It could be possible complete the dialectic of *in vivo* - *in vitro* models adding *in silico* model to increase the resources available to study a complex phenomenon such as the function of male gamete. In addition it could be possible to explain many biological aspects of spermatozoa biology that are out of focus looking at the single molecular determinant, thus overcoming the reductionist approach until now adopted, which did not consider the proprieties that emerge from the interaction among the different molecules involved in capacitation.

4. From the chip to the bench: Experimental validation of a model-based hypothesis

More recently an experimental set-up was carried out to empirically validate this modeling approach. An in silico and in vitro experiment was carried out on an animal model (Bernabò et al., 2011). To this aim the biological network representing boar sperm capacitation was realized, as previously described, and its nodes were separated depending on their subcellular compartment (see Table 4 and Figure 3) using the Cytoscape plugin Cerebral v.2 (http://www.pathogenomics.ca/cerebral/). The statistical and topological analyses of the network were carried out, considering the network as undirected, by the Cytoscape plugin Network Analyzer (http://med.bioinf.mpiinf.mpg.de/netanalyzer/help/2.6.1/index.html).

Parameter	Value	
N° nodes	153	
N° edges	204	
Clustering coefficient	0.056	
Diameter	12	
Averaged n° neighbours	2.654	
Char. path length	4.995	
Most connected nodes (n° of links)	$[Ca^{2+}]_i$	(28)
	ATP	(15)
	Tyr phosphorylation	(13)
	PKA	(9)
	ADP	(8)
	PLD1	(8)
	NADH	(8)
	Actin polymerization	(8)

Table 4. Main topological parameters of boar spermatozoa capacitation network. The number of nodes represent the total number of molecules involved, the number of edges represents the total number of interaction found, the clustering coefficient is calculated as $CI = 2nI/k(k-1)$,where nI is the number of links connecting the kI neighbours of node I to each other, the network diameter is the largest distance between two nodes, the Averaged n° neighbours represent the mean number of connection of each node, the Char. path length gives the expected distance between two connected nodes (adapted, from Bernabò et al., 2011).

From the network analysis it was immediately evident that the "actin polymerization" node has two important and unique features:

- it is one of the most connected nodes (a hub);
- it links in a specific manner all the intracellular compartments.

To best characterize its role in capacitation-related signaling, a computational experiment was performed: the "actin polymerization" was removed from the network and the consequences on its architecture were assessed. It was found that its removal did not affect the global network topology (data not shown) but caused the loss of five important nodes (and among them the "PM and OAM fusion").

The analysis of theoretical data suggested that actin polymerization could be involved in the coordination of signaling among different subcellular districts, and that its functional ablation could compromise spermatozoa ability to complete the capacitation avoiding PM and OAM fusion, without affecting the other main signaling pathway.

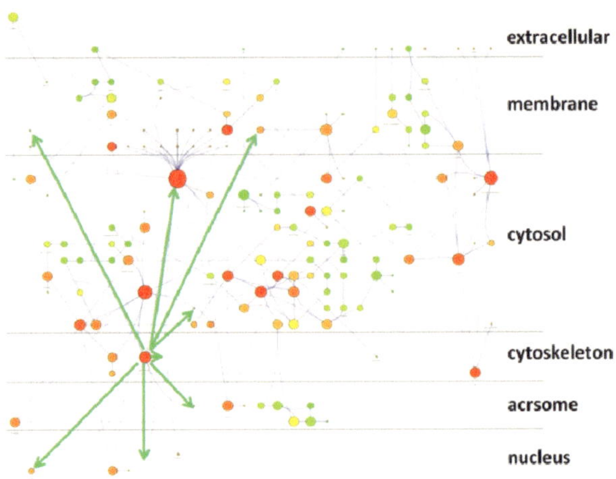

Fig. 3. Diagram showing the structure of the boar spermatozoa capacitation network and the subcellular localization of nodes (see text for explanation). The links of actin polymerization node are indicated by green arrows.

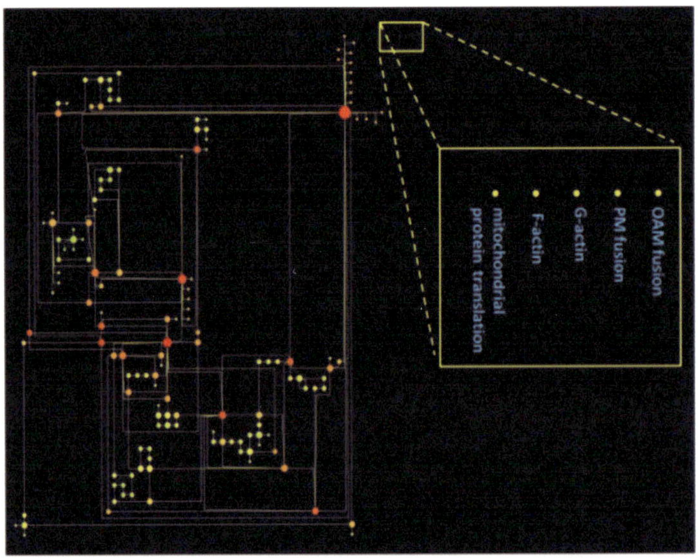

Fig. 4. Diagram showing the structure of the boar spermatozoa capacitation network after "actin polymerization" node removal (see the text for explanation).

To empirically validate this hypothesis an in vitro experiment was performed: the actin polymerization was inhibited, by administrating the cytochalasin D, a specific actin polymerization inhibitor, to boar spermatozoa incubated under in vitro capacitating conditions. Then the effects of this treatment on spermatozoa capacitation status (ZP-induced AR), and on the major cellular events involved in the acquisition of full fertilizing ability, such as membrane acquisition of chlortetracycline pattern C, protein tyrosine phosphorylation, phospholipase C-γ1 relocalization, intracellular calcium response to ZP, were assessed.

To this aim semen samples were collected and processed by an already validated protocol (Bernabò et al, 2010b) and were incubated under control conditions (CTR) or were constantly maintained in the presence of 20 μM of citochalasin D (CD).

The competence of in vitro incubated spermatozoa to undergo AR in response to solubilised zonae pellucidae (ZP) co-incubation was further evaluated as a functional endpoint of the capacitative state. As depicted in Figure 5 it was evident that:

- the percentage of spermatozoa undergoing spontaneous AR was unaffected by the treatment;
- the percentage of spermatozoa able to respond with AR to the ZP coincubation was markedly reduced by the CD administration.

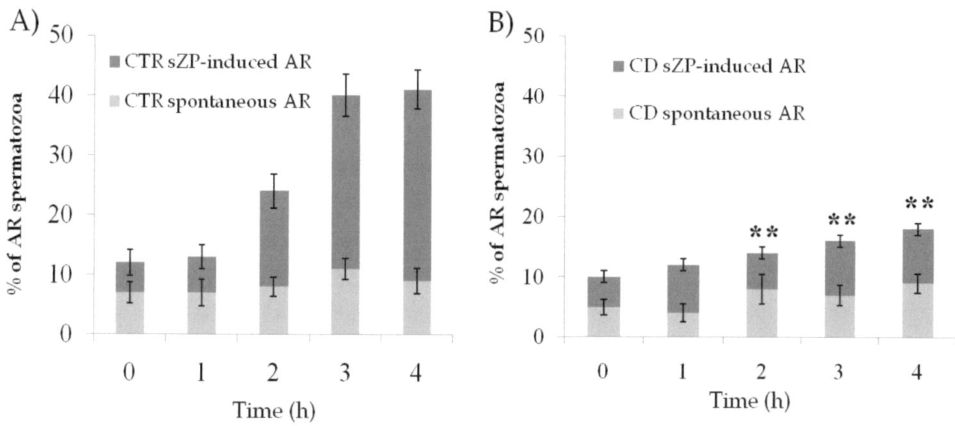

Fig. 5. Histogram representing the percentage of spermatozoa undergoing spontaneous and sZP-induced AR in CTR (A) and CD (B) treated spermatozoa. All the values are represented as mean ± SD. ** = $p<0.01$ vs. CTR, ANOVA test (from Bernabò et al., 2011).

The chlortetracycline stain (CTC) was used to evaluate the completion of calcium-dependent membrane remodelling, in keeping with Mattioli et al. (Mattioli, 1996). For each sample were assessed at least 200 spermatozoa and the percentage of spermatozoa displaying fluorescence pattern C indicative of capacitation (CTC fluorescence over the post acrosomal area) was calculated. As shown in Figure 6 the CD treatment did not affected the kinetic of acquisition of CTC pattern C.

The biochemical and ultrastructural localization of PLC-γ1 was studied by western blotting and by transmission electron microscopy on control and cytocalasin D treated spermatozoa. As a result it was found that this enzyme migrates from cytosol to the active site (the membrane) independently from CD treatment (see Figures 7 and 8)

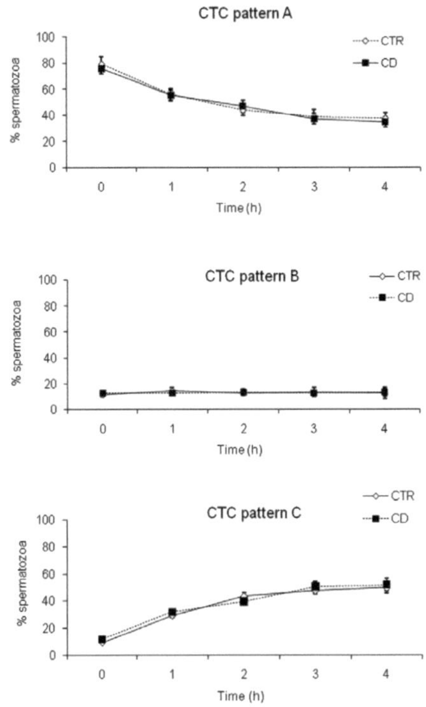

Fig. 6. Kinetic of acquisition of CTC staining pattern A, B and C in CTR and CD treated spermatozoa.
Graphic showing the percentage of spermatozoa displaying the CTC pattern A, B and C, during the 4h of incubation under control conditions (dark continue line) or in the presence of CD (dark dot line). All the values are represented as mean ± SD (from Bernabò et al., 2011)

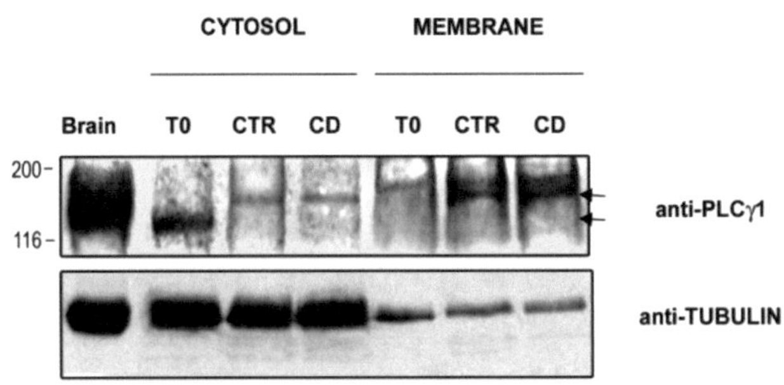

Fig. 7. Capacitation-dependent PLCγ1 relocalization.
Western Blot analysis of PLCγ1 localization in cytosolic and membrane fractions of freshly ejaculated male gametes (T0) or in spermatozoa incubated under control condition (CTR) or in the presence of CD (CD). The data showing the capacitation-dependent translocation of PLC-γ1 (arrows) from cytosol to membrane. Brain proteins were used as positive control. The filter was normalized on Tubulin expression. The data shown were representative of four independent experiments (from Bernabò et al., 2011).

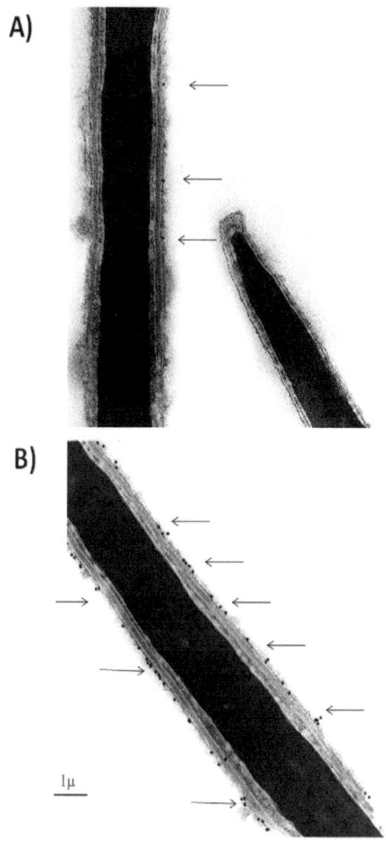

Fig. 8. Transmission electron microscopy pictures demonstrating the topography of capacitation-dependent PLCγ1 relocalization. Panel A): ejaculated spermatozoon displaying few gold particles (arrows) indicative of a low localization of PLCγ1 protein over cell membranes. Panel B): in vitro capacitated spermatozoon incubated in the presence of CD that localized on its membrane several gold particles (arrows) (from Bernabò et al., 2011).

The pattern of tyrosine phosphorylation was evaluated by western blotting on control and cytocalasin D treated spermatozoa. In this case also the CD treatment did not exerted any effect (Figure 9).

The calcium probe fluo-3-AM was used to assess the variations in the intracellular calcium concentration in response to the sZP coincubation and it was found that the physiological agonist of AR maintained its ability to stimulate a rapid rise in intracellular calcium concentration also in the CD treated spermatozoa (Figure 10).

As hypothesized from the *in silico* experiment, the treatment had a duplex effect: in one hand it completely inhibited the acquisition of fertilizing ability, in the other one all the

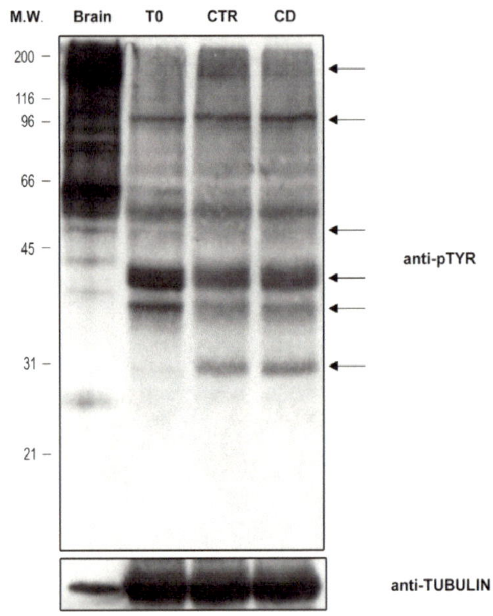

Fig. 9. Western Blot analysis of tyrosine phosphorylation pattern in total lysate of freshly ejaculated male gametes (T0) or in spermatozoa incubated under control condition (CTR) or in the presence of CD (CD). The arrows indicate the capacitation-related changes in P-Tyr. Brain proteins were used as positive control. The filter was normalized on the Tubulin expression (from Bernabò et al., 2011).

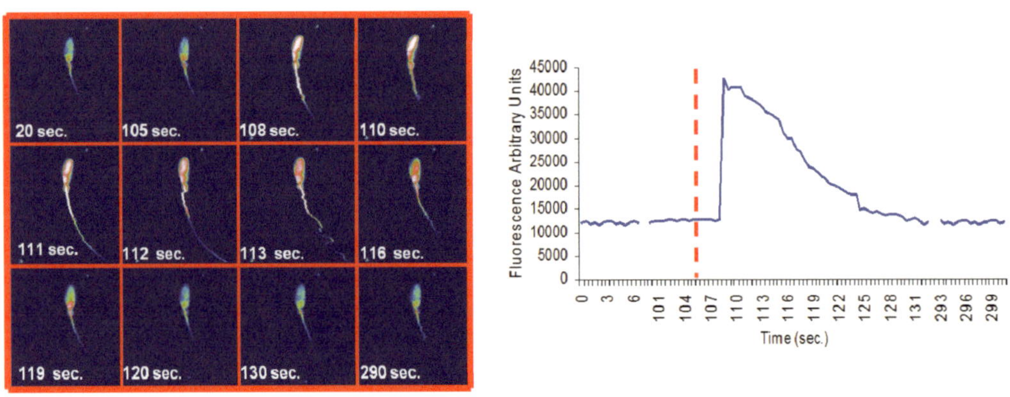

Fig. 10. An example of confocal image gallery of CD treated spermatozoa loaded with Fluo-3AM exposed to sZP (vertical red line). Notice that the rise in the $[Ca^{2+}]_i$ in spermatozoon is evident after <10 sec. from sZP addition, whereas return on the baseline occurs after about 30 sec. (adapted, from Bernabò et al., 2011).

examined pathways seemed to be unaffected by the inhibition of actin polymerization. This finding allowed us to propose some considerations:

- as already discussed the data until now available attribute to the actin dynamics a structural role during capacitation: a network of actin acts as a diaphragm between the PM and OAM avoiding their fusion. At the moment of AR this physical barrier was rapidly removed and the fusion between the two membranes can happen. If this model was correct it was reasonably to expect that the block of actin polymerization (i.e. the treatment of spermatozoa with CD) in early phases of capacitation should lead to the increase in the percentage of spermatozoa undergoing AR because of the inefficiency of PM and OAM separation. In our experiments, on the contrary, it was found that, even in the absence of the actin network, the PM and OAM did not fuse. Thus, it possible to hypothesize that in spermatozoa, as demonstrated in other cells, the role of actin cytoskeleton overcomes this merely structural function, having a more complex role. Particularly in the light of the finding that "actin polymerization" node links three hubs of the system it is possible to propose that this event could play an important role in coordination of information flow. This supposition is in keeping with the newly emerging evidence that in different cellular systems the cytoskeleton is not only a mechanical support for the cell, but it exerts a key role in signaling. As proposed by Janmey, "independent of its mechanical strength, the filaments of the cytoskeleton form a continuous, dynamic connection between nearly all cellular structures, and they present an enormous surface area on which proteins and other cytoplasmic components can dock" (Janmey, 1998). This concept is in keeping with the observation that plasma membrane surface area of a 20-μm-diameter generic cell is on the order of 700 μm^2, in contrast, the total surface area of a typical concentration of 10 mg/ml F-actin is 47,000 μm^2 (Janmey, 1998) and that the diffusion along cytoskeleton tracks could be a reliable alternative to other established ways of intracellular trafficking and signaling, and could therefore provide an additional level of cell function regulation (Shafrir et al., 2000). One implication of this role is that the actin cytoskeleton might provide a signal transduction route and macromolecular scaffold, which, during capacitation, contributes to the spatial organization of signaling pathways (Forgacs et al., 2004).
- the results obtained by the *in silico* experiments are perfectly in agreement with those from the *in vitro* approach. This datum evidences that the model seems to mimic the behavior of real system, in other words it could be possible to assume that the information inferred by the model is correct.

5. Conclusions

In our opinion, the ability to realize a reliable computational model representing main molecular events occurring during spermatozoa capacitation could be an important tool in understanding male gametes physiology and, as a consequence, their pathology. These cells are an ideal candidate to this kind of approach for several reasons:

- one of the most important problems in cell modelization is the continuous modification in cellular protein content and in molecular interactions due to the dynamical regulation of genes expression and protein transcription. The molecular composition of male gametes is stable since they are transcriptionally silent with the exception of the 55S mitochondrial ribosome-dependent protein translation of nuclear-encoded proteins.

- differently from the most of other cellular types, it is possible to empirically evaluate the functional status of the system. In fact it is possible, using for instance an animal model, to verify if the spermatozoa completed their maturation process, testing the ability of spermatozoa to complete the capacitation and, subsequently, to undergo AR by in *in vitro* fertilization assay or by *in vivo* fertilization trials: only the spermatozoa that successfully fertilize an oocyte can be considered fully competent.
- finally the spermatozoa are the only cellular type, produced in an organism, that exert their function in another one. As a consequence they are capable of independent life (unlike the other cells) and it is possible to manage them outside the organism without loss of the cell function.

We think that the adoption of this modelization strategy could be of great importance in the study of capacitation. Sperm cells are complex systems, thus to really understand their behavior it is necessary to consider them as a network of molecules interacting with each other. It is impossible to get complete information on their functional status looking only at the molecular level: the capacitation, as well the fertility, are emergent proprieties of the system, thus it is necessary to study them at a supra-molecular level. As a consequence we propose to adopt, together with the traditional methodologies, a computational-based approach to explore spermatozoa biology and, ultimately, male fertility and infertility.

Ultimately, we fully agree with the WHO statement that "advances in our understanding of the signal transduction pathways regulating sperm function will have implications for the development of diagnostic tests capable of generating detailed information on the precise nature of the processes that are defective in the spermatozoa of infertile men"(WHO, 2010).

6. References

Abou-haila, A. & Tulsiani D.R. (2009) Signal transduction pathways that regulate sperm capacitation and the acrosome reaction. *Archives of Biochemistry and Biophysics,* Vol. 485, No. 1 (May 2009), pp. 485, 72-81, ISSN 0003-9861

Albert, R., Jeong, H. & Barabasi, A.L. (2000) Error and attack tolerance of complex networks. *Nature, Vol.* 406, No. 6794 (July 2000), pp. 378-382, ISSN : 0028-0836

Albert, R. (2005) Scale-free networks in cell biology. *Journal of Cell Science, Vol.* 118, No. 21 (November 2005),pp. 4947-4957, ISSN 0021-9533

Asano, A., Nelson, J.L., Zhang, S. & Travis, A.J. (2010) Characterization of the proteomes associating with three distinct membrane raft sub-types in murine sperm. *Proteomics, Vol.* 10, No. 19 (October 2010), pp. 3494-3505, ISSN: 1862-8354

Austin, C.R.(1951) Activation and the correlation between male and female elements in fertilization. *Nature,* Vol. 168, No. 4274 (September 1951), pp. 558-559, ISSN : 0028-0836

Barabási, A. L. (2003) "Linked: How Everything is Connected to Everything Else and What It Means for Business, Science, and Everyday Life." New York: Plume, ISBN 10: 0452284392

Barabási, A.L. & Oltvai, Z.N. (2004) Network biology: understanding the cell's functional organization. *Nature Reviews Genetics, Vol.* 5, No. 2 (Febuary, 2004), pp. 101-113, ISSN : 1471-0056

Barabási, A.L. (2001) The physics of the Web. *Physics World,* Vol. 14 (July 2001), pp. 33-38, ISSN: 0953-8585

Barabási, A.L., Albert, R. & Jeong, H. (2000) Scale-free characteristics of random networks: the topology of the world wide web. *Physica A, Vol.* 281, pp. 69-77, ISSN: 0378-4371

Barbonetti, A., Vassallo, M.R., Cinque, B., Antonangelo, C., Sciarretta, F., Santucci, R., D'Angeli, A., Francavilla, S. & Francavilla, F. (2008) Dynamics of the global tyrosine phosphorylation during capacitation and acquisition of the ability to fuse with oocytes in human spermatozoa. *Biology of Reproduction,* Vol. 79, No. 4 (October 2008), pp. 649-56, ISSN: 0006-3363

Bernabò, N., Berardinelli, P., Mauro, A., Russo, V., Lucidi, P., Mattioli, M. & Barboni, B. (2011) The role of actin in capacitation-related signaling: an in silico and in vitro study. *BMC Systems Biology, Vol.* 30, No. 5 (March 2011), p. 47, ISSN 1752-0509

Bernabò, N., Mattioli, M. & Barboni, B. (2010a) The spermatozoa caught in the net: the biological networks to study the male gametes post-ejaculatory life. *BMC Systems Biology,* Vol. 4 (June 2010), p. 87, ISSN 1752-0509

Bernabò, N., Pistilli, M.G., Mattioli, M. & Barboni, B. (2010b) Role of TRPV1 channels in boar spermatozoa acquisition of fertilizing ability. *Molecular and Cellular Endocrinology* Vol. 323, No. 2 (July 2010), pp. 224-231, ISSN: 0303-7207

Bevers, E. M., Comfurius, P., Dekkers D. W. C., Harmsma, M. and Zwaal R. F. A. (1998) Transmembrane phospholipid distribution in blood cells: control mechanisms and pathophysiological significance. *Biological Chemistry, Vol.* 379, No. 8-9 (August-September 1998), pp. 973-986, ISSN 0021-9258

Blaustein, M.P. & Lederer, W.J. (1999) Sodium/calcium exchange: its physiological implications. *Physiological Review, Vol.* 79, No. 3, pp. 763–854, ISSN: 0031-9333

Botto, L., Bernabò, N., Palestini, P & Barboni, B. (2010) Bicarbonate induces membrane reorganization and CBR1 and TRPV1 endocannabinoid receptor migration in lipid microdomains in capacitating boar spermatozoa. *Journal of Membrane Biology, Vol.* 238, No. 1-3, pp. 33-41, ISSN: 1432-1424

Breitbart, H. (2002) Intracellular calcium regulation in sperm capacitation and acrosomal reaction. *Molecular and Cellular Endocrinology, Vol.* 187, No. 1-2 (Febuary 2002), pp. 139-144, ISSN: 0303-7207

Breitbart, H., Cohen, G. & Rubinstein, S.(2005) Role of actin cytoskeleton in mammalian sperm capacitation and the acrosome reaction. *Reproduction,* Vol. 129, No. 3 (March 2005), pp. 263-268, ISSN: 1470-1626

Breitbart, H., Rubinstein, S. & Etkovitz, N. (2006) Sperm capacitation is regulated by the crosstalk between protein kinase A and C. *Molecular and Cellular Endocrinology,* Vol. 252, No. 1-2 (June 2006), pp. 247-249, ISSN: 0303-7207

Breitbart,H. & Etkovitz, N. (2011) Role and regulation of EGFR in actin remodeling in sperm capacitation and the acrosome reaction. *Asian Journal of Andrology,* Vol. 13, No. 1 (January 2011), pp. 106-110, ISSN: 1745-7262

Brewis, I.A., Gadella, B.M.(2010) Sperm surface proteomics: from protein lists to biological function. *Molecular Human Reproduction,* Vol. 16, No. 2 (Febuary 2010), pp. 68-79, ISSN: 1360-9947

Bruckbauer, A., Dunne, P.D., James, P., Howes, E., Zhou, D., Jones, R. & Klenerman, D. (2010) Selective diffusion barriers separate membrane compartments. *Biophysical Journal,* Vol. 99, No. 1 (July 2010), pp. 1-3, ISSN: 0006-3495

Chang, H. & Suarez, S.S. (2010) Rethinking the relationship between hyperactivation and chemotaxis in mammalian sperm. *Biology of Reproduction,* Vol. 83, No. 4 (October 2010), pp. 507-513, ISSN: 0006-3363

Chang, M.C.(1951) Fertilizing capacity of spermatozoa deposited into the fallopian tubes. *Nature, Vol.* 168, No. 4277 (October 1951), pp. 697-698, ISSN : 0028-0836

Cohen, G., Rubinstein, S., Gur, Y. & Breitbart, H. (2004) Crosstalk between protein kinase A and C regulates phospholipase D and F-actin formation during sperm capacitation. *Developmental Biology,* Vol. 267, No. 1 (March 2004), pp. 230–241, ISSN: 0012-1606

Florman, H.M., Jungnickel, M.K. & Sutton, K.A. (2008) Regulating the acrosome reaction. *International Journal of Developmental Biology,* Vol. 52, No. 5-6, pp. 503-510, ISSN: 0214-6282

Forgacs, G., Yook, S.H., Janmey, P.A., Jeong, H. & Burd, C.G. (2004) Role of the cytoskeleton in signaling networks. *Journal of Cell Science,* Vol. 117, No. 13 (May 2004), pp. 2769-2775, ISSN 0021-9533

Fraser, L.R. & Herod, J.E. (1990) Expression of capacitation-dependent changes in chlortetracycline fluorescence patterns in mouse spermatozoa requires a suitable glycolysable substrate. *Journal of Reproduction and Fertility,* Vol. 88, No. 2 (March 1990), pp. 611-621, ISSN: 0022-4251

Fraser, L.R., Abeydeera, L.R. & Niwa, K. (1995) Ca(2+)-regulating mechanisms that modulate bull sperm capacitation and acrosomal exocytosis as determined by chlortetracycline analysis. *Molecular Reproduction and Development,* Vol. 40, No. 2 (Febuary 1995), pp. 233-241, ISSN: 1098-2795

Fraser, L.R., Umar, G. & Sayed, S. (1993) Na(+)-requiring mechanisms modulate capacitation and acrosomal exocytosis in mouse spermatozoa. *Journal of Reproduction and Fertility,* Vol. 97, No. 2 (March 1993), pp. 539-549, ISSN: 0022-4251

Gadella, B.M. & Harrison, R.A. (2000) The capacitating agent bicarbonate induces protein kinase A-dependent changes in phospholipid transbilayer behavior in the sperm plasma membrane. *Development,* Vol. 127, No. 11 (June 2000), pp. 2407-2420, ISSN: 1011-6370

Gadella, B.M. & Harrison, R.A. (2002) Capacitation induces cyclic adenosine 3',5'-monophosphate-dependent, but apoptosis-unrelated, exposure of aminophospholipids at the apical head plasma membrane of boar sperm cells. *Biology of Reproduction,* Vol. 67, No. 1 (July 2002), pp. 340-350, ISSN: 0006-3363

Gadella, B.M., Tsai, P.S., Boerke, A. & Brewis, I.A. (2008) Sperm head membrane reorganization during capacitation. *International Journal of Developmental Biology,* Vol. 52, No. 5, pp. 473-480, ISSN: 0214-6282

Goh, K.I., Cusick, M.E., Valle, D., Childs, B., Vidal, M. & Barabási A.L. (2007) The human disease network. *Proceedings of National Academy of Science U S A, Vol.* 104, No. 21 (may 2007), pp. 8685-8690, ISSN-0027-8424

Gomez-Cambronero, J. & Keire, P. (1998) Phospholipase D: a novel major player in signal transduction. *Cell Signaling,* Vol. 10, No. 6 (June 1998), pp. 387-397, ISSN: 0898-6568

Harrison, R.A. & Gadella, B.M. (2005) Bicarbonate-induced membrane processing in sperm capacitation. *Theriogenology,* Vol. 63, No. 2 (January 2005), pp. 342-351, ISSN: 0093-691X

Hickey, K.D. & Buhr, M.M.(2011) Lipid bilayer composition affects transmembrane protein orientation and function. *Journal of Lipids, Vol.* 2011;2011:208457, ISSN: 2090303

Janmey, P.A. (1998) The cytoskeleton and cell signaling: component localization and mechanical coupling. *Physiological Review, Vol.* 78, No. 3 (July 1998), pp. 763-778, ISSN: 0031-9333

Jeong, H., Tombor, B., Albert, R., Oltvai, Z.N. & Barabási, A.L. (2000) The large-scale organization of metabolic networks. *Nature, Vol.* 407, No. 6804 (October 2000), pp. 651-654, ISSN : 0028-0836

Kotwicka, M., Jendraszak, M. & Jedrzejczak, P. (2011) Phosphatidylserine membrane translocation in human spermatozoa: topography in membrane domains and relation to cell vitality. *Journal of Membranes Biology, Vol.* 240, No. 3 (April 2011), pp. 165-170, ISSN: 1432-1424

Krausz, C. (2011) Male infertility: pathogenesis and clinical diagnosis. *Best Practice & Research Clinical Endocrinology & Metabolism,* Vol. 25, No. 2 (April 2011), pp. 271-285, ISSN: 1521-690X

Mattioli, M., Barboni, B., Lucidi, P. & Seren, E. (1996) Identification of capacitation in boar spermatozoa by chlortetracycline staining. *Theriogenolog, Vol.* 45, No. 2 (December 1996), pp. 373-381, ISSN: 0093-691X

Müller, P., Pomorski, T., Porwoli, S., Tauber, R. & Herrmann, A. (1996) Transverse movement of spin-labeled phospholipids in the plasma membrane of a hepatocytic cell line (HepG2): implications for biliary lipid secretion. *Hepatology, Vol.* 24, No. 6 (December 1996), pp. 1497-1503, ISSN: 0270-9139

Naz, R.K. & Rajesh, P.B. (2004) Role of tyrosine phosphorylation in sperm capacitation / acrosome reaction. *Reproductive Biology and Endocrinology, Vol.* 2 (November 2004), p. 75, ISSN: 1477-7827

Nixon, B. & Aitken, R.J. (2009) The biological significance of detergent-resistant membranes in spermatozoa. *Journal of Reproductive Immunology, Vol.* 83, No. 1-2 (December 2009), pp 8-13, ISSN: 0165-0378

O'Rand, M.G. & Fisher, S.J. (1987). Localization of zona pellucida binding sites on rabbit spermatozoa and induction of the acrosome reaction by solubilized zonae. *Developmental Biology,* Vol.119, No. 2 (Febuary 1987), pp. 551-559, ISSN: 0012-1606

Perry, R.L., Naeeni, M., Barratt, C.L., Warren, M.A. & Cooke, I.D. (1995) A time course study of capacitation and the acrosome reaction in human spermatozoa using a revised chlortetracycline pattern classification. *Fertility and Sterility,* Vol. 64, No. 1 (July 1995), pp. 150-159, ISSN: 0015-0282

Saling, P.M. & Storey, B.T. (1979) Mouse gamete interactions during fertilization in vitro. Chlortetracycline as a fluorescent probe for the mouse sperm acrosome reaction. *Journal of Cell Biology,* Vol. 83, No. 3 (December 1979), pp. 544-555, ISSN:0021-9525

Shafrir, Y., ben-Avraham, D. & Forgacs, G. (2000) Trafficking and signaling through the cytoskeleton: a specific mechanism. *Journal of Cell Science,* Vol. 113, No. 15 (August 2000), pp. 2747-2757, ISSN 0021-9533

Storey BT (2008) Mammalian sperm metabolism: oxygen and sugar, friend and foe. *International Journal of Developmental Biology,* Vol. 52, No. 5-6, pp. 427-437, ISSN: 0214-6282

Suarez, S.S. (2008) Control of hyperactivation in sperm. *Human Reproduction Update.* Vol. 14, No. 6 (June 2008), pp. 647-657, ISSN: 1355-4786

Urner, F. & Sakkas, D. (2003) Protein phosphorylation in mammalian spermatozoa. *Reproduction,* Vol. 125, No. 1 (January 2003), pp. 17–26, ISSN: 1470-1626

Venditti, J.J. &. Bean, B.S. (2009) Stabilization of membrane-associated alpha-L-fucosidase by the human sperm equatorial segment. *International Journal of Andrology, Vol.* 32, No. 5 (March 2009), pp. 556-562, ISSN: 0105-6263

Visconti, P.E. (2009) Understanding the molecular basis of sperm capacitation through kinase design. *Proceedings of National Academy of Science USA,* Vol. 105, No. 52 (December 2009), pp. 66766-66768, ISSN-0027-8424

Visconti, P.E., Bailey, J.L., Moore, G.D., Pan, D., Olds-Clarke, P. & Kopf, G.S. (1995) Capacitation of mouse spermatozoa. I. Correlation between the capacitation state and protein tyrosine phosphorylation. *Development,* Vol. 121, No. 4 (April 1995), pp. 1129-1137, ISSN: 1011-6370

Wagner, A. (2000) Robustness against mutations in genetic networks of yeast. *Nature Genetics,* Vol. 24, No. 4 (April 2000), pp. 355-361, ISSN : 1061-4036

Wennemuth, G., Babcock, B.F. & Hille, B. (2003) Calcium Clearance Mechanisms of Mouse Sperm. *Journal of General Physiology,* Vol. 122, No. 1 (July 2003), pp. 115–128, ISSN: 0022-1295

WHO (1986). Consultation on the zona-free hamster oocyte penetration test and the diagnosis of male fertility. *International Journal of Andrology* (Suppl. 6). ISSN: 0105-6263

WHO (2010) *Laboratory manual for the examination and processing of human semen* - 5th ed., pp. 246-152 ISBN 978 92 4 154778 9

Yanagimachi, R. (1969) In vitro capacitation of hamster spermatozoa by follicular fluid. *Journal of Reproduction and Fertility, Vol.* 18, No. 2 (March 1969), pp. 275-286, ISSN: 1470-1626

Yanagimachi, R. (1994). Mammalian fertilization. *In*: Knobil E, Neill JD editors. *The physiology of reproduction (2nd edition).* New York, USA: Raven Press; pp.189–317, ISBN: 0-7817-0086-8

Yook, S.H., Jeong,H & Barabási A.L. (2002) Modeling the internet's large-scale topology *Proceedings of National Academy of Science U S A, Vol.* 99, No. 21 (October 2002), pp. 13382-13386, ISSN-0027-8424